Diary of a Breast Cancer Husband

J. Scott Lyman

• Times Publishing Group •

For Cindy and Matt Johnson and all the gallant and brave victims of cancer that struggle daily in a war that kills, maims and mutilates more victims annually than all the wars in the history of the United States. For my wonderful mom, my dad and my brother Jerry, who I have missed every day of my life since his death.

Acknowledgments

Whether this book turns out to accomplish the purposes, for which I wrote it, remains to be seen. But regardless of the outcome, I could not and would not have attempted this task without the encouragement and help of a number of people. First and foremost, credit goes to my wife, Suanne for allowing and at times encouraging me to write *Diary of A Breast Cancer Husband.* Her comments, contributions and suggestions have been invaluable. She is truly the co-author of the book. I also need to thank Suanne for her extraordinary patience in spending what must have seemed like an infinite number of evenings at home with me glued to my computer. Without the suggestions, contributions and encouragement of Dr. Ellen Mahoney and Dr. Steven Mann I question whether I would have stayed the course to complete the book, or perhaps even have started it. Both Ellen's and Steve's footnoting have provided legitimacy that could only come from dedicated professionals in the field. My partner Pete Mair graciously reviewed any number of drafts and unfailingly encouraged me to continue through to the end of the project. Drafts were read by my publisher, Patrice Edwards, and others on her editorial staff and received enthusiastically, which is always encouraging. Tom Black, my editor, turned the bumps and potholes of the author's rough drafts into the final product that finally went to press. Dr. Susan Love, the renowned author of *Dr. Susan Love's Breast Book,* kindly gave me permission to use the glossary and Resource, References and Additional Reading appendix from the third edition of her book. Simply being able to thank her for this permission was and is mightily appreciated. Finally, I owe a debt of real gratitude to the participants in the case histories chapter for their willingness to participate in this effort by allowing me to interview them and learn the heart-wrenching details of their own experiences.

Diary
of a
Breast
Cancer
Husband

Table of Contents

Introduction
By M. Ellen Mahoney, M.D.

What is it about breast cancer that terrifies women so? If you ask any medical oncologist, surgeon, radiation oncologist or women's primary care physician they will tell you that there is a level of terror associated with this disease that they do not see even with more lethal cancers such as lung cancer. There are several reasons for this phenomenon.

The first is the absence of identifiable risk factors. At present, the only risk factors we are sure of are being female and getting older. Neither of these is effectively modifiable. An additional risk factor is a family history of the disease in a mother, sister or daughter who had the disease before menopause. Women, too, cannot modify this, and even women with this risk factor are likely to die of other causes. The news and scientific literature are regularly peppered with stories of crude epidemiological research pointing weakly to other possible associated factors. Scientists use these results as mere clues to guide the design of the next controlled study. Journalists oftentimes report these results out of context, some in a clumsy attempt to "inform" and others just to sell media. The public, confronted by this unfiltered information, take the reports as exhortations to make lifestyle changes, acting as if the association indicates proven causes, and burn out when confronted by seemingly contradictory reports.

The second factor is related to the first. It is fact that all around us are cases which seem to defy the common wisdom about this disease. Lung cancer has passed breast cancer as the most common cause of cancer death in American women, with 67,600 deaths estimated in 2000 compared to 40,800 deaths for breast cancer. But we can so easily (and not always fairly) blame the victim of respiratory cancers for their own diseases as the overwhelming number of them are smokers. Heart disease, AIDS, cervical cancer and accidents likewise afford a chance to differentiate the risky behavior of the victim from our own model lives. But breast cancer is the perfect equal opportunity killer of women. It strikes young and old, saint and sinner, women with multiple pregnancies and women who have never been pregnant, women with a family history but more women who do not have a family history of disease. Cases that seem to defy the popular concept of risk factors are not rare. Indeed they are observable in every community. The victim in this story is a woman almost devoid of common risk factors.

The third factor that makes breast cancer so terrifying is the uncertainty of the prognosis. There was a rise in incidence in the 1980's as mammography came into common use, but the incidence then leveled off promptly to 180,000 to 185,000 cases in America each year. A prediction was made early in the history of mammography that if early detection made a difference the death rate should begin to decrease in the early 1990's, and this is exactly what was seen. The number of deaths from breast cancer declined from about 46,000 per year to the current projection of 40,800. Another way of looking at these numbers is to say that about 75% of women who contract breast cancer die of other causes. Most of those are actually cured of their cancer. At higher stages of the disease, less than 75% survive, but at lower stages (such as Mrs. Lyman's) the survival rate is 95% and higher. Even at this favorable stage, though, up to 5% die of breast cancer and we cannot account for the difference between them and others like them. This leads to tremendous and persistent fear, which is well described by the author.

The good news is that most cases are cures; the bad news is that we can't say who they are. There is no blood test or scan that can tell us that someone is free of the disease after treatment. The best that we can say is that there is no detectable cancer in a particular patient, and we say this with the knowledge that our detection methods are highly flawed. What we do have are statistics on survival, which allow us to predict those factors with long term survival. Until we have a method of prevention for this disease, our best weapon is early detection, and our best method of early detection so far, however flawed, is still mammography.

The fourth factor, and the one that fills many of the pages of this book, is the realization that this disease and its usually effective treatment affect a woman at every imaginable level of her life. It shakes faith, changes bodies and body image, and rewrites scenarios for the future that have been driving forces in one's life. Health and trust in one's body are difficult and in some cases impossible to regain. Psychological trauma is inevitable. Finances are almost invariably affected as the disease and treatment attack income, savings, insurance prospects and raise expenses both for medical care and for other support.

But this is not just a woman's disease. It is a disease of her partner, her children, her doctors, her co-workers, her family and her friends. This book provides an intimate and poignant glimpse into this extension of the disease as it affects a loving and devoted husband. But not all stories of breast cancer victims end as well as this one, and many marriages are destabilized and destroyed under the many pressures breast cancer visits on its extended range of victims. The knowledge that this can and does happen is another source of stress, and if it does happen, the combination of breast cancer, its treatment, and a tested marriage with all of its associated tragedies is almost unbearable. Others must take up the void, including sometimes the physicians, while family members are further victimized and less available as a source of support. Certainly these new losses can affect the medical care plan and at worst can compromise the outcome.

Long hours, powerful emotions, and (relatively) low pay mark the practice of breast surgery. The reimbursement for doctors was established at a time when there were no options for treatment; biopsy, frozen section and immediate mastectomy without reconstruction was all that was offered. One of the advantages of the field, a distant second to the opportunity to be excellent and thereby make a big difference for a woman and family in crisis, is the enormous advance in the understanding of the molecular biology of breast cancer and the huge increase in the options for management of the treatment. Discussion of these options entails much time and facilitates a bond between doctor and patient that often becomes very intense and reciprocal. It is bad enough to have a friend with breast cancer; it is much worse when their primary supporter is absent without explanation. This book greatly helped me to understand some of the complex dynamics experienced by husbands in this crisis. I shall always be grateful for this insight.

There are about 525,600 minutes in a year. Death, of course, occurs around the clock, so current projection is for a death from breast cancer every 12.8 minutes in the United States in 2002. There are a projected 184,200 new diagnoses in the USA this year, but breast cancer is not diagnosed around the clock. Biopsies are performed and pathologists work over about a 50-hour period each week. Excluding weekends, nights and holidays, this means a diagnosis every minute in the United States alone during business hours. Every minute during office hours somewhere in our country a woman is being told that she has invasive breast cancer, an experience that has been compared to being shot by a sniper. Multiply that by the wounding of all of those who care about her, and the mayhem takes on battlefield proportions. I fervently beg all of you and all the readers of this book to keep up the pressure for the funding for research, for the improvement of our health care system and for the women you care about so that they obtain exams and mammograms in accordance with the guidelines of the American Cancer Society. Support organizations which have been formed to enhance patient education and support, and to mobilize political action.

Although we are making progress against this dreaded disease, much more is needed. If we could end it by virtue of some magic elixir today, there would still be almost two million women in the U.S. who, as we speak, are experiencing changes within the cells of their breasts that will lead to breast cancer in the next ten years. No one who cares about women and those who depend on them can afford to be complacent. The knowledge gained from this book, I am certain, will prove to be a valuable and important contribution to ending complacency and expanding the war against breast cancer.

M. Ellen Mahoney, MD
October 2001
Statistics from CA A. Cancer Journal for Clinicians, 50:1
January/February 2000 (American Cancer Society)

Prologue

It has been said that all true knowledge comes only from experience - from tasting the flavor, feeling the texture, hearing the sounds, and seeing the colors of life's always uncertain and ever-changing journey. True knowledge is rock-hard, vivid in color and shape, unmistakable in the sweetness or bitterness of its taste, and forever deep. Accordingly, all else is but speculation and conjecture; shimmering images that reside just beneath the surface, in the shallows of our minds - surfacing only in the form of abstractions, fantasy or illusions. Perhaps nowhere is this proposition better demonstrated than in the case of men and breast cancer.

We read about it in the newspaper headlines whenever a celebrity or a celebrity wife is stricken with or dies from breast cancer. The names of Linda McCartney, Peggy Fleming, Olivia Newton-John, Kate Jackson, and Carly Simon come to mind. But for most men, our interest in celebrity breast cancer cases quickly wanes and we move on to the sports section, scan the latest box scores and read about which pampered adolescent millionaires committed what crimes, and the names of the breast cancer victims fade into the mantle of their fame. But the celebrity breast cancer cases are just the tip of an iceberg, adrift in a sea of ordinary women struggling daily against this deadly disease.

The celebrity cases do, nevertheless, serve as a lightning rod to focus public attention, including even some men, on the ravages of breast cancer. Many will remember the great impetus given to breast cancer research when former first ladies Nancy Reagan and Betty Ford were diagnosed with the disease. More recently, when Linda McCartney, wife of Beatle Paul McCartney, died of breast cancer, hundreds of hours of media time were devoted to her personal struggle and to the subject of breast cancer. Radio and television talk shows focused on the disease, articles appeared in newspapers and magazines, experts opined on the subject and new studies and strategies were proposed. But even this kind of attention can compete in the media market for only so long before it fades from our collective consciousness into the background din of media marketing priorities.

Closer to home, most of us know or have heard about a woman that has been diagnosed with breast cancer. Perhaps it was the wife of a colleague at work, a neighbor just down the street, or a popular teacher at a local grammar school that died in the prime of her life. Maybe it was an in-law or a cousin. But even when it strikes this close, breast cancer remains a vague distant abstraction for most men; like a civil war or natural disaster in a distant land. As long as the earthquake or insurrection doesn't rock our own personal world, it is someone else's problem. But, in actuality, breast cancer is neither vague nor distant, nor somebody else's problem.

In the 1990s, breast cancer in America reached what some called epidemic proportions. As we enter the 21st Century, over 180,000 women a year are diagnosed with the disease. It kills in excess of 42,000 mothers, daughters, wives and lovers annually. It knows no social, ethnic, racial, religious, economic or geographic boundaries. White, black, brown or yellow; Christian, Muslim, or Jew; rich, poor, middle class; North, South, East or West, it strikes with devastating viciousness and at every segment of our society. Yet, despite all the social, medical and economic havoc it wreaks, for most men the topic of breast cancer remains an abstraction shrouded in mystery, fear and ignorance. This was certainly the case with me prior to my wife's being diagnosed with breast cancer. Even after the diagnosis, for a time I remained somewhat oblivious to much of the burden women carry with the disease. My first real awakening came after my wife related to me the comments of one of her physicians about breast cancer husbands. It was following an appointment early summer of 1996.

As we were pulling out of the parking lot at Dominican Hospital in Santa Cruz, California, Suanne casually commented that Dr. Mann, her radiation oncologist, was happy to see me participating in her care and treatment. I was mildly surprised by this comment, thinking to myself that surely most men would want to be involved in their wife's battle against breast cancer. Not so, I soon learned. According to Dr. Mann, most men have little or nothing to do with any aspect of their wife's breast cancer experience. They do not attend doctor visits, they do not participate in the decision making process, nor do they even elect to inform themselves about the disease.

Upon further inquiry, I learned that it is not uncommon for many men to feel outright resentment against their wives for the intrusion of breast cancer into their own life. They take it highly personally; many affronted, imposed upon and unfairly deprived. And in more instances than I would have ever imagined, men abandon their wives as a result of a breast cancer diagnosis. Although my first response was to self-righteously condemn these unfortunate reactions, within the deeper recesses of my mind, I knew that I had grappled with my own doubts and fears over the prospect of dealing with breast cancer and all of its potentially life-altering consequences.

The first thing that hits you upon learning that your wife has breast cancer is the suffocating realization that, despite all of the modern medical advances in detection technology and treatment, breast cancer remains a vicious killer of women in the prime of their lives. Next, while the shock and fear of the lethal nature of the disease never goes completely away, it does tend to subside in the face of the mind's willingness to be convinced by brilliant physicians and research scientists that a breast cancer diagnosis is no longer a death sentence, particularly with early detection.

But then, after the immediate survival hurdle is crossed (if you're so lucky as in my case) the mind is liberated to wander about in a jungle of very male thoughts and fears motivated at least in part by carnal appetite, deeply rooted male sexual fantasies that headline breasts, and dark frightful body images of what the future could hold in store. Many of these very private, very visceral thoughts can be extremely difficult to deal with, even among the most loving and considerate of husbands and in the strongest of marriages. But to deny them is to deny the reality of the neuro-biological make-up of the male human animal, with all of our evolutionary warts and scars. And while I'm certain there are many men who claim to be free of such blemishes, I, myself, cannot. And frankly, I question the candor of any man who does.

Since we emerged from the primeval slime, the males of our species seem to have been genetically programmed to love, crave, and fantasize about women's breasts. The only reason the word "obsession" (in the pathological sense) is not used is because it is deemed the normal psychological and physiological state for most men to be obsessed with female breasts.

In the early stages of my experience as a breast cancer husband, I found the thoughts welling up out of my own primordial slime at times fairly crackled with the fires of primitive fears and passions. The word "mastectomy" rang dolefully in my ears and the images of going to bed with a pockmarked, moonscape of a female bosom scorched my mind like a funeral pyre consuming the sweetest male fantasies a normal compliment of testosterone ever conjured up.

Where these disturbing thoughts come from is not at all difficult to fathom. Contemporary standards of "political/sexual correctness" to the contrary notwith-standing, it cannot be denied that the visual, tactile and emotional response of the male to female breasts was a survival or mating instinct long before the onset of our social and economic needs and/or monogamy. Did we not all (men as well as women), crave the suckling experience for years before we were even aware of the existence of self? Were we not survivors in a world where only the fittest survived long before we were mechanics, engineers, teachers, lawyers, and husbands? Is it not an incontrovertible fact that we were driven to procreate by lust, passion, and appetite long before we learned to recite the literal "for better or for worse" pledge that many of us uttered when we exchanged marriage vows?

So, I had to ask myself in the throes of my self-righteous indignation over the more "visceral" response some men have to breast cancer, who am I to say that under a variety of different circumstances, my reaction to my wife's breast cancer diagnosis might well have been resentment or flight instead of fight? Who am I to condemn any man for an inability to conquer his primordial fear of breast cancer and its anecdotally predictable consequences? After all, have not the irresistible Siren call of breasts and the compulsion of testosterone proved to be overpowering for more than a few epic heroes? Pretending a noble and virtuous response certainly feels better than being unreasoning and primitive about it, but not if it is contrived for effect or simply to mask one's true feelings, which eventually will rise to the surface anyway. So after hearing about Dr. Mann's observations, I sat back and gave full sway to the unabating emotions and fears I had been feeling over the previous several months. I concluded that it would be useful for me to write about it. And so I have.

My purpose in writing about my experience as a breast cancer husband is neither to condemn nor to pass judgment on any man or what might be viewed as a politically incorrect or "inappropriate" response to breast cancer. Rather, having felt the pangs of my own reactions to my wife's breast cancer diagnosis, having experienced the fear, the guilt and the projecting that goes along with the vicissitudes of being the spouse of a breast cancer victim, and at the same time having done my best to walk the mile in the moccasins of my life-mate, whom I surely love as much as I love my own life, I decided that a frank, unvarnished, unbridled discussion of this experience might contribute to a greater under-standing and participation on the part of men in the war against breast cancer. I also considered that such an exercise might be of some value in exploring some of the male's instincts and habits in the context of the breast cancer experience, as least as seen through my eyes.

I knew from the moment I started writing that exposing my warts and scars would not be easy on my wife or myself. But I also understood from a lifetime of struggling against the demons of catastrophe that were thrust upon me in my childhood that ignoring our frailty and vulnerability in dealing with tragedy and guilt serves absolutely no useful purpose. On the other hand, as my mom and dad and I learned almost 30 years after my brother's violent death at twelve years old, exposing and dealing openly with the horror and the fear that resides within us in dealing with tragedy and guilt is the only path we can take that will lead to some semblance of closure.

I also realized from the nature of the subject matter, that much of this book would deal with the most intimate of relations between a husband and wife, emotional, psychological and physical Even under the most propitious or compelling of circumstances, this is not an easy thing to do. But again, after much discussion between us, Suanne and I concluded that the discomfort of such a self-inflicted invasion of privacy would be more than compensated for by the potential of making a contribution to the war on breast cancer.

It also needs to be acknowledged that the breast cancer experience related in the pages that follow, in terms of the stage of diagosis and prognosis, pales in comparison to most of those that are not so fortunate in cathcing the disease early. But when first confronted with something as fearful and menacing as breast cancer, and one doesn't know where or what it will lead to, the reaction is no different than if the tumor turns out to be a Stage 1 or a Stage 4. Initially, I didn't even know the difference. All I really knew when my wife was diagnosed, was that breast cancer kills tens of thousands of women every year and my wife was a candidate to join that tragic group of women. The fact that our experience seemed to be turning out so positive, only served as further motivation for me to write this book, and perhaps soften the path of those that follow. It is our hope that in the not too distant future, every case of breast cancer will be diagnosed at Stage 1 and every victim will turn out to be a victor.

The book consists largely of an edited and expanded version of journal entries that I recorded from the inception of our (and it was "our") breast cancer experience until the point in time when Suanne and I came to believe and understand that total victory is a realistic goal in the campaign being waged against breast cancer, both within and beyond the walls of our home. We earnestly hope and pray that whatever light (and passion) this book may shed will serve to hasten the heroic efforts being waged by professionals and nonprofessionals alike in the ongoing crusade against this often brutal, always emotion-wrenching disease.

Diary of a Breast Cancer Husband

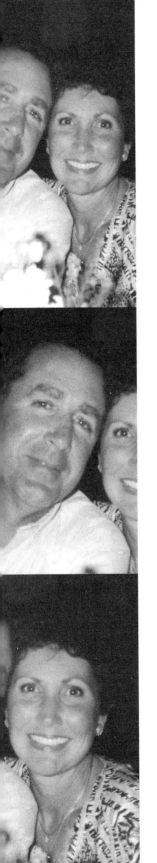

CHAPTER 1
Discovering A Lump

January 16, 1996

There was nothing unusual about the day that marked
the beginning of my experience as a breast cancer husband.
I got up at my usual time, put on the coffee, took the dog
out to pee and picked up the newspapers from the
driveway. By the time the coffee was ready, Suanne had
rousted our son Josh and was in the kitchen preparing
breakfast.

The morning television newscast was telling us that the
Russians were engaged in a full scale assault on Chechen
rebels, that former President Bush was lamenting his error in
judgment about the overthrow of Sadam after Desert Storm,
and that President Clinton received a standing ovation at a
Martin Luther King Junior Day rally in Atlanta for his defense
of Hillary against political attacks for her role in their various
scandals. Thankfully, the long ordeal of the O.J. Simpson
trial was fading into media limbo.

I had a case management conference in Santa Clara
County Superior Court at nine o'clock, so I left directly from
home, giving myself plenty of time to get over the hill to the
courthouse in downtown San Jose. It was raining and
blustery on the drive over Highway 17, one of the last of
California's infamous "blood alleys," but miraculously, there
were no accidents, slides or fallen trees, so I made it to the
hearing with time to spare. By late morning, the rain had
turned to occasional showers and I was back in my office in
Aptos, engrossed in a complicated medical chart on a new
malpractice case that had found its way to my office after
three other law firms had thrown in the towel. And yes, I
am a trial lawyer specializing in suing lawyers, real estate
professionals and occasionally medical doctors. I agreed to
review this case largely because it involved severe injuries to
a newborn with the attendant potential for huge damages
common to almost all "bad baby" cases.

This particular case involved a 31-week preemie infected at birth with genital herpes virus. The medical term for the disease is herpes simplex virus II, commonly referred to by doctors as HSV II. As is dictated by the disease, the medical chart presented a case of terrible complexity, involving over a dozen physicians, a throng of nurses and three hospitals where the mother and her baby had been cared for. The lawsuit had found its way from Santa Cruz County, where it originated, down to a law firm in Southern California and finally back to Santa Cruz. At each stop along the way, there had been the initial gush of enthusiasm for the case (such as I experienced), followed by the grim realization of what it would cost to take the case to trial and prove to a jury that some or all of the defendants had committed malpractice and caused the child's injuries.

It had been dark for an hour when I put down the chart and left the office for home. A chill northwesterly wind was blowing when I walked out to my car. After several hours of pouring over doctor's orders, nurse's reports, progress notes, test results and lab entries, I was just beginning to grasp the extent of the medical mayhem visited upon the tiny little boy shortly after he came into this world. When I got home, I changed into my sweats, fixed myself my favorite Mount Gay rum highball, and sought out some welcome diversion on CNN. I had just settled in to watch Larry King when the cordless phone on the end table next to me rang. It was Nancy, a neighbor just down the street. There was an unmistakable sound of urgency in her voice when she asked for Suanne without so much as extending a perfunctory salutation to me. I immediately handed the receiver to Suanne.

Suanne cradled the phone in the crook of her neck and went back into the kitchen (which is not separated from the family room), to continue getting dinner ready. I often marvel at the natural "multi-tasking" talents women display while cradling phones to their ear or babies on their hips. Moments later she gasped, "Oh no! Oh I'm so sorry Nancy. Are they sure?" At this point my attention was re-focused from Larry King's interview with Jesse Jackson to the one-sided conversation that Suanne was having with Nancy in the kitchen. It was obvious that something was terribly wrong. Moments later, when she put down the phone, Suanne told me Nancy's daughter-in-law, Mendy, had been diagnosed with breast cancer. It was shocking news.

I knew Mendy. As an attorney, I had represented her in a personal injury case several years earlier. The case involved a temporomandibular joint injury (TMJ) that she sustained in an auto accident. She was only 26 at the time of the accident, engaged to Nancy's son, Rob, and working for a high-tech firm in

Silicon Valley. Mendy was very attractive, smart and self-assured. The kind of young woman that turns brains as well as heads. She and Rob were married not long after her case settled and they now had two little girls. Mendy was 33 and her youngest child was less than a year old. Nancy told Suanne that Mendy found a lump while doing a breast self-examination in the shower.

After dinner, I retired to my study, as is my habit, and did some quick Internet research on the demographics of breast cancer. Although I had handled a number of malpractice cases involving various types of cancer, and was familiar with the some of the broader medical aspects of the disease, I had yet to handle a breast cancer case to conclusion and could not claim to have any real familiarity with the origins and course of the disease.

From my cursory research I quickly learned that Mendy was way too young to have a palpable malignant lump in her breast unless it was a highly aggressive form of the disease. Most commonly, breast cancer tumors are made up of slow growing mutant cells that take years and even decades to grow to the size that the lump can be felt by self-examination or even by a trained doctor. This is the reason that the majority of breast cancer cases occur in women in their mid to late fifties and early sixties. When we went to bed, Suanne asked me if my research had revealed what the typical age was for a women to be diagnosed with breast cancer. It's unusual for someone as young as Mendy, I replied.

January 17, 1996

I got to the office about 8:00 am and began plowing through the new medical malpractice HSV II chart again. Just trying to decipher the chart notes was exasperating enough, much less understanding all the medical terminology attendant with a case of this complexity. I had an appointment to meet with the parents of the little boy at nine. Obviously, should I elect to take the case, they would be my clients and I was anxious to see what kind of first impression they would make as juries are always keenly interested in the appearance and person- alities of the plaintiffs.

The young couple arrived punctually and following some preliminary get-to- know-one-another small talk, we waded into the murky circumstances of the care and treatment rendered to their baby after his delivery.

The mother, thin, unadorned and somewhat distant, had understandable difficulty in discussing almost any aspect of what had transpired with her son. The passage of just under two years since the birth had done nothing to blot the inscription of the pain that had been lodged upon her face. The father, no less affected by the enormity of the tragedy, but, not unexpectedly for a male, was very angry and vocal about it. He was angry not only at the medical community for what he construed as a gross failure to read his wife's medical history and diagnosis his son's illness, but also at his prior attorneys for giving up on the case with no resolution in sight. Both parents were terribly discouraged and were seriously considering dropping the litigation altogether after being dropped by three different law firms.

Some lawyers call these kinds of cases "orphans," because they have a hard time finding a good home and end up getting passed from one office to the next. Of course, this doesn't exactly inspire confidence in the fourth lawyer to get involved in the case either. At about 10:30 the receptionist's voice come on over the intercom; Suanne was on the line. I was just finishing up the appointment and said that I'd call her back. "She asked me to interrupt you," the receptionist responded, "She wants to talk to you now."

"Hi." I said, unenthusiastic about interrupting the meeting, "I'm with clients. Can I call you back in a few minutes; we're almost done."

"No, I need you to come home," she said, her voice suffused with palpable anxiety.

"What's wrong?" I asked, my first thoughts immediately turning to our son Joshua.

"I was thinking about Mendy this morning," she answered, "and I realized that I hadn't given myself a good breast examination for a while. Scott, I think I felt a lump in my breast." The word "lump" dangled for a moment in the earpiece of the phone. "It's probably nothing," she added, "but I want you to come home and feel it for yourself."

My office in Aptos is five minutes from our home in La Selva Beach, so it wasn't a big deal for me to run home in the middle of the morning and I certainly didn't panic at the thought that Suanne might have thought she felt something unusual, or even a lump in her breasts. At 51, she was still several years away from the high-risk age category for being diagnosed with breast cancer, and we had already been introduced to a false alarm breast cancer scare back in the late 70's. At the same time, however, I did appreciate the unreserved emotion in her voice.

Suanne was still in her mid-thirties when she first felt something in her right breast accompanied by some intermittent swelling and pain. When she tried to show me what she was feeling, I could barely feel anything. As an aspiring medical malpractice attorney, I took it upon myself to get her to a physician in Palo Alto to check out the lump. At the time, mammograms were not routinely used in younger women to screen for cancer, and for reasons that are unclear to this day; a mammogram was never ordered to diagnose the lump we thought we were feeling. Instead, an outpatient biopsy procedure performed under a local anesthesia resulted in a diagnosis of a non-malignant (benign) condition called fibrocystic disease or mammary dysplasia. Fibrocystic disease, back in the late 70s, was an ominous sounding diagnosis used by gynecologists and surgeons to describe a wide range of symptoms that in reality were nothing more than normal changes and sensations in a woman's breasts as she ages. Today, attaching the label "disease" to fibrocystic is frowned on by most physicians.

The good news for us was that what Suanne was feeling evidently wasn't a malignancy; the bad news was that she was diagnosed with a "disease." Suanne was told that having fibrocystic disease might put her in a higher risk category, at least statistically, for a breast cancer diagnosis in the future. It was a frightening experience, to be sure, but most of Suanne's concerns were allayed when her long time Ob/Gyn told her that the condition was not anything she need worry about. Following her doctor's advice, and believing that she was not a likely candidate for breast cancer, we both soon forgot about this early scare.

My immediate response upon hanging up the phone was that Suanne probably was overreacting to the news about Mendy. But I hadn't eaten any breakfast and avocado on sourdough toast was sounding pretty good about then. After telling the parents that I was interested in further investigating their case and making a follow-up appointment, I told my secretary that I was leaving and would return shortly.

It was raining steadily when I pulled out of our parking lot and on to the freeway. Most of the cars had their headlights on. A flashing yellow light on the shoulder near our off-ramp warned of a minor mudslide spilling onto the road. I barely thought of my conversation with Suanne before pulling into the driveway. In fact, when I arrived, I momentarily forgot why I went home. My mind was completely preoccupied with the neonatal herpes case and the just-concluded client interview.

What I had learned in the meeting with the parents and from my review of the hospital charts was a medical story so horrifying in its aftermath as to leave me almost too stunned to focus on anything else. There had been a complete failure to include an HSV II infection in the infant's differential diagnosis following a Caesarian-section delivery, notwithstanding the mother's documented history of genital herpes and classic signs and symptoms of infection noted in the infant's medical chart within the first 24 hours after birth. The parents also informed me that they had seen a skin lesion on their son's back near his right armpit about two weeks post partum (a telltale sign of herpes infection).

However, not only was nothing done to follow-up, the lesion was not even recorded in the chart. Left undiagnosed and untreated, the herpes virus eventually progressed from what is called the skin, eye, mucosa variety (SEM) to the central nervous system presentation (CNS), and the little boy's brain ended up being ravaged by herpes encephalitis.

Although given a statistical life expectancy of thirty to forty years, the little fellow would live it severely retarded, functioning at no better than the level of an eight-month-old infant. In addition, he was also rendered partially deaf, blind and his immune system severely compromised, among other dreadful medical problems. Having just been made privy to the horrifying details of the neonatal herpes encephalitis disease process for the first time, I felt terribly sorry for the guilt-ridden parents, who struggling bravely, shared with me their solemn and gritty resolve to care for their child at home for the duration. I thought to myself, it was as though they had been consigned to one of the bottom rings of Dante's Inferno where the flames of pain and guilt would forever scorch their daily lives, even though they had done nothing to deserve such a wretched fate.

When I arrived home, I went around back and through the workout room into our bedroom, where my mood and attention immediately changed. The wind chimes were creating a pleasing metallic little euphony, backed by the muffled chorus of rainfall on the translucent corrugated roof of the workout room. I found Suanne lying on our unmade bed wearing the floral oriental bathrobe I had given her for some special occasion. A mauve colored bath towel done up like a turban covered her damp hair. Her skin was still a ruddy pink from a hot shower. Notwithstanding the sober purpose of my call, when I saw Suanne supine on our bed dappled in the gray blush of the dark January morning with one breast barely covered and her left hand cupping the other, she was the very picture of tantalizing sensuality and allure.

A beam of warm light from the bathroom lay like a comforter across the foot of the bed. As I paused at the door I could see her gently massaging her right breast. I walked in and sat down on the bed next to her and watched, feeling warm irrepressible waves of desire roll over me. Was this perhaps but a clever ruse to lure me home for a "morning delight?" For several moments she continued to knead and poke at her breast, saying nothing.

"Here Scott, give me your hand," she said at last, "I'll show you what I'm feeling." Her voice was calm but icily serious. She took my hand and proceeded to guide my fingers to the lateral side of her right breast. All I could feel was the satiny texture of her lovely skin.

"Don't worry," I rasped, "You're probably just having a paranoid reaction to the news about Mendy."

"Maybe," Suanne answered, "maybe not. Granted, I did get a little uptight after talking to Nancy last night. That's why I examined myself so carefully in the shower this morning."

I said nothing as she kept trying to steer my fingers to the spot where she thought she had felt a lump. As she pressed the tips of my fingers into the side of her breast, her nipple rose and fell slightly almost in syncopation with the murmuring wind chimes. It was, I must confess, a most pleasant sight and the urge I was feeling grew in strength and intensity. I made a slight effort to move my fingers in a different direction from where she was taking them, but her grip remained firm and she didn't seem to even notice. I felt a slight hint of personal disapprobation.

"It was eerie," she allowed," I was showering and there it was. I felt a lump. I thought, 'My God, how have I not felt this before?' So then I went felt all around both breasts to see if I could feel anything similar. There! Push down right where your finger is and tell me what you feel."

I gently pushed in and moved my finger in tiny circular motions. Again, I felt nothing but the soft satiny texture of skin. "I don't feel anything," I whispered. "It's probably all in your imagination." I started to lean over to kiss her, having more or less convinced myself of the truth of my reverie about the ruse.

"Don't." She said emphatically, and took my hand again and moved my fingers slightly up and back toward her armpit. "There, push in right there."

Again I pushed delicately and moved my fingers in the same small circular motions, and again I felt nothing. "Push a little harder," she ordered. Then I felt it. A slight shiver reverberated though my body. My fantasy of the ploy vanished instantly. This was not a time for fun and games.

No question, I could definitely feel a small pea-sized lump on the side of her breast at about nine o'clock and back an inch and a half or so from the border of the areola toward her armpit. What exactly did I feel, she asked.

"It feels small, roundish, fairly hard. Bigger than a BB - maybe about the size of a pea." It also felt immobile. Then, without the slightest basis, I added, "It feels just like the last time - like a benign mass." Even as the words passed my lips, I could taste the transparency of them.

"It's probably a recurrence of the fibrocystic disease," Suanne volunteered. "But what worries me is the shape of the lump. It's smooth and round and feels very similar to the lump I've felt on the model breast at Dr. Andrews' office. You know, the one I've told you about that they use to show patients what to feel for during self-examinations." I had no good response. In fact, I had no response at all and just looked at her. The sound of the wind chimes and rain falling on the roof of the workout room grew louder. But now, in the short fifteen minutes I'd been home, the syncopation was gone, the harmony, the rhythm, the romantic blush of the morning, all gone. All I could hear was so much aural clatter.

Finally, I asked, "When are you due for your next mammogram?"

"Three months, but I'm not going to wait. I think I'd better call for an appointment right away and have it checked out." I agreed.

The topic of breast cancer, if not the reality of the threat to Suanne, was not a completely foreign topic in the Lyman household, even long after we had our brush with fibrocystic disease back in the late seventies. Indeed, we had a good friend and neighbor Suanne's age who had been stricken with breast cancer when she was 47. We had followed her progress from discovery through a mastectomy and chemotherapy, all in the span of about two or three weeks. But even with this breast cancer experience by osmosis, literally next door, and our brush with the fibrocystic disease, before Suanne discovered her own lump, breast cancer always seemed to be a remote and abstract threat; it-always-happens-to-someone else type of thing.

Perhaps because of the lack of first-hand experience with cancer in our families and coupled with Suanne's regular checkups and excellent health in general, the act of scheduling the appointment to have the lump examined did not seem at the time to me to be anything to be particularly worried about. Certainly it was not like we were about to cross some medical Rubicon, at least as far as I was concerned. On the contrary, I convinced myself without much trouble that this appointment would be just another preventive medicine measure, much like her annual checkups; nothing to worry about. Suanne herself exhibited a similar confidence. As it turned out, we were both mistaken and about to learn how close upon the sound of distant thunder the storm can strike.

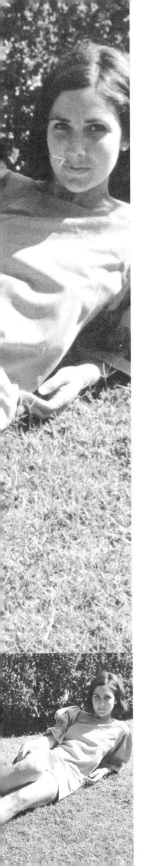

CHAPTER 2
Risk Factors and Mammograms

January 19, 1996

On the theory that if it ain't broke don't fix it, Suanne had been with her same Ob/Gyn since 1965, the year I entered Stanford University as a twenty-two year old Navy vet with a wife and two little boys.

Dr. Andrews was young and handsome, just a couple of years out of his medical residency. Fifteen years later he delivered Josh, our youngest son, at Stanford University Medical Center. In between, Suanne felt that she got excellent care from Dr. Andrews and because of their long-standing relationship she was willing to continue as his patient, even though it meant traveling "over the hill" from Santa Cruz to Palo Alto, a drive of just over an hour, once or twice a year for appointments.

Suanne had known Melanie Andrews, the doctor's wife, since she went to work in the office in the late 1970's as a nurse practitioner. In addition to Suanne's abiding respect professionally for both of them, she also felt a genuine kinship. They were warm and caring people who treated their patients more like family members than as paying customers. It was he that had handed me the powerful shears to "do the honor" of cutting the umbilical cord at Josh's birth at the Medical Center and she who poured the champagne to celebrate the occasion. Unquestionably, moments like these, in addition to the longevity bonds that develop over the years, create powerful doctor and patient relationships.

Suanne called Dr. Andrews' office immediately after our midmorning bedroom conversation and told the receptionist that she had felt a lump in her breast and wanted to have it checked. By now, Dr. Andrews had his own mammography equipment and was holding forth his office as a high quality testing facility for the diagnosis of breast cancer. It was no problem to get her in right away.

Three days later Suanne drove over to Palo Alto for a mammogram and a complete physical examination, fully expecting that what she and I had felt was nothing more than some lumpy breast tissue. Although I wouldn't say that either one of us took the appointment casually, we both felt certain that the results of the examination would be negative, as was the case when she had the biopsy many years earlier. Our expectations were not based on blind faith or some notion of medical hubris, but rather on Suanne's medical history and on knowing that she was not considered a high-risk candidate for breast cancer.

Indeed, she was free of virtually every known variable risk factor. High fat diets are believed to increase the risk of breast cancer. Suanne had always enjoyed a very healthful, low fat diet including plenty of fresh fruits and vegetables. She had never been overweight. Smoking and excessive alcohol consumption are considered risk factors. She had never been a smoker, a drinker, or exposed to any environmental or industrial carcinogens (at least as far as we know).

"Terrific!!" That's the word I would use to sum up Suanne's physical appearance. She is athletic-looking, fairly tall (5'8"), brunette, amply endowed (34D), has piercing hazel eyes, and, at the time this saga began, weighed 148 pounds. Being fairly large-boned, she carried the weight well.

It is generally accepted that female hormones, particularly estrogen, play a role in the most common forms of breast cancer. Suanne started menstruating late, gave birth early, and entered menopause surgically and hence ceased menstruating at a relatively young age. Consequently, she had experienced significantly fewer menstrual cycles (both over her lifetime and between her first menses and her first pregnancy). Consequently, she had been exposed to less estrogen washes than many of her contemporaries. [1]

Perhaps most significantly, to our knowledge, Suanne had no genetic predisposition for breast cancer on either side of her family. Her mother is an extremely active and healthy octogenarian, and there was no history of breast cancer in either her immediate or her extended family. We came to learn statistically, the risk of breast cancer in a woman who has an immediate family history is two times greater than for one with no history.

Suanne's father, although diagnosed with prostate cancer late in his life, died of heart failure. He is the only known familial link with cancer in any form. In short, if risk factors are accurate indicators (as some studies show them to be), Suanne should have been near the bottom of the list of likely breast cancer

[1] - Some studies suggest that modern women (mid to late 20th century) may have as many as 15 to 20 times as many periods (estrogen washes) as their cohorts from prior centuries. During earlier times the average age of menarche (first menstruation) was in the late teens. It is now down around 12 in most western nations. Historically, women would become pregnant around a dozen times and on average deliver 5 to 6 births. They would then nurse for up to two years or longer. Many would then die or enter menopause (stop menstruating). This resulted in many women having as few as 15 to 20 ovulations during their lives, compared to up to 400 for modern women. **JSL**

candidates. The absence of these risk factors, we felt at the time, provided us a reason for our confidence that this scare, and the pending appointment with Dr. Andrews would amount to much ado about nothing. That said, we also recognized that Suanne was not free of all known risk factors and that breast cancer needs no risk factors whatsoever to come knocking.

Thanks to a partial hysterectomy, Suanne had been on hormonal (estrogen) replacement therapy for almost seven years. During the 80's, Suanne was an avid and talented tennis player, and after our youngest son's birth she was occasionally troubled by "leakage" when exerting herself on the court. She recalls one time when Dr. Andrews performed an internal examination, asking her, "Are you having any leakage?"

"Yes," she acknowledged. "Sometimes when I sneeze or when I'm playing tennis. It's really bugging me."

"We can fix that," he replied. "And maybe we'll just remove the uterus at the same time."

"Is something wrong with my uterus?" Suanne inquired.

"No," came the answer. "But it's really not good for anything anymore except growing cancer cells, so we might as well remove the uterus and eliminate the risk. By leaving the ovaries, you will continue to produce estrogen, just not as much as you would otherwise. All that you will miss is having your monthly period." At the same time, Dr. Andrews also said he could tighten her up "here and there."

It all sounded inviting enough to Suanne. It sounded good to me too. She had the surgery and recovered quickly. A short time later, however, Suanne began experience minor anxiety attacks. She would become nervous and hot, and have heart palpitations that would leave her breathless. When she complained to Dr. Andrews about these symptoms, he prescribed hormone replacement therapy (commonly known as HRT), to supplement her now diminished production of estrogen. Suanne wore an Estradiol patch on her abdomen, switching it from one side to the other every 3 days. The HRT took care of the hot flashes and anxiety attacks she had complained about and the only side effect of the HRT was that every six weeks or so, her breasts would become quite swollen and tender. A problem for her; yes; but a visual and tactile delight for me.

Dr. Andrews assured Suanne that HRT would take care of the menopausal symptoms, ward off osteoporosis, keep her heart healthy, stoke her libido and help her feel and look younger than her chronological age (all known benefits of supplemental estrogen). We now know, of course, that the pharmaceutical companies, despite having conducted little research on the long term risks of hormone replacement therapy, did a terrific job of marketing HRT as financial gold mine to the Ob/Gyn establishment. Not only would Ob/Gyns see women of childbearing age, but these same patients/clients would continue to be joined at the hip, as it were, with their gynecologist in managing their hormonal needs as they aged. It was a whole new treatment regimen that could be given to women following their childbearing years.

Before beginning her own treatment, Suanne read the literature provided by Dr. Andrews (in the form of handouts from the pharmaceutical companies), on HRT and was sold on its reputation as a "magic potion" for menopausal and pre-menopausal women, enabling them, if the claims were to be believed, to retain the benefits of youth well past menopause. Supple skin, a strong libido and a wet vagina were certainly advantages that most men, myself included, are apt to "buy into" without hesitation. Sounded like a win-win proposition to me!

Then, in the summer of 1995, some six years into Suanne's therapy, Time magazine ran a cover story on HRT, noting some of the potential risks associated with it, including breast cancer. Reading this article motivated Suanne to revisit the subject with Dr. Andrews. He again assured her that the benefits of HRT far outweighed what he described as a remote risk of breast cancer.

When Suanne inquired of me what I thought about her continuing on HRT, I voiced my unqualified support, notwithstanding that I simply took Dr. Andrews' word regarding the low risk factor at face value. My reasons, of course, were not entirely unselfish. Indeed, my wife was not exactly getting an unbiased second opinion. Enthusiastic, yes; impartial, no.

By the time I turned fifty, Suanne had become the focus of virtually all my sexual fantasies. Belying popular beliefs about middle- aged men, I was still as eager as ever to pursue an active, passionate sexual relationship with Suanne. I had long since graduated from the Calvin Klein inspired youth culture image of bubblegum sexuality and allure. I had moved up to the privilege and reality of being able to spend my life with a beautiful woman whom I truly love and have always lusted after. So if the ravages of menopause and age could be forestalled by hormone replacement therapy, I was all for it. Why would any man really feel differently? The possibility that HRT might marginally increase her risk of breast cancer didn't even enter my mind as a factor to be considered.

Together with the years spent on HRT, Suanne also had taken birth control pills for about seven or eight years in her late twenties and early thirties. Like estrogen replacement therapy, according to some studies, the long-term use of birth control pills (which contain estrogen), may similarly increase the chance of breast cancer. Finally, Suanne had nursed none of our children, which is also thought to increase the risk of breast cancer by eliminating still more menstrual cycles. But compared to the comfort level we derived from knowing that most of the major risk factors were absent, the few modest factors that were present did not weigh in that heavily. **2**

Around 11:30, Suanne called from the Dr. Andrews' office. He had just finished his physical examination. "Charles doesn't seem particularly worried about the way the lump feels. He says I shouldn't be alarmed because most lumps don't amount to anything and that the mammogram will give us a better idea of what we're feeling. I'm going to have it done in a few minutes and then I'm going to the shopping center for a little while. I'll be coming back at the office around four."

I hung up the phone feeling relief and comfort from Dr. Andrews' medical support and Suanne's casual decision to combine the appointment with some shopping. If it didn't feel like a tumor to the doctor, then it didn't feel like one to me either. Little did Suanne know, but her appointment that day was the first, last and only time for several months that she would speak with Dr. Andrews personally about the lump in her right breast; the same lump that would be later be diagnosed as a malignant tumor. Instead, from this point forward, during a medically crucial and emotional period, Suanne would be left in the hands of one of the office nurses or technicians.

Dr. Andrews' radiology technician, had been doing Suanne's mammograms for years, ever since the mammography equipment arrived in their office. I had talked to Stephanie on the phone once or twice, I think regarding an appointment, and I had met her in the office on one occasion when I went in to pick up Suanne. She was tall, thirty-something, brunette, friendly and attractive; more importantly, she seemed to take great pride in her work and as a member of the professional team.

After taking the images Dr. Andrews had ordered, Stephanie looked at the films and told Suanne that she had all the angles needed to fully "see" both breasts. Informally, Stephanie had said that the lump Suanne was feeling did show up on the film but that it looked negative for a malignancy. She concluded by reassuring Suanne and saying that the films would be sent to the Imaging

---

2 - I don't agree with the popular supposition that HRT causes breast cancer, nor do many other experts in the field. Studies do not support this view, and links which have been seen are weak and often contradictory. There is even greater acceptance of using HRT in women who have been treated for breast cancer. I also don't agree that there is a plot by pharmaceutical companies to convince MDs to use the hormones unnecessarily to boost profits. I do believe in environmental causes for breast cancer, and in xenoestrogens like dioxin and organophosphates which can use the estrogen receptor to get into the cell and therein do damage. This is a large and complex topic–estrogen is needed by some who may then become afraid. It is hard to believe even from a Darwinian angle that it is our reproductive hormones which kill us. **EM**

Center for reading by a radiologist and she'd call with the results as soon as they came back.

Suanne called me again while en route home. "Stephanie told me she could see the lump in the mammogram, but to her it does not appear suspect." The relief in Suanne's voice was obvious. I glommed on to Stephanie's off-the-cuff comment as though the Mayo Clinic had just given my wife a clean bill of health. "I knew it," I said, "it's probably just another benign fibrocystic lump." In fact, we were both so accepting of Stephanie's would be assurances that the topic of breast cancer was dropped for a few days. And even though Suanne continued to feel the lump from time to time, she seemed to be pretty relaxed about the whole matter. Case closed, or so we thought.

January 23, 1996

Stephanie called during President Clinton's State-of-the-Union message. I had read a column by William Safire in the New York Times that gave a number of bullet points to look for and I was fairly engrossed in watching. The report from Stephanie was as she had predicted. "Just like I thought," she said, "everything seems to be fine. There doesn't appear to be a malignancy."

"What is it, then?" Suanne asked, almost casually, "What am I feeling?"

"Probably just a nodule," Stephanie replied. "Just some nodule."

"Nodule?" Suanne wasn't satisfied with so vague explanation. "What exactly do you mean by a 'nodule'?"

"It's just a general term we use to describe tissue like your lump that although not suspicious is unexplained," Stephanie said. Up to this point in the conversation Suanne's relief at the delivery of good news completely over-shadowed any doubts she, or I, may have had about the veracity of the mammogram results. But Stephanie's non-explanation of the lump didn't sit well with Suanne. It was like dangling the security of health and well-being just beyond her grasp.

"Stephanie, I really would like to know the exact nature of the lump. If it's not something I should be concerned with, then what–exactly–is it? It seems like you're using a different word to describe the same thing."

"What we mean when we use the word "nodule" is just breast tissue that feels like a lump, but that isn't suspicious," she reiterated. "You don't need to worry about it."

Suanne could sense Stephanie's growing impatience and knew that the phone conversation was taking more of the tech's personal time than she had either intended or wanted to accord. "Perhaps the best thing for me to do is to ask Dr. Andrews to get back to you," Stephanie concluded with a tincture of irritation creeping into her voice.

Suanne thanked Stephanie for calling and hung up, more than a little disturbed by the way the conversation had ended. For one thing, she wasn't satisfied at all with the lack of an explanation for the lump. Neither was she satisfied with the term "nodule" which to her reckoning didn't have any different meaning than "lump."

More than a little curious about the word being bandied about and feeling a bit dismissed, Suanne proceeded directly to our library and looked up the word "nodule" in the World Book Medical Encyclopedia. She became fairly alarmed to read, "Nodules or lumps on the breast should always be seen by a physician, even if they do not change in size."

When we went to bed that night she had me feel her lump yet again. Somehow when I felt it this time, it felt smaller and less distinct than before, perhaps more like a nodule perhaps, than a lump. What did I know? What did either of us know about lumps and nodules? But I did like the feel of her breast.

"Maybe you're just being a little paranoid," I suggested snuggling up to her.

Suanne's response was swift and certain. "Do you think that Tom Grace should have been a little more paranoid when his legs started going numb and the doctor wouldn't do a spinal tap and he ended up a paraplegic? Do you think that Ed Bowles should have been a little more paranoid when the doctor told him not to worry about his elevated PSA and he ended up with prostate cancer? Maybe if Doyle Yancy had been a little paranoid about the injury to his neck, the ER doctors wouldn't have sent him home with a dislocated and fractured vertebra and he wouldn't have woken up a quadriplegic!"

Whoa! Suanne was obviously getting a little worked up. As for me, however, based on the only information we had to go on –a mammogram we were told was negative and a negative clinical impression–I didn't really share her concerns, at least not to the degree she obviously did. But I didn't discount them either. The snuggling came to an abrupt halt.

There wasn't a medical malpractice case I had worked on in the past ten years that Suanne, as my office manager, bookkeeper and sometimes receptionist, wasn't intimately familiar with. Now that she found herself under the medical microscope, the skepticism about medical explanations and judgments was beginning to flow from her mind like sweat from a racehorse. And, as our conversation continued, I could tell that she was becoming frustrated with me, too.

"Look, all I'm saying is that you are not a likely candidate for breast cancer and that both Dr. Andrews and the radiologist think you're fine. Isn't that enough," I asked, somewhat querulously. "Good grief, you don't need, all of the sudden, to think they're committing malpractice because they say your lump isn't suspicious. If there was something to be concerned about they would have said so."

Even though I see the dirty laundry of the medical community hanging out my window all the time doesn't mean that I am suspicious of every judgment or opinion a doctor renders. On the contrary, seeing the small number of bona fide mistakes that are made actually engenders confidence in the medical profession. At least it does for me. I turned over and went to sleep convinced that Suanne was letting her emotions cloud the sound medical advice she seemed to be receiving.

January 22, 1996

Stephanie called early in the morning. I answered, and after calling to Suanne, stayed on the line to listen in on the conversation. "Hi Suanne, it's Stephanie. I spoke with Dr. Andrews about your concerns. He asked me to assure you that the nodule in your right breast does not appear suspicious and that you shouldn't worry about it." There was a long pause.

I knew Suanne was expecting the call to be from the doctor, not his technician, so the conversation didn't start well for her. But like most patients, Suanne found it difficult to be too assertive with her health care professionals–be they doctors, nurses or radiology technicians. But by the same token, she also wasn't ready to simply accept, as an article of faith, the explanation of an unexplained nodule.

"If it's not suspicious," Suanne began, "and I shouldn't worry about it, what does Dr. Andrews think it is? Besides, I still don't understand what exactly is the difference between a lump and a nodule?" I could hear and feel the emotion creeping into her voice.

"The term nodule," Stephanie allowed, "as distinct from a lump, is a catchall phrase used to describe a benign tissue mass of unknown etiology. Breast tissue gets lumpy as women get older and just because you feel a lump doesn't mean it's cancer. It usually isn't cancer. It's usually just a benign tissue mass."

"That's all well and good Stephanie, but the fact that it is unexplained and it feels so much like the 'lump' in the model breast in the mammography room, leaves me feeling very uncomfortable with what you're telling me," Suanne countered. "I need to know exactly what it is, not simply that it is of unknown etiology."

Stephanie, no doubt, was ready to end the conversation. "Let me talk to Dr. Andrews again," she said abruptly, "We'll call you back."

"Thank you," Suanne said with equal abruptness.

When I went back into the family room, I could almost see the frustration oozing out of her pores. She fully expected now that Dr. Andrews, her trusted Ob/Gyn and, mind you, her friend of more than three decades, would in fact return the call as had been promised. He didn't.

Again, it was Stephanie on the other end of the line several hours later. "Suanne, Dr. Andrews says that if you're not satisfied with his examination and the mammography results, and if your concerns about the nodule are going to interfere with your quality of life, then all he can do is refer you to a surgeon."

"Fine," Suanne said, now firmly miffed about not hearing directly from her doctor. "Who are you referring me to?"

Stephanie gave Suanne the number of a breast surgeon in Palo Alto named Ellen Mahoney. "Thank you," Suanne said, slamming the phone down with an audible thunk.

Determined to find out exactly what it was she and I had been feeling, Suanne immediately called Dr. Mahoney's office for an appointment. She was determined to find out exactly what it was she was feeling on the side of her right breast that felt so much like what she had been trained by her doctor to be on guard for. At the same time, she was more than a little disappointed that she had not had the opportunity to discuss this matter personally with the doctor that had been treating her for almost her entire adult life. Plainly, the whole situation, and particularly not hearing from Dr. Andrews directly, was beginning to be very distressing to Suanne and her distress was splashing over on to me.

Following the afternoon conversation with Stephanie, Suanne came storming into my office and demanded to know if I thought she was being hysterical. In truth, my reaction to the medical advice she was receiving and the circumstance of Dr. Andrews not calling, was very mixed. More than anything else, I wanted to believe that what the doctors were saying was true and that Suanne was being unduly emotional. So, when asked to judge Suanne's reaction, I must admit that even in the phone conversation I had listened to with Stephanie, the word "hysterical" had occurred to me. But being careful not to show any insensitivity, I suggested to Suanne that perhaps she might be overreacting, just a little.

"They make mistakes, Scott," she fired back. "You know that better than I do. Mammograms are not always accurate. You can get false negatives; it happens all the time. I can tell you are getting exasperated with me because I can't help feeling the lump without worrying about what it might be. My hand is constantly on my breast feeling the lump. I lay in bed at night and feel it. When I'm in the shower, I feel it. I feel it during the day in my office. It's kind of like when you have a sore in your mouth and your tongue just goes on automatic pilot, seeking it out. I need to see the surgeon. I need to take care of this. Damn it, Scott, you're not the one with the lump or the nodule or whatever it is." I started to get up from my chair to calm her, knowing full well she was right, but before I was upright, she turned abruptly on her heel and was gone.

In the course of dealing with a vast array of medical catastrophes over the years, I had learned to have a well-refined skepticism of the proclamations of doctors in situations exactly like our own. Therefore, I suppose, for us to err on the side of caution made all the sense in the world. Too often patients simply abandon their own feelings and intuition about their health in favor of slavishly believing everything the doctor offers up. Instead of being our own advocates, our own health care champions, we become little more than punch cards for an authority figure's prescriptions of what supposedly is the passport to good health. The consequences of such unthinking abject trust, I have learned time and again, are not always pretty. Even so, for whatever reasons, dealing with a personal circumstance like Suanne's lump seemed miles removed from my professional experience with representing clients in medical malpractice cases. No doubt, it has something to do with the maxim that "the lawyer that represents himself has a fool for a client." The same maxim, in situations involving the first degree of consanguinity or matrimony, probably also obtains.

I did recognize, at least in the back of my mind, that I could be allowing my conscious and subconscious fear of what a positive diagnosis of breast cancer might hold in store for me to override my own better judgment and experience. Having labeled my wife's reaction as "hysterical," I later admitted to myself, it might have been a convenient rug to sweep my own fears under. But whatever sub-currents may have been in play there, I fully supported Suanne's announced vow of self-advocacy and her decision to follow-up immediately with this Dr. Mahoney. [3] The decision was strictly hers and there were no ifs, ands, or buts about it. Suanne was being Suanne, doing her thing, her way. I was there in a supporting role.

---

3 - It is true that many patients are reluctant to express their feelings and concerns about their medical care, particularly if they are hearing what they want to hear. But every patient needs to take a certain amount of responsibility for their own medical just as Ms. Lyman did in this case.

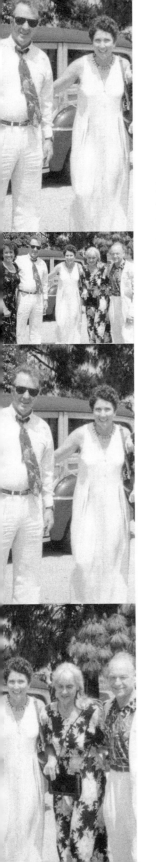

CHAPTER 3
Appointment with the Surgeon

January 31, 1996

Suanne didn't have to wait long for an appointment with Dr. Mahoney. Even though my initial reaction to scheduling the appointment was no big deal, as the date approached, I began to experience an entirely different, but perhaps not unexpected reaction. Until now, everything about breast cancer still seemed distant and abstract, like the importance of opening a retirement account while in your twenties or thirties. But as I thought more about the fact that Suanne was going to see a physician who specialized in breast cancer surgery, my mind started conjuring up images of every form of surgical mayhem imaginable.

My experience as a medical malpractice attorney told me that primary care physicians, in our case Suanne's Ob/Gyn, ordinarily refer their patients to surgeons for surgery. **4** To my thinking, it made no difference that Suanne, the patient, was the one contesting the medical opinions expressed by her physicians and insisting on the appointment with the surgeon. But once I drew the line between the dots connecting "breasts" and "surgeon", it was a small logical step to imagining a radical mastectomy. And think about it I did. Plenty!

Even though I fully endorsed the idea of scheduling an appointment with the surgeon, the more I thought about what might be in store, the more I could feel the roots of fear burrowing deeper and deeper into my psyche. I found myself imagining what it would be like to look at Suanne without breasts, or with one breast, or without nipples, or with nipples tattooed on stretched skin filled with saline

---

4 - When I opened my practice in PA there was no such thing as a breast surgeon - now there is a professional organization - the point is to avoid unnecessary surgery where possible, and if it has to be done that it is done with the least invasion appropriate to the situation. This development also parallels an explosion in the understanding of the molecular biology and behavior of the disease, with resultant complexity of the decision to be made and the surgical skill involved. In the old days when a woman signed a consent for a biopsy it included a mastectomy, and all biopsies were open ones followed by the now-universally recognized notoriously inaccurate frozen section. There was minimal decision-making and minimal surgical skill involved. There also was generally little interest in this aspect of general surgery - it was not macho like vascular or thoracic cases and there is so much emotion to deal with. **EM**

solution and without sensitivity to touch, to stimulation. These thoughts, even though fleeting and spawned by my bloated imagination, were truly frightening.

Another part of the problem I was having with the pending appointment owed to my mistaken belief that mammography and breast examinations by Ob/Gyns were the methods of choice in diagnosing–that is, ruling in or ruling out breast cancer. In most areas of non-elective medicine, surgery is considered to be the treatment of last resort. Here it was being resorted to rather quickly. Or so I thought.

The breast cancer surgeon is the medical specialist most qualified by training and experience to make a definitive diagnosis of a questionable breast lump, or in Suanne's case, a so-called "unexplained nodule." Self-examination, doctor examination and mammography are all merely "screening tests" and nothing more. Since in our case, these tests had failed to provide the definitive answers we were seeking, and despite the fact that Dr. Andrews seemed completely confident that there was nothing to worry about, the surgical appointment was the next step in diagnosing or ruling out a malignant tumor. [5] But even the existence of a "suspicious lump" on a screening test doesn't automatically mean cancer or surgery (and usually does not since only one out of five suspicious lumps turn out to be cancerous), and certainly a suspicious lump doesn't mean an ipso facto mastectomy. However, try telling this to a neophyte husband fresh on the breast cancer track. The images conjured up by the surgical appointment, I have to say, were my first real wake-up call.

Between the time Suanne made the call and the day of the appointment with Dr. Mahoney, I had barely gotten off my own self-imposed breast cancer roller coaster ride. One minute I'd be satisfied that all of the medical judgments that had been made and the advice and opinions we had been given were well founded, supportable and accurate. The next minute, I'd be thinking that the doctors were just flat-out wrong and guilty of the same kind of egregious malpractice on my wife I had been exposed to time and time again in my law practice. To help me cope with my growing fears, I began doing "Suanne" research just the way I would for any client. Much of the information I gathered about the disease gave me ample reason for optimism and hope.

Early on, I learned that many women can develop lumps or masses in their breasts that are entirely harmless and therefore require nothing more than a definitive diagnosis to rule out a malignancy. There are several types of these harmless lumps.

There are cysts, consisting of a semi-soft, squishy, fluid-filled sacks that are similar to a common blister. This benign mass can be found either superficially

---

5 - This is a critically important point – the value of a negative test, such as a mammogram alone is very limited, and should not be relied on if there are clinical signs to the contrary, such as a palpable lump. **EM**

(near the surface), or deep within the breast. Typically cysts occur in pre-menopausal women, but can appear as early as the late twenties. Depending on their location cysts can feel much like a cancerous tumor. Suanne's lump, however, didn't feel soft and squishy. It felt hard and round.

Cysts often can be diagnosed on physical examination and a definitive diagnosis can almost always be made by use of a procedure called a fine needle aspiration, or FNA for short. As the name implies, a fine needle aspiration consists of inserting a very fine needle into the unidentified sac or lump and withdrawing a sample of the fluid. If it's a benign cyst the sac collapses and voila, that's it. You're home free. Case closed.

Another common benign lump found in women's breasts is called a fibroadenoma. A fibroadenoma consists of pieces of breast tissue that closely mimic cysts and cancerous lumps. Because of its hard, smooth, round shape, on self-examination a fibroadenoma can feel very similar to a malignant lump. Usually though, an experienced physician can readily distinguish a malignancy from a fibroadenoma during a physical examination of the breast.[6]

Fibroadenomas can range in size from a few millimeters to a few centimeters. Typically, they are more mobile than a malignant tumor and like malignant lumps can occur anywhere in the breast. Research shows that teens and young adult women are more prone to this type of lump than are older women. When a malignancy cannot be ruled out upon physical examination, fine needle aspiration (FNA) and ultrasound are the methods of choice for diagnosing a benign fibroadenoma lump. If no fluid comes out and it feels like a fibroadenoma, the doctor can usually make the diagnosis. If doubts remain after this procedure, the fluid withdrawn by the FNA procedure can be sent to the lab for definitive testing.[7]

Another category of benign breast masses are the so-called "pseudo-lumps." These are nothing more than exaggerated, albeit normal, lumpiness typically found in pre-menopausal women. Although consisting simply of the predictable alterations in the texture of maturing breast tissue, pseudo-lumps are a constant source of alarm among pre-menopausal women and even a source of confusion among experienced physicians. However, because by their nature pseudo-lumps

---

6 - Don't count on this – cancer should always be in the differential diagnosis. Ultrasound can be very helpful, along with documentation that the lump is not growing, but it is not always necessary. I never thought that this was a cyst. I did think of an intramammary lymph node, which can get larger for all the same number of benign reasons that any lymph node can. **EM**

7 - Plain aspiration using a syringe and a needle is the old-fashioned way of "ruling out" cancer and not all that reliable. Usually we want an ultrasound fist to be sure that there is fluid and the appearance is that of a "simple cyst." Fine-needle aspiration puts the syringe and needle into a special holder so that cells can be shaved off deep inside the lump and brought into the needle by the vacuum produced. The cells are always sent to the pathology lab. Like the previous point, this is very helpful if malignant cells are seen. If there are benign cells or few cells, cancer has not been ruled out and the next procedure is an open biopsy or a short period of observation to make sure that the area doesn't resolve, as "fibrocystic change" tends to do. Even if there is a malignancy, the needle can miss the malignant cells and pull up only the normal cells inside the area of the lump. In many cases, not all that we feel as a lump is cancer – it is a combination of cancer and the reactive benign cells around it. **EM**

tend to change over a relatively short period of time, they can usually be diagnosed in follow-up examinations. This lies in contrast to malignant lumps that do not change markedly in the short term. For this reason, follow-up appointments are the most frequent method of diagnosing either lumpy breasts or pseudo lumps.

Armed with the knowledge I was gleaning from my legal malpractice lawyer research, I began to revert to my initial belief (read, hope), the odds were favorable that the likely end result of the surgical appointment would bring peace of mind to the two of us. However, while I was Suanne's hopeful advocate, supporter and husband, she was the one facing the challenge of breast cancer and no amount of research, support, optimism or love on my part could alter that basic fact.

That said, by the day the surgical appointment arrived, we were both growing a bit more accepting of the medical judgments that had been passed along the way in interpreting Suanne's physical examinations, mammograms, and other diagnostic tests. After all, we tried to assure ourselves, they were the experts weren't they? What did we know? Indeed, what I had learned from my own preliminary sleuthing only seemed to confirm exactly what we had been told first hand by the doctors. Heck, if they weren't alarmed by the lump why should we be?

Even though my professional involvement with medical malpractice precludes me from being the typical patient husband, I must say it isn't easy to resist the appealing authority of medical practitioners and their aggregate wealth of knowledge, training and experience. Perhaps the same might be said of the trust and confidence clients put in their lawyers under circumstances where we are desperately needed. For most of us, it's akin to the tacit, almost unquestioned faith that small children place in the proclamations of their seemingly omniscient and infallible parents.

Even in adults, the mind, prodded by a little motivation, has the remarkable ability to lull us into a sense of accepting as true that which we want to be true, particularly if there is some tangible evidence and authority (credible or otherwise) to support it. In contemporary society this can mean as little as seeing something in print, on television or on the Internet. Among the more obvious examples of how this proclivity is exploited are the TV infomercials hawking physical fitness machines that promise tremendous gains with no pain, skin care products purporting to banish wrinkles and restore the smooth supple skin of youth, health care supplements vowing Lourdes-like cures for maladies ranging from prostate cancer to hair restoration; arthritis and osteoporosis cures to ward off or even reverse the aging process. It goes without saying that I wanted very badly for Suanne to be cancer-free and therefore was ready to believe just about anything and anybody who gave me a semiplausible reason to believe she was.

Although understandably anxious on the day of the appointment, Suanne put on her best game face and went to see Dr. Mahoney feeling more than a little unsettled about the lump in her breast and what she might learn. On the positive side emotionally, Suanne was feeling bullish that here was a doctor who, as a woman, might better relate to her "female" emotions.

Later, I asked Suanne if she noticed a difference being treated by a female, rather than a male, physician. "Yes," she reflected, "I'd say it's a more complete relationship. Maybe better unspoken communication. She has breasts. She's at risk along with the rest of us. I feel more confidence that emotionally we're on the same page."

Believing (read hoping), that there was no cause for undue alarm, I did not go to the appointment. I kissed her goodbye that morning telling her I'd see her at the office afterward. I had a full plate dealing with various assorted medical and legal tragedies at the hands of a variety practitioners in various specialties, including a prostate cancer case, with all attendant deadlines, client calls and research responsibilities, so I busied myself in work as best I could.

At this stage of Suanne's care I was still trying hard to avoid any negative thoughts regarding the quality of her treatment; besides, Suanne seemed very confident and comfortable with Dr. Mahoney. She didn't need me at her first appointment to intrude my medical malpractice mentality into her new doctor/patient relationship, did she?.

Here's how Suanne described the initial visit:

"Dr. Mahoney has a small office on Welch Road near Stanford Hospital. She is so warm and genuine. I just loved her instantly. Probably the most significant and alarming experience of my first meeting with Ellen was that I felt like I had the most thorough breast examination ever performed on me by a doctor. It was remarkably different than any exam I had ever had by Charles Andrews. First, I was lying on my back. Then, I was sitting. Then, I was lying on each side. About the only thing I didn't do was stand on my head. She examined my breasts like they had never been examined before. I got to thinking about how terrible it is that with all the education about the importance of breast exams, it took a physician specializing in breast surgery to give me a really thorough examination. All doctors treating women should do breast exams in this manner! That was the alarming part. How many doctors miss lumps because they don't know how to do a complete and proper breast exam, I wondered. The significant part was that my breast exam gave me tremendous confidence in her as a doctor. I knew I had a personal ally, a champion. At the end of the appointment, she looked me straight in the eye and said, 'Suanne, I'm not going to cut you loose. We're going to find out what this lump is.'"

Returning at about 1:45 p.m., Suanne entered my office and before even sitting down blurted out, "Dr. Mahoney can feel the lump and said we need to find out what it is."

"What about the mammogram?" I asked. "What about the ultrasound? What about what Dr. Andrews and the radiologist said? Does Dr. Mahoney think they're all wrong when they say the lump isn't suspicious?" I could almost hear myself arguing the case against breast cancer.

"Dr. Mahoney said that if you can feel a suspicious lump you should never rely on a mammogram alone to ascertain whether it exists or is benign," Suanne replied. "She says that if you can feel a lump, it's really there and you have to follow-up and find out what it is." There was a bit of bewilderment and unmistakable resignation in Suanne's voice. Still and all, her persistent search for conclusive answers seemed absolutely reasonable to me, both as her husband and as a malpractice attorney.

She sat in the client chair closest to the window gazing out on my garden for a moment before continuing. "Scott, Dr. Mahoney gave me the most thorough breast examination I have ever had. She told me in no uncertain terms that she didn't like the way the lump feels. She said that it doesn't make any difference what you call it, lump or nodule or whatever, it begs to be explored.

"To her it was a lump. She didn't say anything about it, but I could tell she didn't think kindly about the delay in getting me to see her.[8] She said it's a mistake to rely on a negative reading of the mammogram and ultrasound to rule out a malignancy. I think she is probably the most caring doctor I've ever known. She explained all the options that are available to make a diagnosis."

This was the part that I was most eager to hear. "So, what are our options?" I asked.

"There are several and I wrote them down. There's a fine needle aspiration, a needle biopsy, a core biopsy, a surgical biopsy, and a lumpectomy."

I immediately pictured a worst-case scenario of a long incision and a huge lump growing in her breast and tried to shove it out of my mind so that I could concentrate on what Suanne was telling me.

"I can have the fine needle aspiration, which may explain the lump

8 - As with any profession, every physician is not qualified to address all the medical needs of their patients. Just as I would refer a breast cancer patient to a medical oncologist and/or a radiation oncologist (as in Suanne's case), it is critical for primary care physicians to make the appropriate referrals when a definitive diagnosis is need for a suspicious lump. **EM**

immediately. If it doesn't give us the needed information, we can wait and have a follow-up mammogram in three months and then reevaluate the situation. Depending on if there's been any change, at this point I could have a surgical biopsy. Otherwise, I can go ahead right away and have the surgical biopsy. Dr. Mahoney didn't recommend the core biopsy."

"Why would you wait three months if the needle biopsy is inconclusive?" I asked. It sounded like such a long time.

"Dr. Mahoney said that although it would mean a lot of waiting and anxiety for us, it wouldn't really change the outcome should we learn the lump is malignant. At my age and given the small size of the lump, she said two or three months won't make a difference one way or the other."[9]

"Are you okay with that?" I asked.

"Yes," Suanne replied, "I trust what Dr. Mahoney is telling me."

"What do you want to do?"

"I think I'm going to do the needle aspiration procedure. Dr. Mahoney is comfortable with that. I have a lot of confidence in her strategy. Also, I don't want to miss our river boat trip if I don't have to."

Suanne had scheduled a steamboat cruise up the Mississippi from New Orleans with her mother and two sisters. They had been taking short trips like this since Suanne's father had died, and she really looked forward to them. This excursion was especially anticipated as it took Suanne back to her family roots in the Louisiana Bayou country, where she was born, and I emphatically wanted her to go.

Despite Suanne's confidence in Dr. Mahoney and her plan, my knee-jerk reaction was to return my focus to the mammograms since it was they that were yielding the most desirable results. "So, Dr. Mahoney is saying that the mammograms are false?" I asked.

"She said that Dr. Randolph (the diagnostic radiologist at the Imaging Center) is excellent and that the films probably justified the conclusions he reached.

"But, she also said the films could be wrong. She said that it is not unusual for surgeons to find malignant breast tumors following negative mammograms. What if that's the case with me? What if the mammogram and ultrasound reports are incorrect? I've read statistics somewhere that say that twenty or thirty percent of mammograms interpreted as negative are actually positive. And some reports that read as positive are actually negative. All it is, is a picture that somebody is interpreting and describing. I can feel the lump, and it feels exactly like the one in the model at Dr. Andrews' office. I can feel it, Dr. Mahoney can feel it and she says there's no way we're going to treat it as if it's not there. If we don't get

9 - The idea here is to avoid the unnecessary biopsy, and not incur any extra risk. I didn't have the long history with the lump that Suanne had. I always offer an open biopsy, and sometimes patients just want to go straight ahead. **EM**

something done soon, I'll probably worry myself to death before they find out I don't have cancer. Scott, Do you still think I'm being overly paranoid?"

"No, I don't. We, of all people, know that doctors aren't gods and that, indeed, they do make mistakes. That's why we sue them. But then there's the matter of medical judgment. When a radiologist says that the mammogram is negative, all he or she is really saying is that based on their knowledge, training and experience, your mammogram looks more like the thousands of ones that turn out to be negative than the ones that turn out to be positive. As long as the doctors' judgments are accurate, they're hailed as gods, but if they're wrong, they're only human and it was just an unfortunate judgment call. I think you ought to heed your own inclinations and instincts regarding what's best for you."

Suanne opted for the fine needle aspiration, and wanted it ASAP. I agreed with her decision, but for probably the "wrong" reasons. We both had the impression that a fine needle aspiration could be an effective means of ruling out a malignancy even though it sampled only a tiny amount of tissue from the lump. Our thinking, after weighing all the options and probabilities, was that the other surgical procedures were significantly more invasive and perhaps unnecessary. Why opt for more if less would do the job? At least we were doing something immediately.

Suanne finally slumped back into her chair and stared off into space, looking resigned to accepting whatever the future might hold in store.[10]

As she sat there in front of my desk, lost in her fears, the late afternoon sunlight streamed into my office, creating one of those radiant, sun-filtered kind of scenes that we used to see in old Doris Day movies.

Throughout our just-ended conversation about her appointment with Dr. Mahoney, I kept thinking to myself what a truly remarkable and courageous wife I was blessed with. It was always easy for me to love Suanne. Even during the protracted years of my youth when I imagined myself standing in the bow of my literary whaling boat, knee braced in the nook, singing "a dead whale or a stove boat" at the top of my lungs, she always pulled at the strings of my adventuring heart.

Deep down, I always knew that Suanne would be the one true love of my life; the unshakable foundation upon which my understanding of love and truth would be built. She was always one of the most beautiful and alluring women I have ever laid my eyes on. But her physical beauty and allure was only the portal through which I ultimately gained access to the spirit and courage she possessed in the face of adversity and challenge, measures of which I had

---

10 - There is a tiny false-positive rate and a larger false-negative rate of 5% in experienced hands. No definitive operation should proceed without a larger biopsy. Without the trip, I might have gone straight to the excision when the FNA came back negative. But waiting for the trip was not dangerous – remember that we are dealing with a multi-year process and a statistically improbability of metastasis with such a tiny size. **EM**

unstintingly supplied in spades. She valued her role as a wife and mother above all else and she was willing to give the last ounce of her patience and commitment to ensure success in those roles. Now, as I watched the silent questions raised by the threat of breast cancer threaten her faith in her body, I could not imagine my life–past, present or future–without her. There was no one else in the world like this woman; there was no one like Suanne.

I got up from behind my desk and gave her a long, languorous hug. "Don't worry," I said, "everything will be all right. You'll be fine. I have confidence in Dr. Andrews and Dr. Randall's assessment of the films, and the biopsy will confirm what they've told us. You'll see. Everything will be okay." Although the odds were heavily in her favor that all would be well, as I hugged Suanne tightly I could feel the fretful pounding of her heart, the ponderous weight of her resignation, and her desperate need for all the aid and comfort I could lend.

Notwithstanding my sanguine prognosis and Suanne's best efforts to maintain a positive mien, it was obvious that, with the very real prospect of a breast cancer diagnosis looming straightaway before us, the atmosphere changed in our household.

There was, of course, a new found interest in the subject of cancer in general and breast cancer in particular. Suanne took to scanning the vital statistics in the obituary column related to cancer and sought out news and magazine articles dealing with breast cancer. I found myself spending more and more time researching breast cancer, everything from cause, to treatment, to mortality rates. There was no shortage of material on the subject. It was like the change in perception one experiences when buying a particular type of car that you've never really noticed before. Once it's parked in front of your house, suddenly you see it everywhere.

CHAPTER 4
The FNA

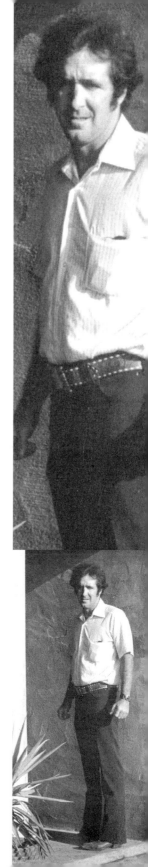

February 7, 1996

Suanne's appointment for the fine needle aspiration was scheduled for Thursday morning. After the two of us discussed the options the doctor had presented, I did some further research on mammography and the several methods of obtaining tissue for a pathology study. I learned that short of doing a biopsy of some sort, the odds of diagnosing or ruling out a malignancy were not as encouraging as I had previously believed.

Yes, mammography is an excellent screening tool, but a negative mammogram reading, as Dr. Mahoney had informed Suanne, ought not be construed as a clean bill of health if there are other clinical signs such as a suspect lump that can be detected upon physical examination. It is reported in the medical literature that nearly ninety percent of lumps that prove to be malignant tumors are discovered by self-examination.[11] Most physicians concur that self-examination is right up there with mammography as a critically important screening tool in the fight against breast cancer.[12]

The truth is that some women discover lumps upon self-examination after having received a negative mammogram. In Suanne's case, she was lucky that the lump was close enough to the surface as to be detectable to touch. Not always the case. Indeed, I came to learn that because of the anatomical configuration of the breast and surrounding structures, it is not uncommon for a lump in the breast to be shielded from both physical and radiographic discovery.

Because Suanne's mammogram results were interpreted as negative by Dr. Andrews and the radiologist, the chief

11 - While I am aware of such reports, I disagree. Happily, in my experience, most lumps are discovered by mammography – I don't have exact numbers and it is a bit dependent on education, but the BCEDP (breast cancer education and development project) in California has reduced access problems for most over-40 women. **EM**

12 - True, but many physicians, including Susan Love, feel strongly that the typical self examination is worthless. My feeling is that it is certainly cheap and immediately available, but needs to be taught properly – it is not a "search and destroy" operation, but a means of gaining confidence in knowing what one's own tissue should feel like. **EM**

source of worry for her was in feeling the lump everyday. As many women do, she might have simply dismissed her own intuition and fears as so much emotional overreaction and instead relied on the professional opinions of her doctors and nurses. But, convinced as she was of the suspicious nature of the lump, Suanne was determined to find out for herself exactly what it was that she was feeling. Dr. Mahoney had made it abundantly clear to her that the only truly accurate way of ruling out a malignancy is to go in and take out some tissue and examine it under a microscope.

Suanne and I felt justified in opting for the fine needle aspiration for a variety of reasons. Principal among them was that, besides the less invasive nature of the FNA, the lump was well defined, palpable, near the surface. This combination of factors, we concluded, militated in favor of the FNA as opposed to one of the more invasive procedures.

We had the negative readings on the mammograms and the stated opinion of Dr. Andrews was that he wasn't worried about it. We had also had the one previous experience where the doctor had done a biopsy (the results of which were negative), that had left a scar of about half an inch on Suanne's breast. I could remember the raised (keloid) scar that appeared prominently above her tan line before she had it revised through plastic surgery. The scar wasn't a big deal to either of us, but the idea of avoiding more scarring struck me as desirable, particularly since Suanne had such deliciously beautiful breasts. Did it mean that at this stage, I was already entertaining visions of the cosmetic effects of the various options? Although I might not have been willing to admit it, even to myself, the answer was "Yes." [13]

Because I had to take the deposition of an emergency room doctor in a medical malpractice case on the day of the biopsy appointment, I was unable to go with Suanne to the procedure. Although I felt bad about not attending, Suanne assured me that she would be fine, and we wouldn't know anything immediately anyway, so I was not to worry about it.

I certainly hadn't related to Suanne any of the more grotesque images that had been plaguing me, so I just agreed– treating the event as casually as possible. And because the FNA is a relatively simple in-office procedure that requires only a local anaesthetic and the insertion of a small needle into the breast, I took Suanne at her word that she didn't need my company. Further, we were told that the procedure wouldn't impair Suanne's driving faculties at all, so there wasn't any real need for me to go other than to provide emotional support (not to say that this is a minor matter). Likewise, I also had convinced myself to a certain degree that there was nothing wrong, so why make a big deal of it by

---

13 - One of my vows was to be skillful and careful enough that no one would refuse a biopsy on the grounds that they or someone they knew had a poor cosmetic outcome – I always closed wounds like plastic surgeons do. This is something that should be discussed between doctor and patient prior to surgery. **EM**

tagging along like some toad.

There are two kinds of fine needle procedures. As described earlier, in one of them the needle is inserted directly into the suspicious lump to see if fluid can be withdrawn. If it is discovered that the lump is filled with fluid, it is almost always a benign cyst and nothing further is done. The other procedure is the one most commonly referred to as fine needle aspiration (FNA) and uses a very large syringe attached to a very small needle. The purpose of using the large syringe is to create a suction powerful enough to withdraw a sufficient sample of cells through the needle which is inserted into the lump from several angles. The cell sample withdrawn is then examined in a laboratory by a cytologist (a scientist trained in the examination and analysis of cells) to ascertain whether it contains cancer cells. The analysis, assuming that the needle biopsy produced enough tissue cells to study, takes about a week. Despite the simplicity and the safety of the procedure, my rationalizing, and our best game faces, neither one of us slept well the night before FNA day.

It's the free floating thoughts that attend situations like this that are so difficult to deal with–like blue water sailing in hurricane season. Once in your mind, you turn the corner from abstract doubts to discernable, discrete fears, one's thoughts run amok and fear teeters on the dual edges of terror and desperation. There is a child-like, almost autonomic simplicity to the thought processes that take place, or take over, once the fear invades your mind. Darkness brings out goblins; sickness and disease result in agony and death; distant sounds of thunder mean a force 10 storm is approaching. Fear exaggerates everything. And everything echoes the thoughts of fear.

Remember when you were a kid and would always be asking stupid "what-if" questions, such as if you had to be paralyzed or blind, or if one of your parents had to be killed, which would you prefer? The very word "cancer," like some thematic projection test in Psychology 101, conjures up immediate thoughts of despair, decay, and hopelessness. You ask questions like When and How? Sooner or Later? Quickly or Slowly? The abstract and the macabre seem to materialize out of the shadows and enter into a slow, sad dance with reality.

Then there are the variations on all these themes that arise from subconscious coping mechanisms stimulated by fear of the unknown and by mundane issues of self-preservation. What will it be like living alone? What will it be like living with someone other than Suanne? Some thoughts are so tangled and menacing that you prefer not to remember that they ever resided in your mind, even if on a transient basis. Images of mutilation handed down through anecdotal accounts of unknown breast cancer victims from times past replay over and over in your mind. I felt anxiety and even shock at some of my responses to these images. I even began to engage in the accounting of opportunity costs (What will I do if Suanne dies?) for every scenario that dread and hope can conjure up.

As I lay awake the night before the biopsy, drifting in the nether world between sleep and wakefulness, these bizarre thoughts seemed to take flight and flutter about in my mind like so many frantic gulls fighting over fish offal at the end of some long, long wharf. I couldn't tell if I was the hunter or the prey. Maybe I was both. I didn't know; I wasn't sure of much of anything, other than that I loved Suanne to pieces and that I was scared shitless.

Then there's the image of every smile and every look of love Suanne and I ever shared. Every adventure we'd ever participated in together: the soda fountain at McIntosh Pharmacy where we met when in high school; seeing her lying on a beach towel beside a pool under a full August moon, clad in nothing but a flimsy wet tee shirt while I was home on leave from the Navy; winging my way back home from Washington D.C. During law school, knowing that by some miracle or the grace of God, she would be waiting at the United Airlines gate at San Francisco International Airport, to cart me back to hearth and home and into her loving arms. It is in the irrepressible power and attraction of these latter thoughts that the perfection of an otherwise imperfect reality is accomplished. It is in the perfection of these all– consuming, all– encompassing feelings of love and belonging that the purity and absolute uniqueness of the bond between two human beings can manifest itself. The sensation of the feeling is as full and warm and complete as an equatorial sunset. Your skin fairly tingles with the heat and kinetics of love.

What, I wondered, would life be like for me without the daily touch and feel of Suanne's presence? Without the daily sight and sound of her, what would happen to all my memories? What would my bed be like at night without her redolent smells and her soft sweet touch? Who would there be to tell me, by word and by deed, that it's okay for me to be me?

In a veiled vision,
I peer out unto eternity,
Through eyes not yet awake,
And not awakening,
Asking blind men to explain
The hues of my thoughts and dreams,
Is passion pure and holy,
Is love a quantum thing,

Or do we wander throughout life,
Excluded from such mysteries,
Denied the knowledge of the once sweet knowing,
Some have glanced, some have felt,
If but for a moment,
Into the ponderous majesty of those mysteries,
And the knowledge of that fleeting knowing,
Lays low the simple heeding of that hoary calling,
But a low deep pain will often follow,
As now it has,
And men of vision may rend their eyes,
To seek refuge in the dark side of the mind,
While blind men all around,
Dance a happy song,
In the comfort of the darkness,
In the denial of that once sweet knowing.
So now I gaze into your eyes,
In a veiled vision of eternity,
Lost forever, is it not,
But still in the keeping of one gentle glance,
Along the road that led into these mysteries,
Now the pain I must burden upon my soul,
Is a gift of life and love,
Bursting with light, color and fantasy,
Like the beauty of the sunset,
The coming of the dawn,
Is lost forever to our eyes,
Yet blind men stop in awe,
So let those misty shadows,
Cloud my memory of the mystery,
Let capsuled time fade into eternity,
My soul cry out in anguish just and deep,
There is a beauty in the knowledge of the knowing,
That the passion and the love,
Was sand and feeling,
That the time amongst the shadows,
And that beneath the moon,
Is a gift from God all knowing,

That life will end too soon,
So I embrace the fleeting beauty,
Of that soft sweet gentle motion,
That speaks of love and glory,
In the sun that comes with morning,
And life, I love you.

But no matter how bizarre, melancholy, passionate or emotional my thoughts, I was not the one lying there in the darkness wondering if the dawn would bring a diagnosis of breast cancer. I was just the one threatened ultimately with morbid and mortifying thoughts of the possible loss of the woman that had been the one true lodestar of my life since adolescence. It is so easy to engage in self-pity at times like this. It is so difficult not to do so.

February 8, 1996

I had to leave the house at around five to do some final preparation for the deposition of the ER doc, which I'm sure also contributed to my shortage of sleep. The case involved a spinal cord injury. My client was a young man who had been in a solo vehicular accident striking his head on the roof as the car rolled over. I'll call him Doug Yancy.

Doug was returning from a day of fishing with his brother at a reservoir east of Madera when he missed a turn and lost control of his car, causing it to leave the road and roll several times. He had a pre-existing condition known as ankylosing spondylosis, which means that his neck was stiff and bent due to the idiopathic fusing of the cervical vertebra. At the scene of the accident, Doug had been put into full C-spine precautions by the attending paramedics, who later testified in deposition that they feared, from the nature of the accident and his pre-existing condition, that he could have suffered a spinal cord injury, even though he was able to move all extremities without limitation. There were empty beer cans in the car and Doug admitted to having been drinking out at the reservoir. He remained immobilized and secured to the C-spin board in the ambulance on the way to the hospital.

At the hospital, the full C-spine precautions remained in place when he was transferred from the ambulance gurney to the ER examination table. After the ER doc performed a cursory neurological examination, Doug was freed from the restraints and allowed to sit up on the examining table. He was then allowed to get off the examining table and was sent to get X-rays in a wheel chair. The ER doc noted in the chart that Doug appeared to have ETOH (alcohol) on his breath and was loud and verbally abusive.

In the x-ray lab Doug was transferred from the wheel chair to the x-ray table with the assistance of the lab technician and his brother, who had accompanied Doug to the hospital in the ambulance. Of course, his brother was trained better in fishing hole beer drinking than he was in Boy Scout first aid. After the X-rays were completed, Doug was helped off the table by his brother and returned to the ER in the wheel chair. The report issued by the radiologist indicated that Doug had sustained a fracture and dislocation of the C-7 vertebra. Then, for reasons that gave rise to the claim of malpractice, the attending ER doc sent Doug home with instructions to stay off work for a week. He managed to get out of the car, walk into his house, get himself into bed and go to sleep.

In the course of the ensuing twelve hours, the dreadfully predictable outcome came to pass. Doug Yancy, a young man of thirty-nine years old woke up a quadriplegic. He was poor, partially disabled due to his ankylosing spondylitis condition, not even a high school graduate, and now relying on me, his attorney, to provide him with the few meager creature comforts allowed by California's perverse tort reform system that protects physicians and other health care providers from responsibility for their own negligence.

I think I fell asleep around 1:30 or 2:00 a.m. engulfed by fears of what the dawn might hold in store for Suanne and amplified by my knowledge that, to this day, medicine remains an inexact art, subject to the same failure and malfeasance that plagues all human endeavor. Only in medicine, mistakes and misjudgments can have immediate and catastrophic results, as was the case with Doug. Most other areas of professional negligence have the luxury of time to repair their misdeeds.

I woke up about 4:30. Through the open sliding glass door that leads to the back deck, I could hear a light rain falling on the roof of the workout room. The only illumination came from the courtyard, where a faint crimson tinged fountain light undulated off the water and bathed our bedroom in the melancholy glow of my nocturnal fears. I slipped out of bed, trying to be quiet as I moved about, pretending that Suanne was sleeping, even though I knew better. She was lying there in bed listening to the rain, probably engulfed in thoughts similar to those that exercised my mind throughout the night.

Would the little needle that Dr. Mahoney was going to insert into her breast withdraw some innocuous fluid from a benign cyst or microscopic samples of tissue containing lethal little cells that had overcome the myriad safeguards provided by our bodies to ward off cancer? Was that tiny pea sized mass on the side of her breast malignant and already invading surrounding tissue? Had rogue cells already broken loose from the tumor and penetrated the lymph system or nearby blood vessels? Were these deadly cells being ferried to distant organs in Suanne's body to start new cancer colonies? If there is a malignancy, how long has it been there? Was it one of the variety of cancer cells that is so virulent and aggressive that it can accomplish in a matter of a year or two what other less aggressive types takes a decade or more to accomplish? In the rain broken silence of that February morning, we both knew that in the answers to these questions hung the balance of our lives.

When I was ready to leave, I turned out my bathroom light, walked quietly to Suanne's side of the bed and sat down next to her. She raised her arms to me and we embraced for many long moments. I held her tightly, saying nothing, as our bodies melded together in the fervent hope that the day would produce nothing more than evidence of one of the benign types of lumps that showed up as a small pea-sized lump in the left side of her right breast.

"I love you honey," I said, "Everything's going to be all right." I tried to sound strong, but the timbre of my voice had the shallow ring of hope and little more. With the reality of the biopsy upon us, I was starting to get very scared. As I drove away from the house I forced my thoughts to the upcoming deposition and the respite the exercise would provide from the increasingly morbid thoughts now plaguing my every waking moment. Concentrating on the task at hand, I knew, would not be easy.

When I got home that night the news was not what either one of us had expected. The bad news: No fluid was withdrawn that might have signified a benign cyst. Dr. Mahoney, Suanne related, ruled out a fibroadenoma and was skeptical that it was a pseudolump. She was also doubtful whether the FNA had produced a sufficient sample of cells in which to do a reliable study . Dr. Mahoney had tried several times to get into the lump, but was not optimistic about the results.[14] While we both took this as a good sign, we had to wait almost two weeks to find out that all that had been withdrawn was a tiny amount of bloody fluid with no tissue cells showing anything, one way or the other. But by this time the "no news is good news" syndrome combined with the lingering effects of negative mammograms was beginning to take hold on us.

The deposition of the doctor in the ER case also had not gone as I had expected. When I asked the doctor to explain what the x-rays had shown he acknowledged, as of course he was constrained to do, that the C-7 vertebra was dislocated and fractured. This was clear from the x-rays. What I hadn't expected was the graphic display put on by the defendant doctor to demonstrate the extent of the dislocation. He described the spinal column as being like a series of blocks aligned one on top of the other vertically in a straight line. He pointed

14 - There's good and bad news here. The good news is that Suanne's lump was tiny, which means we caught it very early. The bad news is that its tiny size made it hard to hold still for the several shearing passes that had to be made.

to the x-rays showing the C-7 vertebral body misaligned to the right of both C-6 and T-1. Next, the doctor put one fist on top of the other to illustrate how the proper alignment should be and then slide the top fist almost completely off the bottom fist.

"What happens to the spinal cord," I asked, "when this type of dislocation occurs?"

"Well," the doctor responded, "the space within the vertebral bodies accommodating the spinal cord is rather small, maybe about half an inch or so in diameter. So when the one vertebra is dislocated (at this point he held his fists up horizontally in front of his eyes in the manner of looking through a telescope), it pinches off the space occupied by the spinal cord and can injure the spinal cord." As he was carrying out his demonstration, he slowly slid his fists apart creating an aperture-like effect within the space he had been looking through, with the setting finally closing down to zero.

"If you were aware," I asked, "of the fact that he had this fracture and dislocation of his C-7 vertebra, and you knew that it could result in a permanent injury to the spinal cord, why did you send him home with instructions to stay off work for a week?" The doctor's answer, quoted here almost verbatim, was enough to strike terror into the heart of even the most parasitic of defense lawyers.

"Because," he declared dryly, "he seemed knowledgeable and sounded like he knew more about his medical condition than I did, so I took him at his word."

Suanne went on the river boat trip on the Mississippi River with her mother and sisters in March. They all had a great time. Following Dr. Mahoney's advise, we decided that she could wait until after her regularly scheduled annual physical in April before deciding further what to do. Her next scheduled appointment with Dr. Mahoney was for a week after her annual check up. That date became our new "D-day." [15]

---

[15] - I was very committed to the idea of taking that lump out of there if it didn't disappear by the next visit.

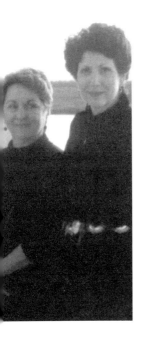

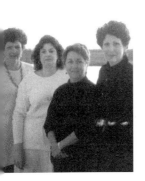

CHAPTER 5
The Second Round of Tests

April 17, 1996

In the weeks following the unproductive FNA, Suanne and I tried to let the topic of breast cancer recede from the flood tide that had inundated us during the frantic months of January and February. Spring was in full bloom, trials were looming immediately ahead and Josh's high school baseball games were affording us a welcome distraction. Almost every evening, however, whether she was watching television, needlepointing or reading, I would see her left hand unconsciously exploring the locus of the lump on the side of her breast. One might never have guessed from her outward appearances, but it was clear to me that the lump in her breast was never far from her mind.

The Mississippi River trip in March had been a great distraction, even though with a cousin's physician husband along, the topic of breast cancer remained somewhat on the itinerary, even though Suanne did her level best to avoid the topic as much as possible.

Through most of her life, Suanne's habit had been to endure most of her mountains and valleys as a solitary traveler. Whether it be problems in our marriage, my penchant for irresponsible and reckless conduct, or her own insecurities, Suanne was never one to pour her heart out to friends or even family members about intimate matters. Instead, she would typically look inward, to a deep and placid reservoir of personal and spiritual strength enabling her to redouble her efforts to find solutions, protect her family and clear the obstacles leading to her vision of a healthy and secure future. Predictably, she dealt with her fears of a possible breast cancer diagnosis in a similar manner. On the trip she did share some of her concerns and fears with her sisters, but had resolved not to let it hover over the river trip like a dark ominous cloud. Upon returning home, Suanne resumed her regular workout

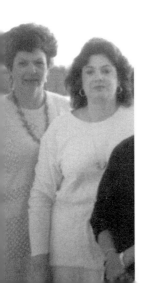

program, which included stretching, strength training, the Versaclimer, skipping rope, the Stairmaster and bicycling. After years of rigorous training, in most of her exercises Suanne was performing at the levelof a college athlete and was not backing off one iota. Whatever stress she was feeling from the lump, she tried to smother under a blanket of sweat, hope and optimism. From her responsibilities as my business partner to her role as a homemaker, she continued to function almost without missing a beat.

In April, however, with the approach of her annual appointment and the follow-up scheduled with Dr. Mahoney, the floodgates opened anew, spilling out her pent-up fears of what the lump in her breast might portend. The first follow-up visit was with Dr. Andrews for her annual physical. After the experience in January and February with the mammograms, the bewildering explanations and Stephanie's phone calls, Suanne was hoping for a rekindling of the relationship she had enjoyed in the past with Dr. Andrews. She was genuinely relieved when it was Dr. Andrews doing the physical examination and not his nurse practitioner.

After examining Suanne's breasts, Dr. Andrews told her that there may have been some change in the way the lump in her right breast felt, but he adhered to his original assessment that it did not feel like a cancerous tumor. He added, however, that they would perform another mammogram and see if any change showed up on the film. Dr. Andrews knew, of course, that Suanne had pursued her own follow-up with Dr. Mahoney. He made mention of this and expressed confidence that she was in good hands. After her physical examination, Stephanie performed another mammogram, but this time assiduously elected not to opine at all on its significance. All she said was that she'd get the film over to the radiologist that same afternoon and call with the results. Suanne sensed there was a change in Stephanie's attitude toward her. Just prior to this appointment, I had called Stephanie and requested that I be informed of any changes in the appearance of the lump. From my brief conversation, I felt certain that Stephanie was aware or had been made aware of the nature of my law practice. I admit to wondering if perhaps they were circling the wagons.

When Suanne returned home from the appointment, she conveyed that Dr. Andrews had said that there was a change in the way the lump felt to him. She was nervous about the pending results of the mammogram. Stephanie called late in the afternoon. She said the radiologist also saw what appeared to be some slight changes in the lump and ordered a follow-up ultrasound. When Suanne related all this to me, I could hear a resignation creeping into her voice that had not been there before. Never in her life had Suanne been under the kind of medical pressure she was now confronting. And understandably, she was beginning to stagger a bit under the strain. But even at this point, resignation, stress and all, her attitude remained what I would describe as defiant and positive. For my part, I was trying, but with only limited success, to let the weight of medical authority convince me that I should not spend all my time worrying about it. Suanne's appointment with Dr. Mahoney was the following week, so she scheduled her ultrasound on the same day.

Tuesday, April 23, 1996

The ultrasound examination was at the Imaging Center just prior to Suanne's appointment with Dr. Mahoney. While we were hoping this test would provide good news, the ultrasound, as with the mammograms before it, proved inconclusive.[16] Dr. Randol (not a real name), the radiologist, put the film up on the light box and pointed out to Suanne the area of concern. She could see what looked like two tiny tentacles coming out of the lump. When asked what they were, Dr. Randol acknowledged there was some change in the appearance of the nodule, though nothing clearly suggesting a malignancy. He offered that the change might be attributable to scaring from the recent needle aspiration procedure, which was not uncommon.

As to the curious tentacles, he said he didn't know what they might be, but indicated that a core biopsy might provide a definitive diagnosis. He offered to perform that procedure right then and there in his office. Suanne agreed that something needed to be done, declined Dr. Randol's offer, and went directly from the Imaging Center to Dr. Mahoney's office. She did not take kindly to the proposal of the core biopsy by the radiologist, feeling that she was being "sold" a procedure that might, or might not, be necessary. The two physicians she had been seeing, both male, unquestionably had left her frustrated and upset. By contrast, she viewed Dr. Mahoney as her refuge, if not her safe harbor.

Arriving at her office a short drive later, Suanne felt at once fearful and relieved. Fearful because there had been an apparent change in the lump over the past three and a half months (certainly not a good omen), and relieved because there was now at least a general consensus among the primary care physician, the radiologist and the surgeon that it was time to get a definitive diagnosis on the lump.

Dr. Mahoney explained the difference between a core biopsy (a procedure similar to the needle aspiration only using a much larger needle that mechanically samples the core tissue in the lump as opposed to the much smaller amount of tissue aspirated in the FNA), and an excisional biopsy, which she

---

16 - The previous mammogram was not just inconclusive, it was really benign-looking with very defined margins, indicative of something that is growing and staying self-contained while pushing surrounding tissue out of the way. Cancer tends to "infiltrate" or grow by slithering into surrounding tissue – as I recall, the only change was that one edge of the lump now had a more indistinct border. It was OK to have these extra studies, but not critical for me – it was going to come out if still there. The core biopsy has a false negative rate, and if positive, still requires excision – so I was going straight to the excision.

described as similar to a lumpectomy, depending on whether all or part of the lump is removed.

The excisional biopsy, or lumpectomy, the doctor explained, would consist of making an incision of approximately one inch in length at the site of the lump and removing the mass along with some of the tissue around the periphery (margins) of the lump. The procedure, to be done on an outpatient basis under a local anesthesia plus IV sedation, would take a half-hour to forty-five minutes. She was to arrive at the hospital two hours before the surgery and would have to be driven home once the anesthesia wore off.

Suanne liked Dr. Mahoney a lot. More importantly, under her care she seemed to be regaining some of her confidence in the medical establishment. This was a welcome change since for a while she had begun to feel as though she was giving orders to the coxswain while manning the laboring oar of her care. After weighing the options afresh, Suanne elected to go with the excisional biopsy. It was scheduled for the following Monday. ,

In contrast however, by now I was beginning to feel like a yo-yo on a string. One moment I'd feel confident in the benign nature of the lump and the next moment I'd feel my confidence eroding.[17] My emotions were beating me down and boxing me in. I was the fox hearing the baying of the hounds grow louder and louder, and realizing that there may be no place to hide.

---

17 - So was I – that's why I didn't want to do a core – we all didn't need another test with a false negative rate – I wrestled with just doing it when she got back from her trip, and made it clear that she could always call me and get in sooner if she wanted too– I had no idea that there was so much suffering going on. Had I known, I would have urged that we do it sooner. There is no breast lump worth much worry – if there is anything like "minor surgery" this is it. Which is not to say that it can't be done exquisitely to reduce scarring and maintain the contour of the breast.

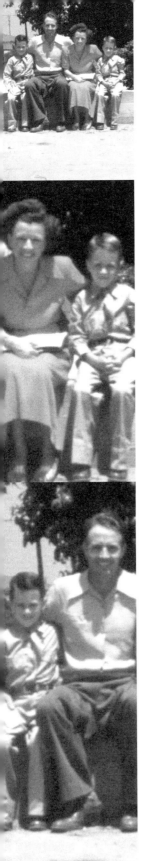

CHAPTER 6
Weekend Interlude

April 26, 1996

Long before we had any idea that the specter of breast cancer had invaded our lives, we had plans to attend a family wedding in Southern California, where both of us had grown up. We hadn't seen my maternal cousins for several years and now, with the lumpectomy looming, the weekend trip gave us the opportunity to spend some time alone and perhaps distract ourselves before the surgery the coming Monday. To say the least, we were both nervous, and with good cause. Was the proverbial "other shoe" about to drop?

There was a time, not too long ago, when women, upon entering the hospital, not even knowing whether what they were feeling in their breasts was just normal lumpiness or a malignancy, went home without any breasts at all.

These women, and there were thousands of them, would go to the hospital and sign a routine consent form acknowledging and agreeing that their breasts could be removed during the biopsy procedure if a malignancy was found. The patient would then be put under general anesthesia, go to sleep, and if the tissue was positive for malignancy, radical mastectomies were performed right on the spot. Only upon awakening would she discover whether both breasts, one breast, or neither breast remained. And while this was happening, there were countless false positives, misreadings, and diagnostic and typographical errors made by the pathologists and technicians in analyzing and reporting on breast tissue tests for cancer cells. Alas, in some areas of the country, and in some communities, this is still true.

Whether it was a latent fear of these antidotal accounts of breast cancer treatment or simply the imminent possibility of Suanne being diagnosed with the disease, neither of us felt in much of a mood for celebrating at the wedding, but we didn't feel like sitting around sulking either.

While packing and getting on the road, we said little to one another save for some perfunctory remarks about what clothes we were taking, the weather, and if we'd left food out for the dog. Our teenage son Josh would be looked after, staying with a friend. By the time we passed the power plant stacks at Moss Landing, the gloom hanging over the trip was still as thick as the chilly morning fog that shrouded the coastline. I rotely pushed the radio button looking for some news. The Chechen rebel leader had been killed in a bombing and Mexico was accusing U.S. police of brutality against immigrants. Hardly the sort of news I wanted to hear, so I flicked it off.

We were both lost in a maze of anxiety and fear that left us silently groping to find our way out and put the best faces we could on the trip. It promised to be a long journey. But as we turned inland at Espinosa Road just south of Castroville, the temperature warmed and the fog surrendered to bright cozy sunshine. Suddenly, it was a beautiful day with Spring in the air and we were going to visit my cousin Gary, one of the great icons of the Southern California hot rod and surf culture of the fifties and sixties.

Because I hadn't seen Gary since building my latest automotive creation, and I was eager to show off my wheels, we took my '55 Chevy 210 four-wheel-drive ('82 Blazer running gear) station wagon, a frame-up restoration project that I had been using as my daily driver for several years. As we pulled on to Highway 101 and motored down the Salinas Valley, I stuck in a Janice Joplin tape, turned up the volume and by King City our spirits had begun to climb. In almost every car we passed or that passed us, people would crane their necks to look at the gleaming white kick-ass '55 Chevy that looked like a drawing board prototype of the first suburban ever made, only cooler, much cooler. Little kids would wave, teens would give us the thumbs up or "V" sign and truckers would honk approvingly. Around Paso Robles, a California Highway Patrol officer, upon overtaking us in the passing lane, blared out "Nice '55 Suburban" over his loudspeaker. Even Suanne had to laugh over that one.

Ever since I was a teen myself, driving around Pomona and La Verne with Gary and his hot-rodding friends in their coupes and roadsters, I have always found driving down the highway in a well-tuned, smooth running hot rod to be a balm for whatever troubles might be ailing me. And yes, despite the passage of years, I admit to remaining chronically afflicted with that well-known ailment known as the "California hot rodder."

The first car that Suanne and I went on a date in during my senior year in high school was a '34 Ford five-window coupe that my dad and I built in the shop at our ranch near Thermal, a little desert town in the Coachella Valley, 137 miles east of Los Angeles. When we were married, Suanne drove us to Las Vegas in an immaculate canary yellow '51 Merc Tudor that my parents gave me for my twentieth birthday.

My '55 Chevy is a genuine work of art, with all the creature comforts of a modern vehicle. It sits up high on nine by fifteen-inch rims and oversized tires. It has tilt, cruise, power windows, power disk brakes, power steering, reclining buckets, and a high-end Sony stereo with eardrum-rattling Altec speakers: the works. The power plant is a 350 cubic inch Chevy, fresh out of the crate, that makes 300 plus or minus horsepower. For me this was about as fine a ride as anybody ever created. For what it cost to build–close to 40 grand for the whole make-over–Suanne reminds me, twittingly, it damn well ought to be! By the time we had gone through Jefferson Starship, Dire Straits, two Van Morrison tapes and a Billie Holiday, we were past Santa Barbara and finally somewhat distracted. We had even managed a laugh or two after the CHP officer's public prodding.

As had been our habit for many years in our trips back and forth from Southern California (we both grew up in the Coachella Valley), to break up the trip south we stopped in Ventura at a hotel just off the Highway 101 called the Country Inn. Among the charms of the Country Inn is its proximity to a great point break where I have indulged another chronic California affliction, surfing (as on a surfboard), for many years. The Inn also has a complimentary cocktail hour with hors d'oeuvres, clean large rooms and serves a palatable buffet breakfast made to order; so it was always a no-brainer to stop there.

We planned to dress the next morning and drive directly to the wedding after helping myself to an early surf session. That night, after I spent an hour enjoying the evening glass at California Street, we went to the complimentary cocktail hour at the hotel, managed a few laughs with a group of compatible strangers, and then decided to take in a movie. Presented the choice between the lugubrious-sounding, *Dead Man Walking* and the more uplifting, *Mr. Holland's Opus*, we opted for the latter.

Afterwards, we stopped by a little coffee house for a latte and then strolled hand in hand back to the hotel, looking, no doubt, to all the world like a love-struck couple enjoying the pleasures of a weekend getaway. Suanne was wearing a white linen tank top with matching shorts. She was tan and hard and looked absolutely stunning. The combined distractions of the trip, the surf, cocktail hour and the movie had lightened my spirits considerably.

The setting, notwithstanding Suanne's upcoming appointment on Monday, was made to order for one of my favorite indulgences of middle-aged married life–the intimate occasion, where sensuality and allure are the prime and dedicated focus of both participants. I slid into the prospect like I didn't have a care in the world. Back at the hotel, with Suanne in the bathroom getting ready for bed (and me), I had visions of erotic sugar plums dancing in my head.

I have always had this ability to put things out of my mind, or to use a contemporary phrase, "compartmentalize," particularly when responding to my primal instincts, and on this evening I wanted very much to put whatever Monday's appointment held in store out of both of our minds. But while waiting for Suanne to emerge from the bathroom, I began to have second thoughts. Hitting me square in the face was the gnawing realization that this weekend could be the swan song to every titillating fantasy I had ever conjured over the lovely breasts that had nurtured my carnal appetite since my youth. But I fought it off. I couldn't say for sure that the sun was going to come up in the east the next morning, but by the time the light went out in the bathroom and Suanne emerged, I definitely could say that I had let my primal instinct overcome my fears and felt like making love and savoring her delectable breasts, possibly for the last time. I was primed .., I thought.

I looked up from the bed as Suanne came strolling out of the bathroom. She was wearing the same gossamer Oriental gown that she was wearing when I went home to feel her lump back in January. It was a thin veneer of a silk gown that did little more than slightly diffuse the lovely refractions of light that defined the outlines of her breasts, her tan lines, and her nipples. As she approached the bed, she looked as lovely and alluring as she had since I had fallen in love with her when we were both still teenagers.

Suanne returned my look of anticipation with a timid mixture of hope, fear and allure. It was one of those looks that I could read like a book. I knew she was trying, probably with less success than I was having. She then turned out the light, allowed her gown to drop to the floor with some ceremony and got into bed, docking up against me in the posterior-anterior manner that enabled our bodies to lock together from head to toe, a well-practiced prelude to our love-making.

But on this night of irrepressible apprehension, as I cupped her breasts in my hand and began to give expression to the fantasies frolicking in my head, in a screeching turn of anticipation, my sexual reveries congealed into the ghastly image of a headstone with Suanne's name on it. Along with this macabre scene that was assaulting my imagination, I could hear the sounds of a New Orleans brass band playing the mournful strains of a funeral dirge from the movie we had just seen. Then I began to hear the words: "...Run, Fly, Hide/In desperation/ Search, Find, Kill/ In desperation;... Run, Fly, Hide/ In desperation/ Search, Find,

Kill,/ In desperation ..."

I couldn't really place the words or the circumstances of their origin. At first I thought they were from a song, but that didn't seem right. They were too familiar. Then they became an uncontrollable mantra. As I lay there trying to banish these words and images from my mind, no matter how hard I tried, the sound of the brass band and the refrain wouldn't stop. " Run, Fly, Hide/ In desperation/ Search, Find, Kill/ In desperation ..." My lust-laced fantasies for the evening dissolved into the dissident sounds of freeway traffic, distant sirens, and hotel noises. Finally, I began castigating myself for being selfish and insensitive.

How could I be thinking of sex at a time like this, at least in the context of the prominent role that Suanne's breasts played in our sexual rituals and conventions? How could I be slow dancing with my libidinous fantasies when the greatest love I would ever know in my life was threatened with a potentially fatal disease. The silent soap opera being played out in my mind sapped every ounce of desire from my body. I pulled Suanne closer, fighting back the grim emotions and images that were overwhelming me. Her touch and smell engulfed my senses and I wanted nothing more than simply to never ever let her go. Stroking her hair and rubbing her back, I whispered in her ear that I loved her more than life itself and promised with all my heart and soul that everything would turn out alright. I never meant anything more in my life.

April 27, 1996

I was awakened before daybreak by the sound of waves breaking beyond the freeway. I got up quietly, threw on my sweats and Uggs and drove over to California Street where a few surfers were already out on dawn patrol. I donned my wetsuit and waxed my board while surveying the various breaks. The waves were almost head high and the parking lot was beginning to fill up when I paddled out to a break about mid-way out to the point where there were only two other surfers, both on longboards. They looked to be in their late thirties, maybe early forties, and were obviously surf bros. Between sets, we struck up a conversation about the usual things surfers talk about while waiting in the line-up to catch a wave: things like booze, dope, boards, shapes, the swell, and of course, tits and ass. Their names were Carl and Jason.

Over the next hour and a half, I learned that both guys had grown up surfing together here in the Ventura area. Carl was a software salesman, recently divorced with three kids and had come up from L.A. to see a woman he had lusted after in high school but hadn't seen until their twentieth class reunion in 1995. From Carl's brief narration, the divorce sounded acrimonious, replete with all the usual bitter custody and support pills that he had to swallow. The other guy, Jason, sounded like, and I must say, surfed as if he'd never left high school and didn't do much of anything but surf and smoke dope.

From the conversation, I surmised that Jason was on his third marriage, and about to throw in the towel on that one for various and sundry reasons all of which were attributed to having a bitchy wife. Between dominating every wave other than when he was riding in or paddling out, Jason recounted for his buddy and me a litany of extravagant sexual conquests that had occupied his time over the years, seemingly always supplemented by a pharmacopoeia of drugs and alcohol that were not unfamiliar to me. Except now Jason's stories all sounded so barren and hollow that all I could think about was how thankful and fortunate I was to have survived my own escapades and could share my life with Suanne and our boys in an intact family.

Like so many men, young and not so young, Jason and to a lesser degree Carl, seemed trapped in the present by their appetites, their chemically maintained immaturity and their indivisible bond of selfishness. They seemed to have little regard for any personal responsibility, respect for the institution of the family, or to what tomorrow might bring. While I resist such categorizing, the thought did occur to me that without the structure and conscience Suanne and our boys had provided, I very well could have ended up like either one of my surf companions that morning. In between the stories, I managed to get position to drop into a few nice head-high waves with long vertical sections that carried me almost all the way to the beach. Each one provided a most welcome respite from reality, as perhaps it did for Jason and Carl.

One of the great joys of surfing is that it completely takes you away from the trials and tribulations of work-a-day reality. On dawn patrol, you're out on the ocean with the sun usually rising over the coastal mountains. You rise and fall on the swells in a rhythm as ancient and dependable as the watery world we occupy. When a set approaches, you paddle forward as the wave builds and finally humps up behind you and pushes your board forward and down the steepening face of the wave. You then slide forward gathering speed, energy and adrenaline, pop up and make the drop.

Dropping down the face of a head high wave, unbeknownst to all non-surfing denizens of our aqueous little planet, puts you into almost perfect symmetry with nature. In the moment of the drop–believe me–you are freed from all worry, all anxiety, indeed, almost all aspects of rational consciousness; you become a part of the perfection and balance of nature. Few surfers can ever actually remember the moment of the drop off the crest of a breaking overhead wave down into the trough. In that moment, you are at one with the wave, sliding down the blurred face, carving a deep slicing bottom turn into the trough and ripping back up into the breaking lip before whipping back down the face again and racing across a long steep section of emerald green water before it crashes onto the shore. It is truly a kind of re-creation, an incredible rush.

This session at California Street that morning was one of the best I can remember. It is not difficult to understand why some people can become addicted to surfing to the near-exclusion of all else in their life. After kicking out on my last ride, I paddled in and trudged up the beach to the car, strapped my board and the respite it had provided on the roof racks and headed back to prospects of a reality that more than ever seemed totally out of kilter with anything I had ever thought about or imagined.

It took us close to two hours to get to the city of Claremont from the Country Inn. Even though I had left directions to the church at the hotel, we managed to get to the general vicinity of where the wedding would take place in an area up near the foothills of the San Gorgonio Mountains. Then, as we were driving down a street with a familiar sounding name, we encountered a beautiful crimson red '48 Ford Woody station wagon headed in the opposite direction. "Bingo," I said to Suanne, "we found it." I made a quick U-turn and followed the woody down the street and into a short driveway to a lovely chapel surrounded by lawns and well groomed trees. There in front of the little chapel was a forest green '40 Ford Woody station wagon and a '55 Chevy Nomad. With Ernie Artunian behind the wheel, the crimson red '48 pulled into the line behind my cousin's '40. I pulled in behind the Nomad as though I'd been invited.

Moments later Suanne and I were mingling with the old group of guys who had been my heroes as a boy growing up in Southern California in the late fifties. I soon learned that the '55 Nomad was owned by Kent Brownsberger, one of Gary's friends who years ago, when I was small, had taken me under their wings and let me tag along and ride around with them in their hot rods.

Samantha's wedding was one of those beautiful affairs that provide the opportunity for old friendships to be renewed, for families to come together and reminisce about bygone times, and for celebrating renewal and the endless, if serpentine, circle of life.

, everyone went to a reception at Gary's house. Like almost everything in Gary's life, his house stood as a shrine to his creativity and individuality. Adapting a plan drawn by no less than Frank Lloyd Wright that he found in an antique shop in Santa Barbara, he built this beautiful two story Spanish style home with a large courtyard, red-tiled roof and expansive grounds at the end of a long private driveway, ideal for large gatherings like Samantha's wedding reception.

Everywhere around the house and grounds there were reminders of the far distant past our families had shared so intimately forty and fifty years ago. An old faded yellow Caterpillar farm tractor that Gary and his brother David drove as kids in their orange groves around La Verne was parked behind the house. There was a saddle hanging in the garage that I remembered from the old tack room next to the horse corrals behind the house in La Verne. I leaned over and breathed in the aroma of old leather and accumulated sweat from long forgotten rides in the foothills of the San Gabriel Mountains. In the den there was a wall of pictures, many of them depicting family gatherings back when we were kids. After spending the afternoon laughing and talking to Gary and David, Ernie, Kent and Joe Alercon, I found myself back in Gary's den with Suanne scouring over the scads of old family pictures.

Our parents were all young and beautiful and beaming with pride, faith and hope for the future. The Second World War was still a fresh biting memory and the kids in the pictures look pressed and clean as if they had just returned from Sunday school. The scenes depicted in the photographs seemed to harken back to a different age–an age not so much of innocence or purity, but of closeness, stability and small fraternal towns with fresh mowed lawns and back yard clotheslines. It seemed so very long ago.

And there in almost every picture where I appeared with my cousins, was my brother Jerry. Jerry with the raven black hair, the radiant smile and the sparkling blue eyes. Jerry at five years old under the Christmas tree, at eight on a pony in full cowboy regalia at nine sitting on the old yellow farm tractor out in the orange grove with Gary and David; at ten or eleven in trunks down at my cousin's beach house on Balboa Island during summer vacation. Then suddenly, there were no more pictures of Jerry, and life, as I had known it ended in my narrow cloistered little rural world. At the age of twelve Jerry was killed in a horrible horse accident at our ranch.

As I toured this faded Kodak museum of my youth with Suanne at my side, the trembling pulse of old family ties began beating the melancholy refrain again, "Run, Fly, Hide/ In desperatio,/ Search, Find, Kil,/ In desperation ..." Then everything came rushing in on me in a torrent of stinging memory.

The pictures, the mementos and the wedding day had parted some long drawn curtain on the events that had caused me to write the words that had been plaguing me since the night before at the hotel in Ventura. Standing before the pictures beckoned me back to my long suppressed memories of the bitter time of my brother's death. I remembered exactly were I was when I wrote the poem that contained the words, "run fly hide, search find kill, in desperation." I remember the events that were captured in the poem as though it were yesterday. I remembered that Gary was with me on that September day so long ago. I had not peered into the abyss of the details of that day in over thirty years.

As the memories multiplied and evolved into the scenes of that terrible time, I could feel the tightening in my chest, the throbbing of guilt and fear gripping my emotions–my eyes began to sting and glisten. The pictures, the joy of the occasion, the reminiscing over old times with my cousins and old friends and the imminence of the lumpectomy had taken its toll. I felt the need to leave, almost to run away.

It was a long drive back and I suggested to Suanne, with as much decorum as I could muster, that it was time for us to say goodbye. As I hugged my cousins goodbye, I felt a tenderness, love and longing for old family ties that I hadn't experienced in countless years. As we parted I said, "I love you Gary, we mustn't let so much time pass without seeing each other. We are family. We never know what tomorrow holds in store." Then I turned and hurried off so as not to let everyone see the tears streaming down my cheeks from beneath my dark glasses.

As I sat in the car waiting for Suanne to finish her goodbyes, the thought of not seeing her for the rest of my life seemed a burden greater than I would ever be able to bear. My chest heaved, tears poured out, and my mind was engulfed once again by the terrible refrain from the tragic poem of my childhood; "Run, Fly, Hide/ In desperation/ Search, Find, Kill,/ In desperation ..." But now, no longer an abstraction, it was a score accompanying real scenes being replayed in my mind.

CHAPTER 7
September Blood

By the time the hunt had ended, the shadows of late afternoon had begun to stretch their dark purple fingers across the valley floor. It was opening day of quail season in the desert–and for me, a very special opening. For my eleventh birthday my dad had given me an early present–a brand new Stevens-Savage 20 gauge double-barreled shotgun he had ordered from the Sears Roebuck Catalogue. It was the kind of birthday present that made even an undersized prepubescent boy feel the tinge of impending manhood. Back in the early fifties, guns and hunting were still part of the growing up process for farm boys. Thus, it was common to get a .22 rifle or a shotgun when you became an adolescent. In fact, it was almost a desert-culture, ranch-culture ritual. A rite of passage, if you will. We were taught by our fathers, brothers, uncles and (male) cousins to ride horses, hunt and fish, and the art of cleaning and cooking what you killed over an open fire or maybe in the tack room, after the hunt.

The opening day of quail season and the "feed" afterwards was almost as traditional on the ranch as Thanksgiving and Christmas. For almost as long as I could remember, every September, friends, family, and neighbors were invited to the almost day long celebration at the ranch. At the end of the day, the birds were cleaned and skewered on long spits of green mesquite wood with potato, bell pepper, and onion stuffed in between and cooked on an outdoor grill made from a 50 gallon oil drum. There was fresh tomato and onion salad, Jell-O, corn on the cob, corn bread, and gallons of fresh lemonade and sun steeped tea. Usually the adults would square dance on the slab in front of the shop after the dishes were cleaned up.

Having my own shotgun made me feel every bit the big hunter. All the other boys were very impressed as they passed the double barrel around approvingly before we all

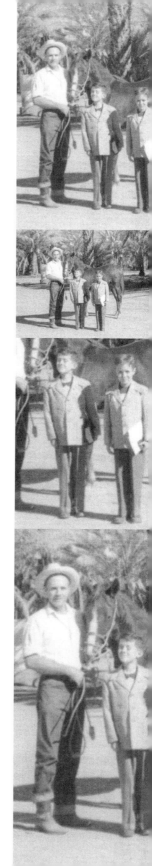

headed out to the fields in several pick-up trucks. The grownups all went off in one direction, and us kids, with the older boys in charge, went off in another. After a few hours of trampling over sand dunes, through mesquite thickets and along ditch banks, everyone had bagged several of the plump game birds that would be cooked for dinner that evening. Everyone, that is, except me. I couldn't shoulder, aim and shoot fast enough with the heavy double barrel to take one of the birds out of the air and to shoot a bird on the ground was considered unsportsmanlike if not downright illegal. With the old single shot 410 gauge that I learned to shoot with and shared with my mother, maybe, but the new double barrel was very different. It was hard to aim and kicked like a mule.

My brother Jerry and I and cousins Frankie and Gary were trudging our way back toward the pickup—all of them with a full larder and me with most of my shells unspent and, far worse, an empty pouch. It was not the ending to the hunt that I had envisioned when we started that morning.

Suddenly, in the mesquite ahead there was the unmistakable sound of a flurry of wings beating the air as a covey of quail rose in front of us in a desperate bid for the reprieve offered by the approaching shadows. One, two, three shots rang out and three birds fell, then a fourth shot, mine, yielding nothing more than the empty bark of the Stevens-Savage. Moments later, as I was grimacing at my failure, my brother pointed excitedly to a spot in the mesquite brush no more than fifteen yards away where a fat guileless quail was scurrying about on the ground trying to get away.

"Shoot," Jerry shouted, "shoot, you'll get a quail."

I raised the double barrel 20 gauge shotgun to my shoulder and took aim at the hapless bird scrambling for its life. I hesitated.

"Fire," screamed my cousins, almost in unison, "fire, Scottie, fire!"

Looking down between the tubes of blue metal, over the bead that was following the bird in and out of the tangled brush, my heart raced and I held my breath until it seemed my lungs would burst. My trigger finger felt as if it were pressing against the string on a 180-pound bow. Then suddenly an explosion and the hard kick of the butt against my shoulder responded to the shouts. When the smoke and dust cleared I saw the gallant bird still trying to drag its bloodied body to cover. It made a strange little peeping cry and shuddered violently as my cousin Gary picked it up and with a swift flick of his wrist cracked the quail's head against the butt of his gun. He sauntered over, handed me the dead bird and said "Real hunters never shoot birds on the ground."

I looked down at the mangled remains in my hand, still quivering and warm with blood oozing out of it. I dropped the bird and plopped down on the desert sand in the failing afternoon sun. My eyes filled with tears and I began to cry. I wanted it to be someone other than me who had shot the beautiful plumed bird futilely running for its life. I wanted it to be someone else sighting down the double barrels at the quail and wanting nothing more than to bag a kill, before squeezing the trigger. I found that the reality of the killing was much different than the fantasy of being a big hunter. Now, the deed done, there was nothing I could do. I took aim, I pulled the trigger, I killed the bird. Jerry put his hand gently on my shoulder.

"Pick up the bird, Scottie." He said. " Let's go. Let's go get in the truck." Sitting remorsefully in the bed of the pickup, I cried all the way home. To make matters worse, Gary and Frankie made fun of me every wheel-bounce of the way.

A few days later, on a hot, still Saturday morning, Jerry and I saddled up our horses, Rusty and Amber, to move a few head of cattle from one field to another on the home ranch. Donnie, a neighbor, tagged along on another of our horses. Rusty was well-broke, but still a colt. We had raised Rusty on the ranch, and after he was broke, my dad gave him to Jerry. Amber was an older mare that we had bought from the same cowboy down in Calipatria who had broke Rusty.

After moving the cattle, the three of us rode off into a date grove to practice roping a dead offshoot stump. Having just roped the stump, Jerry dismounted Rusty to remove his lasso when from somewhere, for some unknown reason, a dry root cracked, spinning my universe out of control.

I was sitting on Amber no more than thirty feet away awaiting my turn at the stump. Rusty bolted at the sharp report of the crack. The bitter end of Jerry's rope was tied hard and fast to his saddle horn and the loop he had just taken off the dead stump was lying on the ground beneath his boot like a spring-set trap. What was I to do?

Although he was only 19 months older, Jerry was my Kit Carson, my George Washington, and my Buffalo Bill, all in one. Before my eyes Jerry's legs were violently jerked from underneath him. After a short charge through the orchard in which I failed to overtake Rusty, on that hot, still September morning in 1953, at twelve years old, my brother was gone forever. It was bad enough to have my brother taken right before my eyes; yet infinitely worse, I was left with the torturous memories of my failure to save him. September blood was on my hands. Shortly after, sitting alone at my desk, with Jerry's identical empty desk just across the room, and before the shadows of that time had become lost in darkness, I wrote this poem:

In another moment, another life,
In another time,
a hunter stalks the land,
He is an Indian,
A warrior, a trapper,
All the things and everybody
He wants to be,
The silent prey
Moves with the early autumn wind,
In tangled bushes, brown from summer's sun
And the thirsty land,
Who knows not of the other now,
He or me,
When the dry root cracked
And drums echo back across the hungry ages,
In desperation,
Run, Fly, Hide,
In desperation,
Search, Find, Kill,
In desperation,
The moment is now upon us,
Lungs screaming,
The heart stands still
As a shot and echo
Answers the hunter's prayer,
Commending unto eternity
The September blood of the prey,
Who died in the hands of a warrior,
Trembling and afraid,
Beckoned from beyond,
In the failing light of an early autumn,
Who knows not of the other now,
He or me,
Did I live or die in desperation?
Unknown to me until today,
In another moment, another life,
In another time, I died,
As September blood fell upon the land.

Were these my words? Who knows? Perhaps they were Jerry's words, speaking to me from his grave? My life and the life of our family, I knew, would never be the same. This much I do know. Who's to say how and why any little boy might react to being confronted with a tragedy on the scale of participating in a life and death race to catch a horse that is dragging his big brother to his death, and losing. Who's to say what causes any of us to react the way we do to many of the challenges of life? Particularly ones that grind down through the strongest fibers of our beings, down into the inner sanctum of our psyches, down to the tun where all of the fears, doubts and frailties that afflict us pool in a suppressed quagmire of vulnerability. It all was coming back:

Run, Fly, Hide,
In desperation,
Search, Find, Kill
in desperation...
Run, Fly, Hide,
In desperation,
Search, Find, Kill
in desperation...

I tried hard, desperately hard, to win that hopeless race of so many years ago. I would have wrestled my brother's horse to the ground with my bare hands if I could, but even in my dreams, which would plague me for months after the accident, I could never catch Rusty in his headlong flight. All I could do was stay close enough to bear unbearable witness to the calamity unfolding before my eyes and be there beside Jerry when it ended.

And, to this day, I wonder still, who I might have been, had the rope not been tied hard and fast to the saddle horn, had the dry root never cracked, or had the loop settled elsewhere than beneath Jerry's boot. It is a certainty, however, that we respond to such events in ways we never know and never learned and will seldom figure out, and that these responses, and the emotional fallout, stay with us and influence us throughout our lives. All we can do is attempt to recognize the influence of such events and struggle to overcome their hurtful influences. Indeed, not just a few times after the wedding reception at Gary's house, did I recall in all its vivid horror that September morning of long ago and ponder how this new specter of tragedy and loss would affect me and the life of my family. September blood does not soon fade away.

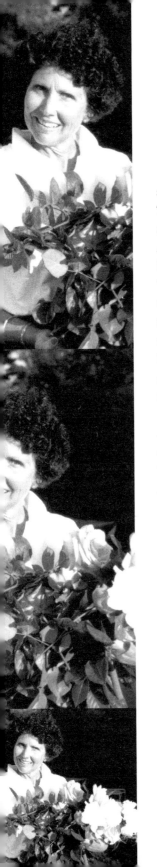

CHAPTER 8
The Lumpectomy

April 29, 1996

The morning dawned bright, sunny and warm with only a hint of the usual marine layer drifting up from the beach. The surgery was scheduled for 10:00 a.m., but we were supposed to be there by 8:00 for the check-in and pre-op. After getting Josh up and ready for school we prepared our bedroom for Suanne's convalescence upon returning home. There wasn't much conversation, just a mechanical touching up of details like turning down the bed, defrosting a chicken that I would cook on the Weber for dinner, and making a list of "things to do" for me for the next couple of days. Just before leaving I went out in the back yard and cut a red rose from the garden, wrapped the stem in a moist paper towel and gave it to Suanne to hold when we got in the car.

On our ride over Highway 17 from Santa Cruz we didn't say much about the procedure. The car radio was reporting on the president's four and a half-hour deposition at the White House by prosecutors in the Whitewater investigation. Although usually deeply concerned about such matters, listening to the news didn't seem all that important at the time. Too much else was on my mind. As if wishing to avoid Topic A altogether, we talked instead about Josh's Wednesday afternoon baseball game, his grades, and the usual things parents of young adolescents are involved in or concerned with.

Josh was a freshman at the time and showing signs of being an excellent left handed pitcher, even if his batting average wasn't exactly ready for ESPN film clips. Suanne loved going to Josh's games and never missed any school meetings or activities. After a while the conversation about Josh dwindled down, perhaps muffled under the blanket of anxiety we were both feeling. The thought of Suanne's absence from Josh's games flickered though both of our minds as we both pondered the common, if mistaken, conception of that a positive diagnosis of breast cancer is, for all intents and purposes, a death sentence. In such circumstances the mind tends to zoom in on extremes, whether warranted or not.

Approaching the Santa Cruz Mountains summit we ran into a couple of sand trucks holding up traffic in the slow lane and checked the time: 7:10. We were in good shape, a little slow-down wouldn't hurt. We continued to creep along in silence, as if sitting in a mausoleum. The thought of the mausoleum seemed macabre and ghoulish. "Shame on me," I thought. But I couldn't help it. The mind oftentimes does what it wants to do.

A little ways past the summit, in trying to refocus my thoughts, I looked down at the rose Suanne was holding in her lap and started thinking about her rose garden. To the casual, and even not so casual, observer, Suanne's rose garden was simply a magnificent display of color, sensuality, fragrance, and romance, all of the things roses connote; but I knew it to be so much more. Suanne had picked out each variety of rose bush in her garden, some from a catalogue her sister had sent, some from a local nursery called Roses of Yesteryear, and a few others she had received as gifts from friends and family. She had cleared a spot for the rose garden on the western side of our house in an area bordered by a long redwood walkway with good morning and afternoon sun exposure throughout the year. She had tilled the beds by hand mixing over two yards of topsoil into the harsh coastal caliche indigenous to our neighbor-hood and then meticulously arranged the garden, giving careful attention to the spacing and size of the bowls. Hard physical labor was not something Suanne ever shied away from. When it was all laid out to her satisfaction, Suanne had me dig the two foot by two foot holes and install a drip irrigation system, retaining for herself the job of sculpturing the cones where fresh potting soil would be placed in the bottom and, of course, planting the bare root rose bushes.

There was the wedding trio of Love, a luscious bright red and pure white reverse grandiflora; Honor, a white to pale yellow hybrid tea; and the soft breezy coral pink floribunda, Cherish. Then there was the passionate Intrigue, the warmth of Summer Dreams, the serenity of Sheer Bliss and Peace and the rapture of Perfect Moment. Suanne's rose garden, like the rest of our home and yard, was not only a reflection of her character and personality, it was also a perfect reflection of how she lived her life. Whether pruning, watering, fertilizing or cutting, Suanne tended her rose garden in much the same manner she had nurtured her family and home: with an outpouring of affection, love and vigilance that never lost focus of the thorny commitment necessary through the months of winter to see her roses through to the blooms and beauty of the spring and summer. As I drove I had visions of what her rose garden might look like if she were not here to attend to it.

I recalled one particularly foggy early spring several years before, when Suanne had asked me to spray her rose garden with an insecticide to control an infestation of thrips along with some aphids and rust that were turning the foliage from lush green into a sooty brown and desiccated yellow. Knowing of my penchant for relying on intuition rather than written directions for many things in my life, Suanne specifically asked me to carefully follow the mixing directions on the container, which I did to the letter. A couple of weeks later we noticed the condition of some of the rose bushes seemed to be deteriorating. Within a month Sheer Bliss, Peace and Perfect Moment were all dead or dying; all victims of the sprayer I had previously used to apply a systemic herbicide like Roundup to the weeds in our side yard. Even the residue in the sprayer from the prior use was enough to provide a lethal dose to some of the rose bushes. When I went back to look at the instructions on the insecticide container, I noted under "Warnings," (as opposed to "Directions for Use" which I had carefully read), "Do not use the same sprayer for applying both pesticides and herbicides."

Around the Lexington Reservoir and after a long silence Suanne asked me if I was okay. "Yeah," I said, "I'm fine. I was just thinking about your rose garden."

Fortunately there were no major traffic tie-ups on our trip over Highway 17, and once we hit the new 85 freeway it was a straight shot to Stanford. I pulled into the parking lot at the Medical Center at 7:55 and we proceeded to the check-in desk. I was sweating by the time we got inside and I wondered if it was my nerves heating up the morning. We were soon on our way to the second floor Outpatient Surgery Center. It's in a relatively new wing of the Center that has grown over the past forty years into one of the great teaching and research hospitals in the world.

The first time I ever saw the Medical Center at Stanford was when I was in the eighth grade. My dad, who was appointed to the Colorado River Board by Governor Goodwin Knight in the 1950s, was attending a water conference at Stanford and we stayed in a sorority house on campus. The medical center was just being built at the time. There were big cranes around this huge building that was being built out in the middle of nowhere. My mom, a kindergarten teacher, had lectured to me on the importance of academic excellence every morning for years on the way to school and took the opportunity of our visit to show me around the sprawling Stanford campus.

One morning after we had walked down to the Stanford family crypt and were walking back to go into Memorial Church (Mem Chu), we passed the part of the Memorial Quadrangle (Mem Quad) that housed the Stanford School of Law. We stopped and my mother took a picture of me in front of the Law School. As we continued our walk, she reminded me that if I studied hard in high school, maybe someday I would go to school at Stanford and become a lawyer. I didn't study that hard in high school, but at least subliminally, I never forgot her admonitions, and the next time I saw the medical center was during my first year as an undergraduate at Stanford, when I got involved in the "big brother, big sister" program which was run out of the Medical Center. Mothers indeed have powerful influences on their sons.[18]

At the check-in desk Suanne was asked a few questions, gave the receptionist our insurance card, signed some forms, and had the obligatory plastic I.D. bracelet put on her wrist. We were then directed to the waiting room and told it would be a few minutes. Before long, a nurse came out and called Suanne's name. She got up to go and I started to follow her until the nurse stopped me, saying that I could come in in a few minutes. I returned to my seat and began looking around at the people that were there, wondering how their lives might be affected by the outcome of their, or their loved one's outpatient surgical procedures.

Names were called and one by one the people got up and passed through the door on their way to a pre-op gurney. Because of the business I am in it was difficult to contain my imagination. Medicine in the era of the health maintenance organization (HMO) is a mass production, profit oriented business that some describe more as managed costs than managed care.

Like many aspects of modern urban society, the necessity of mass production in virtually every aspect of our lives has been accomplished at the cost of individualized personal attention. Mass production requires an assembly line, mechanization, set routines, clock work, standardization, and cost cutting - all characteristics that give rise to opportunities for error and mistake in the practice of medicine. Perhaps worst of all, it also gives rise to and even requires the depersonalization of the doctor patient relationship. Someone whose name I heard called, I imagined might go in for some simple procedure and not even come out alive. Someone else might get the wrong diagnosis, the wrong medications, or the wrong operation and end up tragically disabled for life, like my little HSV II client. It happens more frequently than most people think. My ruminations were interrupted when I heard a voice say, "Mr. Lyman, you can come in now."

At the Stanford Medical Center, the outpatient pre-op room consists of about

18 - I remember the first time I saw it too – I was 18, hoping to get into Stanford undergrad, and the Medical Center rose all alone in a huge field, now long gone. There were many years (including 2 when I ran the trauma program) when I trained residents and operated at very high volume – There many long days and nights on the surgical service when I remembered that first sight of what was to be my future professional home.

nine or ten stations that are enclosed by white curtains running on gleaming chrome rails. Bright light, polished metal and chrome are the first things you notice in the pre-op room and then the antiseptic smell. The gurneys are all lined up with patients in various states of repose, most with someone attending to them, some being wheeled out, others in. The curtains are drawn on some of the patients, while others are open. I walked up to Suanne in the number 6 station while her anesthesiologist was talking to her. Suanne was dressed in the familiar light blue hospital gown with the initials S.U.M.C. stenciled on the front. The anesthesiologist was a young Asian guy, no doubt an intern or resident. He was explaining the procedure and asking her questions.

"What is your name and address?" Check. "What procedure are you here for?" Check. "What previous surgeries have you had?" Check. "Have you had a general anesthesia before?" Check. All questions intended to elicit knowledge-able responses from the patient so that the doctor knows that they are doing the right procedure on the right patient before the patient becomes comatose from the anesthesia and can't answer any questions.

The setting where all this is taking place, of necessity I guess, is both sterile and intimidating. Unlike the legal setting where the lawyer's judgment can be questioned, debated and approved or disapproved by the client at virtually any stage of the proceedings, the medical setting and particularly the pre-op room, is a place where the patients abandon to their keepers virtually all aspects of the decision making process. Any decision that the patient might want to participate in has already been made; all other treatment options have been ruled out, and with the chemically induced coma arrives the point of no return. As I stood beside Suanne's gurney holding her free hand, the starkness of the scene began stoking the fires of my frayed emotions.

Before I arrived, someone had already inserted the needles in the back of her left hand, one of which would be hooked up to the anesthetic in the operating room. Her mood was probably better than mine. She smiled weakly, happy to see me. I smiled back, weakly, and leaned over and kissed her. At this stage the questions in my mind had been stacked on top of one another like so many bankers boxes, the contents of which was a jumble of distant and immediate threats to the life I had been living for the past thirty years. Suanne looked a little wan, perhaps doubt harboring the same fears that I was trying to suppress. I attempted to make some light conversation, but it fell as flat as the questions asked by the anesthesiologist as soon as the words left my mouth. Suanne took my hand and tried to say something encouraging.

"Everything will be fine Honey, don't worry." I could feel the tears instantly welling up in my eyes, so I glanced away and forced a perfunctory response.

"I know, I know." I said with more volume than necessary in an effort to shake off the emotion I was feeling. My voice broke only slightly as I looked up and greeted Dr. Mahoney for the first time. She approached from the double doors leading to the operating room, clad from head to toe in her surgical ensemble, her cap and mask in place. At this point, the refrain was pounding in my head, "...Run, Fly, Hide, In desperation, Search, Find, Kill, In desperation..."

Dr. Mahoney was all business. She explained to me what the procedure consisted of, how long it would take, and when I should return. That was it. She was like one of my petty-officers in the Navy giving the orders of the day: "The work party will begin at 1030 hours, it will be over by 1200 hours. Report back here by 1400 hours." It was 10:17 a.m. when Dr. Mahoney turned to Suanne and said she'd see her on the other side and walked back toward the operating room.[19] By then the orderly was coming to roll her away, so I leaned over and kissed Suanne and told her I knew that everything would be fine. Suanne's eyes were already beginning to glaze over as the first drips of analgesic started to work its way down into the cerebral cortex of her brain. As I watched her gurney disappeared through the automated swinging doors into the operating room, I had the feeling that none of this was real - that it was all a dream. Breast cancer was something that happened to other men's wives, not mine, not to Suanne.

There are times when the emotions seem to act independently of surrounding events and circumstances. This was one of those times. As I walked past Bay Five, then Four, then Three, then Two and One, and back out into the waiting area, the past came cascading in upon me in great pounding emotional waves. I felt numb and disoriented, almost like I was in a trance. My surroundings seemed like it was all a set with actors moving around and saying their lines. And yet at the same time I felt completely consumed by one of the most powerful feelings of love I think I had ever experienced. Perhaps only during the birth of our sons did I experience anything like it.

My heart pined and my mind reeled in a profusion of love, hope, commitment and fear. I walked outside of the medical center and sat on the same little patch of lawn where I sat while waiting for Joshua to be born in 1980.

19 - In the office I take all kinds of time because I am in control of the time there. In the OR, the nurses are in charge, and they are extremely efficient. Stanford (and especially my anesthesia team) has unheard of short "turnover times" – usually less than 10 minutes from the he end of one case and the beginning of the next. During this time I have to do the paperwork for the case just completed, talk to the family, and hopefully have time to greet the family of the next patient. I do a lot of the paperwork the night before in an attempt to spend more time with the families, but it is not always possible. When I get the chance to meet them beforehand I always warn them that chatting time will be short and that I have a "game face" all day when I am doing a large number of cases. But I leave open the time for chatting in the office. Given the choice, I really like to meet the family and/or friends in advance, esp if I suspect a malignant diagnosis. I am very maternal/protective about my patients and always interested in knowing who will be taking care of them when I'm not. If I have to choose, I lavish the attention on the patient and I do short the family. Lesson to the spouse: bond with the surgeon prior to the procedure. **EM**

Finally alone, my chest heaved, my eyes glazed over and I began shedding a torrent of tears. I allowed myself to wallow for a few moments in the agony of being able to do nothing but sit and watch as a biological process as ancient as life itself dictated the future course of my life. After pulling myself together, I went back up to the waiting room and let my fingers drain the day's emotions into the C-drive of my laptop computer.

CHAPTER 9
Men and Breasts

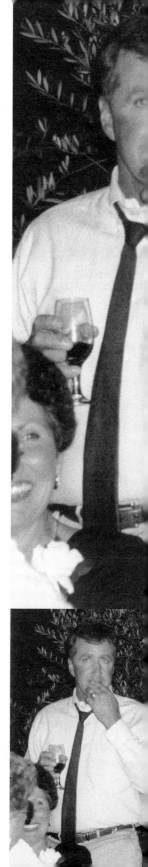

After an hour or so of pecking vacantly at the keyboard on my laptop, I drove over to the Oasis in Menlo Park to get an "LA Well;" which, for the uninitiated, is a well-done (making it hotter), Louisiana (not Los Angeles) hot sausage sandwich. The "O," a renowned Stanford hangout since the Twenties is located just up the El Camino (a major surface road) from the Stanford campus on the north side of the Stanford Shopping Center.

From the outside, the "O" is just another nondescript relic of a commercial building nestled between a gas station and a little retail area across the street from a sprawling Chevrolet dealership - Anderson Chevrolet, named of all things for its owner, John Anderson. John was pursuing an MBA a Stanford about the time I was chasing my J.D. Bright guy, from a car background, major car buff, just like me.

Inside, the "O" is the exact Aristotelian "form" of what a traditional college bar should look like: all manner of Stanford sports paraphernalia and memorabilia; sports posters and vintage photographs; strategically placed TVs always on ESPN or whatever "Game Day" happened to be in season. There are booths, pillars and old redwood tables with initials, monikers, troths, class years and other assorted graffiti carved into every surface accessible to a pocketknife. The lighting is dim, the smells redolent of beer and burgers, and the ambience definitely fraternal, as in fraternity. The place was almost empty with the exception of two college-age looking guys at the bar and two weathered and worn old guys, both of whom I had known since my undergraduate years, perched at the island across from the bar. These two are as much fixtures at the "O" as the pillars and booths.

Both these characters had attained notoriety, if not celebrity status in the early years - one as a popular bartender at the Oasis and the other as a "respected" drug dealer (at a time when many of us were deluded into thinking it was still a cool thing to be). In the intervening 25 to 30 years I must have been in the Oasis at least ten to fifteen times annually, and on virtually every occasion, one or both of them were there. More than once did I wonder what the Oasis must have meant to them for them to have established such an enduring relationship. It had to be like family, or at least like a social club that contributed something important to their lives - a real-world "Cheers" kind of place.

The three of us always engaged in some light banter about the old days, the old "O" crowd, Stanford sports, etc. When I came in this day they invited me to have a beer with them. I obliged and bought a small pitcher of Anchor Steam beer, a San Francisco micro-brewery favorite. When one of them asked me how my family was, the words that emerged from my mouth might as well have come from a prepared script.

"My wife's having surgery right now at Stanford to find out if she has breast cancer; a lumpectomy."

There was a moment of awkward silence, like when you ask about someone and learn that they've died. Most casual conversation is meant to be like social grooming - soothing rather than content seeking; like a ski report: fair to good. I'm sure neither of them was expecting a headline. Then Bob, the former drug dealer, noted that I'd been married a long time.

"Yeah, we've been married for almost more years than I can remember. Since a couple years before I met you guys." I responded.

"My mom died of breast cancer." Bob went on. "I went through the whole thing with her. She died when I was a kid still living at home. By the time they found out, the tumor was the size of an orange and had spread all over the place. But that was a long time ago, things have improved a lot since those days. Today, I understand if they catch breast cancer early, you can beat it. Your wife will be fine." Frankly, I was grateful for the kind and sincere thoughts Bob expressed. I certainly wasn't alone in my experience.

Mark, the one-time "O" bartender, added his two-cents' worth: "I've been there too. I had a girlfriend that had breast cancer about ten or fifteen years ago. By the time they discovered it, it had spread. She had to have a mastectomy and some other stuff on one side removed. God she had great tits. She had the greatest tits I've ever seen. But I couldn't take it. We didn't last a week after she got out of the hospital."

Mark hesitated, perhaps coming to realize the context of his remarks. Then he added, "The last I heard though she was doing okay though. She still had one of her tits. I think she's doing fine." The perspective Mark shared gave me pause, but I didn't respond and thankfully the subject moved to other matters.

"Well," I said, after eating my LA Hot and helping my two buddies with finishing off the pitcher of beer, "I've got to get back to the hospital. We won't know anything for a few days. All I can do at this stage is hope for the best. I'm sure I'll see you guys the next time I'm in town."

Walking to my car, I remembered a day from thirty some odd years earlier when I was an undergraduate. It was a Thursday or Friday afternoon and some of my fraternity brothers from the ATO house and I were getting an early start on the weekend. My companions, as I recall, were John Barnard, Tony Joseph, and Hal King. As we sat at a well-hewn table, this forty something, executive-looking guy, probably from a graduating class of the early 50's, came in and plopped himself at the bar. He was wearing an expensive, tailored suit and had a purposeful, meticulous air about him, but ordered casually without looking at the menu, like a "regular."

"Look at that fucking suit." I said. "Can you imagine dressing up like that every day, going to an office and kissing somebody's ass until someday when you get to have your ass kissed?"

"No fucking way," somebody obligingly agreed. "Who's got the next pitcher?"

Now, settling into Suanne's car, with her smells, habits, and accouterments all about, I wondered if that guy at the bar from thirty years ago was spending his advancing years with the same woman that had given him his kids; the same woman who had struggled with him through their good times and bad; the same woman whom he had fondled, caressed and made love to a thousand times and more; or if, perhaps, for reasons similar to what I was now facing, he was alone, slowly being dispossessed of even his memories. I wondered what memories some day I might have of this time of my life and if I might be soon dispossessed of all the memories I shared with Suanne.

Yesterday, yesterday,
Does it seem a thousand score and more
Since old yesterday,
Or is tomorrow's yesterday
The role I play today
I am,
Am I,
A memory,
Hush now old yesterday,

Lie still,

Breathe not today,

For even now my sun rises upon tomorrow,

Unknown to me, for

I am,

Am I,

A memory.

I stopped by a little flower shop at the shopping center on the way back to the hospital to get something to put in our bedroom for Suanne's convalescence. As I walked into the plant shop (which is partly indoors and partly outdoors), I couldn't help noticing a woman unloading some plants from a truck parked in front. She looked to be a few years younger than Suanne, maybe late thirties, early forties and very attractive. She had dark hair, full lips, a robust complexion and perfect melon-sized breasts. I self-consciously caught myself beginning to fantasize, but continued.

She was wearing a rather gauzy white cotton blouse with what must have been well-worn sheer bra underneath because it looked almost as if she was back in the Sixties going bra-less. Her legs, covered only by a pair of teal running shorts were sinewy, lean and athletic looking. She had a look I always found very, very appealing. The top buttons were open down to her cleavage, which was substantial enough to qualify as a furrow. She had beads of perspiration on her forehead and her blouse was clinging to her collarbones, upper pecks and shoulder blades from the effort of unloading the truck out in the sun.

Remembering Jimmy Carter's famous lines from an interview in Playboy magazine about God forgiving us for looking at strange women with lust, and considering it nothing short of an absolution, I granted myself the pleasure of being visually distracted. In a ritual as natural as dogs sniffing one another at the beach, my eyes (from behind my dark glasses) locked on to her breasts as she went about her business. I looked for a ring on her left hand. None. A saleslady inside asked if there was something in particular I was looking for.

"No, I'm just browsing," I answered, oblivious to the double entendre. "Staying out of the heat. If there's anything I like I'll let you know." I was hoping that I might draw the attention of the unloading lady, if she worked there. I continued to browse. Indeed! Maybe "visually graze" is a better description. She finished her task and signed for the delivery, then turned to take refuge under the awning near the check-out stand. Ah, good, she worked in the shop; not the truck driver.

"Excuse me," I said in a very business-like tone, "What kind of plants are those with the purple flowers you've just unloaded?

"They're Mexican Sage," she responded smiling pleasantly, wiping her forehead and neck with a small white hand-towel she picked up off the counter. "Are you looking for something for indoors or outdoors?"

"Hot out there." I mumbled before answering her. "I'm not sure. Either, I guess. I'm just enjoying looking around." This time I did appreciate the hidden meaning. "You work here, I take it?"

"Yes, you could say that. I'm the owner."

Out of habit I started to tell her my name, but caught myself. "I'll just continuing browsing," I said again, "if there's anything that interests me I'll let you know." This time I almost laughed out loud to myself. As she turned away to attend to business, I unleashed my fantasizing about her.

From one perspective, inside the roofed display area looking out under the awning into the sunlight, I could see the silhouette of her breasts as she stood by the cash register. The lovely sight of her breasts played up, down and across the vitreous chambers of my eyes before communicating with the optic nerves that so stimulate carnal appetite. Her breasts had the mature appearance of having been swollen at one time or another with mothers' milk, a shape (and condition) I find particularly alluring (and appetizing).

From a closer perspective and out from under the shadows of the awning in the sunlight, I could see the outlines of her almost discernable be-jeweled areolas. She was very attractive - a totally gorgeous babe, as they say. I busied myself amongst the plants and flowers making sure I afforded myself the maximum visual advantage. When she finished with one customer, I would move as unobtrusively as possible to her immediate vicinity and ask the identity or price of whatever plant or flower was closest to her. ("Oh, a rose. I guess I should have known that, shouldn't I?") I was trying to be subtle, or at least not too obvious.

I have always had this deep, (some might even say, obsessive) appreciation of breasts, and for more than a moment or two, there in the flower shop, I was transported away from the task at hand, to that place of testosterone induced reverie that only such a visual feast can provoke. The magnetic power and allure of breasts is difficult to overstate. For me anyway. They are a Siren call so ravishing and enchanting that under the right circumstances (or maybe I should say wrong) few men can resist their attraction. Indeed, if I said that a sweeter sight God did not create for man on this whole dang planet, than a gorgeous woman with beautiful breasts erotically displayed, I doubt I would not be seriously challenged in even the most refined of fraternal circles.

I wondered if she noticed me, found me attractive, or if perhaps all she noticed was a middle-aged man making an ass of himself? About the time I was mentally disengaging the top button on the saleslady's blouse and preparing to ravage her, there was a breaking news report coming from a radio somewhere in the shop about a gunman in Australia killing scores of people. I was jolted from my reverie and the scene in the flower shop evaporated in a blizzard of chilling thoughts rooted in the reality of the moment and the ephemeral nature of all life.

"My God," I asked myself, "how can this be happening? What am I going to do if Suanne has breast cancer? How will I react if she has to have a mastectomy?" Mark's comments about not being able to take his girl friend with one breast came flittering back. Though ill-timed and crude, his comments reflected an aspect of the male human condition that is no less real, no less undeniable, no less irrepressibly real than estrus is in dogs and cats and elephants.

I had seen a picture of a woman with one breast on the cover of *New Yorker* magazine and tried to push a mental picture of Suanne with one breast out of my mind. I then began contemplating what the owner of the shop would look like with one breast and what it would be like to fondle or suck on a single breast. "God, what if Suanne has to have a double mastectomy and ends up with no breasts?" How could I face the rest of my life without breasts? "What if I could never get an erection again if Suanne doesn't have breasts?"

By this time my own shirt was sticking to my collar bones and shoulder blades, but I managed to get out of the flower shop without making a spectacle of myself, despite the fact that I was again beginning to reel anew from the emotional eruptions I brought on myself. As I drove away I tried to collect myself.

Hell, Suanne was having a lumpectomy and based on everything that we had been told up to now, chances were that a malignancy would be ruled out, not in. Everything favored a benign outcome, didn't it? Surely I was again letting my imagination and emotions get the best of me.[20] I decided that instead of just giving Suanne flowers, which, as everyone knows, we send for funerals as well as weddings, I stopped at a book store and bought *The Horse Whisperer.* Is it not a known, indisputable, incontrovertible fact that a positive attitude, reinforced with fond hopes, fervent wishes, and a book about a man who could whisper sweet nothings to horses and make them behave well, could never cause a lab test for breast cancer to turn out positive?

It was about 1:30 p.m. by the time I got back to the hospital and proceeded directly to the pre-op room, which was also the recovery room for procedures as

20 - This demonstrates exactly why it is important for a husband to develop a relationship with the physician as soon as possible. I knew early on that even if this was a tiny ugly cancer there was no way a mastectomy would be necessary, especially given the location. **EM**

short as Suanne's lumpectomy. Suanne was still in repose on a gurney, resting under the lingering effects of the general anesthesia. She looked serene, peaceful, and, to my unfaltering eyes, not an iota less beautiful than the day I first saw her, nearly four decades ago, when she was all of fifteen.

"Honey," I whispered in her ear, "you're all done. I love you. Look, I bought you *The Horse Whisperer*." She moaned faintly, opening her eyes but not seeing me. I squeezed her hand and she squeezed back.

A nurse came over and said it probably would be another half-hour to an hour before she would be ready to leave. I repaired to the pre-op waiting room, pulled out my laptop once again and tried to work while waiting for Suanne to shake off the effects of the general anesthesia.

By 3:00, Suanne was pretty much fully recovered and ready to leave, or so it outwardly appeared. The same nurse as before came out to the waiting room to tell me that I should go get the car and meet her out front. I packed up the computer and went to fetch the car.

A different nurse brought Suanne down in a wheel chair and we got her buckled into the passenger seat. She snoozed most of the way home and then went directly to bed. "All" we had to do now was to await the results of the pathology report. As we prepared to drive off the nurse handed me an appointment slip for the following Thursday at 1:30 p.m. "D" day was fast approaching.

The period between 3:30 p.m. on Monday and 1:30 p.m. on Thursday is almost exactly three days - by most people's conception a relatively short lapse of time. But here again, we must view things in context. Seventy hours. That's plenty of time for a man in combat to be driven insane by the sheer horror of the experience. Four-thousand two-hundred and thirty minutes. That's plenty of time, particularly if you're sleep deprived, to cause hallucinations and severe mental disorientation. Two-hundred and fifty-three thousand eight-hundred seconds, each one of which to me was consumed by alternating spasms of hope and fear with prolonged interludes of fervent prayer. I confess that I did a lot of praying, even though I'm not ordinarily given to praying for good fortune. But this was no ordinary circumstance and God seemed like a good place to turn. It was a hellishly long time to wait.[21]

---

[21] - Some hospitals do it faster, but the information lost if the cells are not "fixed" properly in the pathology study can never be recovered, so it is of critical importance to get it right the first time. **EM**

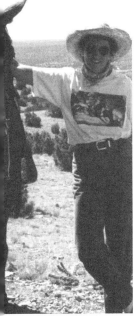
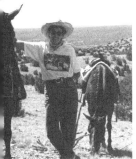
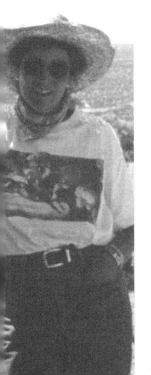

CHAPTER 10
The Breast Cancer Diagnosis

May 2, 1996

The day of the biopsy report arrived. Finally. I was scheduled to be out in the San Joaquin Valley for the deposition of an expert witness in the quadriplegic case, so attending the appointment in Palo Alto with Suanne posed some daunting calendaring problems.

True, I could have changed the date of the deposition as I had done on a hundred other occasions for as many trifling reasons as a creative trial lawyer can dream up to accommodate his schedule, or family matters such as this, but this time I didn't. I ignored the conflict until it was too late to change. I think it was a combination, largely subconscious, of superstition, faintheartedness, and the real pressure of a rapidly approaching trial date in the quad case that pushed me to skirt the appointment and instead attend the deposition.

My going meant Suanne would need me for comfort and support. Not going, I rationalized, was a tacit statement of my unwavering confidence that the biopsy would prove negative, as the mammograms, the ultrasound and Dr. Andrews himself had all indicated it would be. However inventive or legitimate the "excuse," it was a mistake that to this day I sorely regret, and one the likes of which I vowed I would never repeat, for any reason.

I left for the office before sunrise, telling my unconvinced pretend self for the umpteenth time that everything would turn out just fine, hence no compelling need for me to go along. My mood was what I might now describe as "improvised" confidence.

I told Suanne that I would keep my cell phone with me and to call immediately with the news. As I drove away from the house though, I struggled to parry the jabs from my honest (uncontrived) self that kept landing on the unarguable fact that I had left Suanne to go to Palo Alto alone for the appointment with Dr. Mahoney and her unknown medical destiny. After the results were know, no contrived rationalizing on my part could alter this fact, or ever explain it away.

The deposition was in Madera, a small town in the San Joaquin Valley about 20 miles north of Fresno and two hours from home. As I was asking the defense expert witness a carefully constructed hypothetical question, my cell phone rang. I could feel the blood in my head suddenly rush to my stomach as if my brain were a holding tank on a toilet and the ring of my cell phone the flush lever. I'm sure everyone in the room noticed.

Without even finishing my question to the witness, I darted from the room. Whew! False alarm. The call was from another client asking about her case. My heart was pounding so hard that I could hear it over the phone as I fairly screamed HELLO! I returned to the deposition and apologized for the interruption, without further explanation. The doc's answer to my carefully constructed hypothetical question was as transparent as my reasons for being there. I heard nothing by the time the deposition ended, so after packing up, I immediately called the office. It was a little past three.

No one at the office had heard from Suanne either. As I hung up the phone I could feel my defenses crumbling. My premonitions were all bad. It was unlike Suanne not to call with good news. I immediately thought of the way I feel after a jury comes in with a verdict against my client. You just want to go dig a hole and hide in it. I think we all have a tendency to trumpet good news from the highest mountain top, but we are inclined to wander silently on the desert floor with our own doubts and insecurities when the news is bad.

I hesitated calling Suanne's car phone. Doing so, I feared, might put flesh on the bones of my haunting premonitions. Maybe, I thought as I left the court reporter's office, Suanne just wants to surprise me with the good news when I get home. We both kinda like doing that. But I knew I was kidding myself. It was now a waiting game and the tables now seemed to be turning.

On a long straight stretch of Highway 152 between Chowchilla and Red Top, my cell phone rang once again. I had it set on a "William Tell" ring tone. It seemed to capture the entire scene, with the apple squarely on top of Suanne's head.

It was a little before four o'clock in the afternoon. The sun was still high in the western sky announcing the approach of summer. Shimmering phantasms of heat arose from the black macadam on the road ahead. The top of my '67 Camaro convertible was down and I knew the wind noise could prevent me from hearing much of anything at the speed I was traveling. Probably more of my improvising. But I heard "William Tell" loud and clear. As I reached for the phone, the foreboding that had been slumbering restively in my mind rose up like a flock of angry ravens circling overhead. I eased off on the gas and began to look for a place to turn off the highway and stop.

Suanne was sitting in a parking lot off the Highway 85 freeway in Cupertino, crying; and asking in utter disbelief, why and how could this happen to her? She asked all the questions that have no rational answers, but rather languish in a morass of genetic, physiological, environmental, and medical factors so complicated that few if any satisfactory answers reveal themselves, particularly at times such as this.

"Scott, I have breast cancer." In the time it took her to utter those five words, I knew that our lives would be changed forever. My heart began beating so furiously that I thought it was going to jump through my chest wall. The refrain, "Run, Fly, Hide/ In desperation/ Search, Find, Kill/ In desperation!" rang in my mind like a disaster warning.

"Where are you Honey?" I asked. I could feel her words being transformed in my brain into the maws of raw emotion. My questions just tumbled out. "Where have you been?"

She said that after the appointment with Dr. Mahoney, she'd been interviewed for a study seeking reasons why the incidence of breast cancer in the Bay Area is among the highest in the nation. She had been called shortly after her first appointment with Dr. Mahoney and had given her consent to being included in the study. The person conducting the interview met Suanne after the appointment and upon learning the outcome offered to defer it, but true to form, Suanne went ahead, suppressing her dread long enough to deal with the questioning.

After the interview she sat in her car in the parking lot for some time trying to come to grips with the diagnosis. She'd tried to call me on my car phone, but there was no answer (I must have been out of signal for a short while), so then she called her mother. After talking to her mom and still not being able to reach me, she headed for home, alone with the burden of all the grim and grisly prospects that accompany a breast cancer diagnosis.

By the time she reached Cupertino she succumbed to her emotions. She pulled off the freeway near the Apple Computer campus, and tried my number again. This time, she reached me.

No matter how much preparation you make, no matter what you do to steel yourself against the possibility of this kind of medical calamity, no matter where your imagination takes you in morbid apprehension, there is nothing that adequately prepares you for the reality of hearing your wife matter-of-factly declare, "I have breast cancer."

Hearing these words puts you into an entirely different reality, transforming abstract fear of what might be into the terror and panic of what is.

I could feel the dread and hear the trembling in Suanne's voice and wanted nothing more than to hold her close and tell her that I would make sure that everything would be okay. But as these thoughts formed in my mind, I could feel the whetted edge of panic severing away the last sinews of hope I had been relying on to satisfy myself that the whole episode would ultimately amount to nothing.

Now, hearing the fateful words, I was helpless to lift even a single care from the burden Suanne carried, sitting alone in her car, off the 85 Freeway, in Cupertino. I couldn't even speak.

Instead, I was in my car, a hundred miles away, trembling with fear and foreboding, like a lost child in a storm. I finally managed to tell her I was pulling off on a side road and I came to a stop on Road 12 in Madera County, beside a ditch next to an alfalfa field. I reached down and turned the ignition key to off. In retrospect, the gesture now seems symbolic in that the world Suanne and her husband Scott had known and loved and embraced and reveled in had come to a screeching halt. What lay ahead, down the proverbial road, was anyone's guess.

Suanne broke the two-way silence by saying that the news was not all bad. The doctor said we'd caught it early and she had a good prognosis. She used words like "cure," "early discovery" and "fortunate," all of which seemed at the moment indistinguishable from all the optimistic predictions and pronouncements we had heard and I had believed during the waiting period.

Now all I could hear and imagine was the deadly specter of cancer invading every aspect of our lives. I pushed myself back against the headrest, listening numbly to the sounds emanating from the earpiece, not knowing what to do or say.

Listening to her pained words, I wanted badly to say something; I wanted to tell my wife of almost thirty-four years how much I loved her that I would gladly substitute myself in her place if I could; but the words remained stuck in the muddle of my swirling emotions. Finally I managed to blurt out, "Are you sure they didn't just make a mistake? Maybe they've misread the report, like with the mammograms."

"Don't worry Scott," she said, "Everything will be all right." She could tell from the plaintive tone of my inquiry the dread I was feeling and the emotional quagmire my words were floundering in.

After more long, seemingly interminable moments of silence, I managed to tell her, with some semblance of conviction in my voice, that I knew everything would turn out fine and that I would be home as quickly as possible. I hung up the phone with one of the emptiest, most vacant feeling I had ever known. Now indeed, the medical Rubicon had been crossed.

Before starting the car, I closed my eyes and thought, "Shit, here's my wife, just diagnosed with a tumor that could end her life, reassuring me that everything will be alright." I could barely think outside the box of self-flagellation I found myself in. "What kind of man am I that in her hour of need, I'm nowhere to be found? All my proclamations of love and support, and I'm out here in the valley hiding under a deposition rock." There are times when the mirror of our lives does not reflect well on us. For me, this was the worst of those times.

Out in the field on the other side of the ditch, a swather was slowly passing up and down the checks leaving great windrows of alfalfa to dry in the warm spring sun. I watched it, feeling almost frozen in that moment in time. The smell of fresh cut alfalfa flooded me with old memories.

Our first job out on the ranch when we were in grade school was walking up and down the borders of alfalfa fields setting gopher traps for twenty-five cents a tail. We were all of seven and nine. Jerry and I would ride a school bus to the old Foster Ranch out on Avenue 62 three days a week and set our traps and collect our tails. In junior high, after Jerry was gone, I bucked and hauled hay with Willy White off ranches that my dad had claimed in the years after World War II from raw desert a few miles southwest of Thermal, California.

Then, one day, after several years of bad farm prices in the late sixties, the bank foreclosed and overnight, the ranch he worked so hard to build was gone. History. Just like that. A lifetime of my mom and dad's blood, sweat and tears vanished overnight, as if someone had perversely pulled close the curtain on a long-running Broadway play. Not long after, Dad went into a hospital up in LA for a while to get over it. My mom never said it, but losing what he had worked for all his life caused him to have a nervous breakdown. Another major "shit" episode in my life. Now yet another? How cruel fate can be, I told myself. I was reminded of the bumper sticker that seemed to sum it all up so succinctly, "Life is hard, then you die."

Taking a deep breath, I started the car and headed back out onto a new and undefinable road leading to the rest of my life. The highway before me quickly filled with the glistening of my tears and the parade of horribles that I had been suppressing for the past few months came winging back into my mind like a swarm of disfigured harpies.

My thoughts were erupting in blistering torrents of guilt and repentance as I sped up to over 90 mph in a vain attempt to outrun my fears. I couldn't get out of my mind all the grief and torment I'd inflicted on Suanne over the years. Every personal failure, every cruel word, every connivance and contrivance I had ever cooked up seemed to be integral parts of the ingredients that had brought Suanne to this terrible moment. Breast cancer! How could this be happening to her? Maybe the answer, I thought, lies all about me.

All I could do was hope and pray that Suanne would be one of the lucky ones and survive. In tune with the rhythm of my tires on the road, once more, the silent refrain crept into my mind: "Run, Fly, Hide,/ In desperation,/ Search Find Kill,/ In desperation." No matter how hard I tried, I couldn't stop the words from repeating themselves over and over in my mind. It was like an old 33 rpm record stuck in a damaged groove. In an effort to escape the refrain, I picked up the first tape in the console that my hand fell upon and stuck it in the tape deck. It was Dylan. Good 'ol Bob Dylan. Poet, philosopher, and, oh yes, musician. But the hoped for respite was not to be.

For some reason, whenever catastrophe strikes, regardless of whether it's personal, societal, financial or political (which probably accounts for most of the occult proclivities of our kind), the very stars in the heavens seem to re-align in some sort of coalescing support of the event, for good or for ill. And true to form, almost as if on cue from a Father confessor's pulpit, Dylan wailed:

I kain't see my reflection in the water,
I kain't speak the sounds to show no pain,
I kain't hear the echo of my footsteps,
Or remember the sounds of my own name...

God, how could this happen to Suanne? If there is any justice or order in the universe, it should have happened to me, or anyone more deserving of such an awful fate - but not her, she doesn't deserve this. No one deserves this!

There's beauty in that silver singing river,
There's beauty in that rainbow in the sky,
But none of these and nothin' else can touch the beauty,
That I remember in my own true love's eyes...

When I ejected the tape, KCBS news came on reporting that Timothy

McVeigh and Terry Nichols had been connected to the Oklahoma City bombing by dint of a traced credit card. There were 168 people killed ranging in age from Charles Hurlburt, seventy-three, to little Gabreon Bruce, only four months old. Why? Why? Tragedy builds upon tragedy. Malevolence and disease frolic together on the graves of our fondest hopes and dreams. Life, it seems, is turning dark and bleak. Is it all just capriciousness, arbitrariness, the hazards of fortune? Or do we reap what we sow?

Driving down the highways and by-ways of the Great Central Valley had always been a time of reflection and introspection for me. I knew the twists and turns of almost every back road and forgotten highway in the valley from years of traveling between Sacramento and Fresno, San Francisco and Sonora, trying whatever cases and clients came my way.

I remembered a curmudgeonly old duck hunter who had sprayed a kid with No. 9 pellets for invading his blind; an Aryan Brotherhood drug-lord who had spent 23 of his 37 years behind bars; sundry cattle rustlers and trespassers on farms and ranches; a greenhorn Portuguese dairyman whose cows had been killed on Southern Pacific tracks; the successors to the Miller and Lux cattle kingdom, and a young wife and mother whose husband had been killed by the rear view mirror of a motorhome while bicycling down a rural road, among dozens of other cases. These trials were the rites of passage for a young lawyer seeking to earn his courtroom spurs.

Outward bound, after I had loaded up all my trial exhibits, books, briefs and wardrobe, regardless of the case or the destination - Fresno, Modesto, Sacramento, Merced, Madera, San Jose or San Francisco - I always felt an air of excitement, adventure and conquest. The case, the jury, the town, the bars; an opening statement and closing argument; waiting for the jury to return its verdict. Always, in my younger years, no matter the destination, I had a weather eye out on the horizon looking for the adventure of a new dawn:

Springs brooks streams,
Lakes rivers oceans,
Universal calling, mighty joy,
Dawn, dawn first light,
I love you,
Now rushing madly,
Into a new dawn,
Shadowy mystery of the coming,
Driving fury inside me,
Little like a child,

Perhaps not yet a man,
Sun filled shadows,
Those amber shafts of honey and gold,
Drive on thou passion for madness,
Through all but dreary death,
Drive on!

The fantasies I associated with a given destination were usually (but not always), more exciting than the reality to come, except in the winning. As in most great contests, the "rush" of winning trials was like a narcotic to me; always heady and exhilarating, bordering on the euphoric. The axiom "to the victor go the spoils" was more than a metaphor to me, it was an entitlement. And it meant more than just garlands of flowers and booty. Victories in the arena of the trial lawyer are the foundation blocks upon which reputation is built; and on reputation rests the rewards of professional standing, respect in the community, and financial security.

To the exclusion of nearly all else, and for too, too many years, victory in trial was my Holy Grail, or perhaps an excuse for my Holy Grail. I was seldom in a hurry on the homeward bound leg of my journeys, especially if I was flush with victory. I needed to savor my victories, to bathe in the afterglow of the just deserts due me from my Homeric endeavors.

I had stopped at virtually every back-road bar, grocery and liquor store within a two hundred-mile radius of the ranch to cut the dust of the road and to "buffer" the drive home with a bottle or few of Coors and/or an occasional joint, until I suffered the bitter lessons of the example I set for my sons with my flamboyant, balls-to-the-wall, self-indulgent and praetorian approach to life. On these wayfarings my thoughts and reflections almost always revolved around one thing: ME!

Always something involving "ME." J. Scott Lyman, Stanford Doctor of Jurisprudence, Hero and Savior of the Downtrodden, Injured and Oppressed. The feared, swashbuckling courtroom warrior. Mr. Hot-Shit in a three-piece suit. Don't mess with me man, or I'll plant my brand on your pitiful, fucking feckless forehead, quicker than you can say "I stipulate!"

Other times I would sit back, stick in a tape and let my fantasies of Suanne or white whales entertain me. Probably the worst thing I thought could happen to me during those years was losing a case, getting busted for drunk driving or getting caught by Suanne in some, let's say, "compromising situation."

Never once did I give serious thought to what my life would be like without my Suanne. Notwithstanding my own loss, never had I considered what it would mean for the boys to lose their mom, or for Suanne's mom and dad and brothers and sisters to lose her. Realistically, why would I? How many of us really ponder such possibilities?

Yes, intellectually and emotionally, I knew what it was like to lose someone that you hold so dear and close that you question your ability to go on without them, but I had spent a lifetime struggling to put such agony out of my mind and behind me. Blotting it out had been something of a "Holy Grail" in itself. After all, I had managed to cope with the horrific death of my brother, hadn't I? He died right there in front of my own eyes; almost in my arms. I couldn't save him, my own brother. What could be worse than that? Why wouldn't you push it as far away from your memory as possible?

As I sped past Volta Road west of Los Baños, I looked north across the corner 40 to the little ranch a quarter mile up the road where we had sequestered ourselves for ten years, largely as a hedge against the environmental and social Armageddon that, from my years in the academy, I just knew for certain was coming.

The first crop we planted on the ranch was alfalfa. I liked the idea of the thick dark green carpet of alfalfa surrounding our little farm house. The reality was that the front half of the field was somewhat of a sump and thick with salt, so the carpet once laid, appeared tattered and worn. By the end of the season we'd harvested barely over a bale to the acre, but I still felt like we were on our way to being big farmers again. We even started using my dad's old brand. What that first crop failed to yield in bales per acre, I made up for with a productive imagination.

All those years out in the country and I never knew, or cared to learn, the names of the rose bushes Suanne had planted next to the driveway in front of our modest little remodeled farm house. Nor did I know the name of the pattern of her china that she displayed in the kitchen wall cabinet, or her favorite pieces of Roseville pottery that she so ardently collected.

We ate off a kitchen table that Suanne fashioned from an old cable spool and lovingly sanded and lacquered to a shinny ebony finish, yet I didn't even know where or how she got it. Or how much blood, sweat and tears she put into it. It just "magically" appeared one day and became the fitting centerpiece of the kitchen were she practiced her renowned Cajun culinary art. And what art it is.

Indeed, unbeknownst to me (or perhaps just ignored), for all too many years, the entire rhythm of our days on the ranch, from the drop-calves being bucket fed in the wet predawn darkness, to the completion of the boys homework in the late hours of the evening, and everything in between, was arranged, managed and directed by this truly remarkable woman. This remarkable Superwoman! And where was I?

The fields, the corrals and the barns were my domain, or so I imagined; as were brandings in the hills, my jaunts on the other side of the coastal mountains, and my law practice. Ditto Carlo's, Danny's, Espana's, and the rest of the bars in town, where I could prolong the vanishing ambience of fraternity.

While her touch, her smell, and the sound of her voice were as much a part of me as the fields and dreams of my childhood, the delicate contours of her emotions and the hues of her thoughts and dreams for too long remained a mystery to me, buried under some romantic fantasy I maintained of my life as a poet, a cowboy or gunslinger with a cowhide briefcase. Now on this day of terrible awakening, as I sped past the San Luis Reservoir, up over the Pacheco Pass, and down the other side into the lower Santa Clara Valley, the bitter thoughts rising from the inferno in my mind hung over the road ahead like a thick pall of smoke from a funeral pyre of my own making.

Who am I really? Am I a real husband and father? Or, am I an arbitrary, an imaginary me? Am I who I really want to be? Am I the person my parents raised me to be? Or, am I merely a product of instinct and fantasy, being buffeted, pushed and pulled by the winds of fad, change and temptation?

I remembered a passage from Moby Dick (my post-adolescent Bible), where Ahab was explaining the meaning of the hunt for the White Whale to his First Mate:

> All visible objects, man, are but pasteboard masks. But in each event - in the living act, the undoubted deed - there, some unknown but still reasoning thing puts forth the mouldings of its features from behind the unreasoning mask. If man will strike, strike through the mask! How can the prisoner reach outside except by thrusting thought the wall?

I do not want to wear the unreasoning mask. I want the mouldings of my features to be clear and understood, particularly to those that I love and that love me. Why did it take me so long to strike through the wall of selfishness and self-indulgence that separated me from Suanne? Why did I wear the pasteboard mask like a badge of honor for all those years? What have I wrought?

Thoughts of guilt and responsibility are attracted by tragedy and calamity like the swallows to San Juan Capistrano. Sometimes these thoughts of guilt are well deserved, other times they are not so well deserved. In my case, I knew they were more than just well-deserved. My guilt was posted on the signs of my passing everywhere I looked. Now, with Suanne's breast cancer diagnosis, my feelings of guilt enveloped me like a tightly woven cocoon that I couldn't wiggle out of.

Not only in the words and titles of my music did I find reminders of my guilt and unvarnished selfishness, but almost everywhere I looked there was an etching - from the substance abuse and risk taking I engaged in during my twenties and thirties and the extravagant fire-breathing hot rods I have always driven, to the hieroglyphics in my old address books that I could never bring myself to throw away.

What role, I speculated, had I played in causing Suanne's cancer? How many violations of love, devotion and trust does it take to throw the autoimmune system out of kilter? How much stress at the hands of someone who avers to love, cherish and care for you more than anything or anyone else in life does it take to cause healthy systems to go haywire and allow for the cell mutations to spin out of control and show up as a bodily malignancy?

I knew to, for a certainty, that the amount of stress I had cased Suanne would have shattered most wives and families and that it was only her inner strength and devotion to her own personal and spiritual values that had saved us from such an awful fate. I knew for a certainty that I didn't deserve such a rare sweet gift of life.

In the deeper recesses of her mind, I wondered, what kind of man, what kind of person, does Suanne really think I am? What would her last thought be of me if she were to die from this disease? Would she blame me? Resent me? Would our sons blame me for her death? What would their most private thoughts be of me? Would they see me for my successes or failures; for the real or the buffered, rationalized me?

On the other hand, what if the tables had been reversed? How much abuse could I take before the weakest link in my physiological and psychological armor would fatigue and break? I thought about what I told our older boys while they were growing up: "You're going to make mistakes. You're going to stumble and fall. Just try to avoid stumbling and falling over a cliff." Now, all I could do was hope and pray that I hadn't pushed Suanne over a cliff.

As I raced west past the Four Corner's Market on Shore Road, south on Highway 101 and then along side the Pajaro River on Highway 129, I tried to steel myself against the possibility that I had done exactly that. "Jesus Christ!" I heard myself bleating. "She can't die. Please, God, I'll do anything, anything. And I don't care if she has to lose her breasts, I won't care God, really I won't! Please don't let her die!" And I did mean it? Truly I did. The real me meant it.

CHAPTER 11
The Pathology Report

By the time I got home, both of us had regained at least a measure of our composure. Suanne was sitting on our bed reading *Dr. Susan Love's Breast Book*, which she had just bought at Dr. Mahoney's suggestion.

Before saying a word, I sat down beside her and gently kissed her lips. I touched her chin to tilt her head back so I could look into her eyes. I wanted her to see the torrent of love that was flooding through me. I wanted it to cascade over her and wash away her fears, her pain, and her anxiety. Silence. Finally, after many moments, Suanne related to me what she had been told by Dr. Mahoney.

The tumor was small, less than one centimeter. She said that Dr. Mahoney felt very positive about her prognosis and did not think she would need any type of mastectomy or even chemotherapy. "We caught it early, very early."

The pathology report indicated that the right breast biopsy specimen showed an infiltrating ductal carcinoma with poor tubule formation, moderate cytologic atypia, and a low miotic rate. The tumor was classified as a grade two or intermediate grade. Here's what all this means.

First, at .8 centimeter in diameter (.315ths of an inch) the tumor was barely the size that is considered palpable, even by physician examination. Most breast tumors can't be felt until they're much larger, at least a half inch in diameter. The size of a primary tumor is generally considered one of its most important attributes. The smaller the tumor the better the prognosis, and of equal importance, the less likely it is that the tumor has metastasized (spread) .

Infiltrating ductal carcinoma is the most common breast cancer, accounting for 86% of all breast cancers. The tumor originates in the epithelial cells that line the milk ducts of the breast that lead from the lobules deep within the breast where milk is produced, to the nipples. Usually, a ductal tumor is characterized by a stony hardness on palpation.

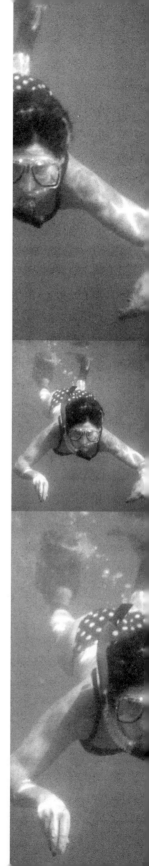

After they reach a critical size, ductal carcinomas often metastasize to the axillary lymph nodes.

The infiltrating characteristic means that the tumor has infiltrated or invaded the fatty tissue immediately surrounding the duct where it started. When the tumor has not infiltrated any surrounding tissue (that is to say, it is confined to the duct or lobule where it originated), it is called *in situ*, and usually has a better prognosis than an infiltrating tumor.

"Poor tubule formation" refers to the visual appearance of the cancer cells. A "tubular" appearance is highly unusual (involving only 1 to 2 percent of all breast cancers), and is usually less aggressive than most other types of cancer cells. Less aggressive, of course, is good.

"Moderate cytologic atypia" means that the cancer cells are moderately atypical or "moderately differentiated" in appearance. Cells of the breast ducts are distinct (differentiated) in appearance from, for example, liver cells or kidney cells or hair cells. This differentiation is what makes each cell suitable for its job. The closer the cancer cell looks to normal (healthy) cells in the organ or tissue where it is situated (described clinically as "well differentiated"), the less aggressive it is deemed to be. More good news.

On the other hand, cells said to be "poorly differentiated," (that is, bearing little resemblance to the healthy neighboring cells,) are typically much more virulent.

The "low miotic rate" means that the nucleus of the cell is dividing (undergoing mitosis or cell division) at a slow rate, which is also good news. Then came the really good news.

The report concluded that there was no definite evidence of what is called angiolymphatic (AL) invasion! The presence of AL invasion can be a major factor in metastasis. The absence of AL invasion can mean that no cancer cells had managed to migrate beyond the primary ductal tumor into any of the surrounding blood vessels or the lymph system. It can also simply mean that the cells that migrated into blood vessels or the lymph system weren't picked up.

From my own research, I knew that if the cancer was confined within the boundaries of the tumor itself and had not yet sloughed cells into the lymph system or blood vessels, there was a good chance Suanne's breast cancer could be eradicated. Completely cured!

Yes, cured. Not simply "treated," or "arrested," but actually cured! It was about as good news as we could possibly have hoped for in the initial pathology report on the biopsy. In addition, the tumor showed a positive response to both estrogen and progesterone staining. This suggests that by chemically blocking or reducing the positive effects of the estrogen and progesterone on cell proliferation, the chances of spread or recurrence could be reduced. Hell, I was so pumped up by all this news, I was ready to go dancing! But my jubilation did not last long.

Suanne now informed me that another surgery had been scheduled three weeks hence to remove more breast tissue around the margins of the tumor and an unspecified number of axillary lymph nodes. The total specimen removed in the lumpectomy, she explained, was only a spherical fragment of 1.8 cm. In other words, the total size of the tissue cut out was just under three fourths of an inch. So the pathology report didn't cover that much tissue from the lump.[22] Even with a tumor as small as this one, it was possible that malignant cells had escaped and spread to other sites.

The next test of whether there was cell migration or metastasis would come from the exploratory surgery being scheduled.[23] Despite the need for more investigation, more surgery, and more worry, I drank long and deep from the well of good news contained in the pathology report. Cancer, I was beginning to learn, was not totally omnipotent in the face of modern medicine. Still and all, we realized that it was going to be an uphill battle and the war long and hard.

Dr. Mahoney told Suanne that the most likely course of treatment would consist of radiation therapy for six to seven weeks and an extended course of tamoxifen therapy, an estrogen blocking medication to reduce the influence of female hormones on the growth of cancer cells.

Suanne concluded by telling me that Dr. Mahoney qualified her sunny prognosis and conservative treatment plan with the proviso that it would apply only if the biopsies of her margins (the area of tissue immediately surrounding the tumor site) and lymph nodes after the second surgery showed negative for cancer cells.

I was holding both of Suanne's hands tightly in mine when she finished. Afterwards we sat there in a long silence, both of us trying to come to grips with the numbing burdens we had been carrying for several months, and wondering if the doctor's lush promise of a full tomorrow would fulfill our most fervent prayers.

"I love you Suanne," I said, "I love you with all my heart and soul." She nodded, as if to say, "I know you do." That was all the acknowledgment I needed. I kissed her gently on the lips.

22 - Actually it was enough as it turned out – I just wanted more and I knew I could get a wider margin without compromising the cosmetic result. I wanted the same wide margins around all aspects of the tumor. **EM**

23 - It's one test, but again, the value is in a positive result – a negative result does not mean that the cancer has not spread – it can go by bloodstream or other nodes. Same comment for the point about angiolymphatic invasion – just because it isn't seen doesn't mean that it isn't somewhere in the specimen.

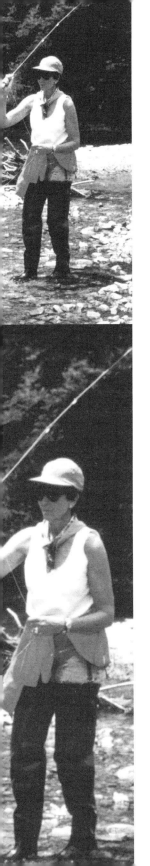

CHAPTER 12
The Surgeon Speaks

May 6, 1996

I told Suanne that I wanted to talk with Dr. Mahoney about her prognosis and the treatment plan being contemplated. Hearing it from Suanne was one thing, but having the opportunity to "cross-examine" the doctor and learn the basis for her prognosis first hand, in a one on one discussion, was quite another.

I had read an article suggesting that claims of both the "epidemic" proportions of breast cancer cases and new "cures" were usually gross oversimplifications and to be viewed with skepticism. In truth, even without the benefit of the information I gleaned from the article, I was wrestling mentally with what I was hearing about the likelihood of a complete cure. To me the word "cure" rang hollow; it seemed too good to be true. Suanne conveyed my message and informed me that Dr. Mahoney would be calling. I took the call at home at 7:45 on Monday evening. I was sitting at my computer reading a report out of Switzerland suggesting a strong causal relationship between breast cancer and smoking. No surprise there.

I had never heard Dr. Mahoney's name before the referral by Dr. Andrews. At the time she performed Suanne's lumpectomy the only thing I knew of her was that she was an assistant clinical professor of surgery at Stanford Medical School. Beyond that association (which to me said a lot), she was "simply" a surgeon and the woman behind the mask that artfully wielded the surgical blade on my wife. I didn't know whether she specialized in breast surgery, or even if there was such a specialty.

As a medical malpractice lawyer, I had sued scores of physicians just like her over the years for a myriad of acts of negligence in a wide array of specialties. In advance of receiving the call, however, I had inquired of a physician friend in Palo Alto about Dr. Mahoney. I wanted to have more than a vague idea of who the doctor was behind the surgical mask. From him I learned that she held herself out as a breast surgery specialist. Moreover, I was told that seventy-five percent of her practice involved breast cancer patients. To my mind, this was most reassuring. And not only did she commit the bulk of her professional practice to helping breast cancer patients, but she was a co-founder and a volunteer medical director of the non-profit Community Breast Health Project in Palo Alto.

My physician friend further told me that Dr. Mahoney was a renowned and highly respected advocate for breast cancer patients, for public education on breast cancer and a tireless champion of breast cancer research.

I came to learn that the Community Breast Health Project of Palo Alto is recognized as one of the most respected and most successful community based breast cancer organizations in the country. Here, I concluded, was a practicing professional whose actions spoke far louder than words ever could; a rare breed of an individual whose commitment to excellence and good works surpassed her need for fame or fortune. So, when the call finally came, I felt humbled, and a bit embarrassed that she took the time out of her work or rest to speak with me.

Over the phone the doctor's voice was warmer and more pleasant than what I remembered from the hospital; it conveyed, I thought, an almost light and cheerful tone, plainly upbeat.

The report I got from Dr. Mahoney was essentially a corroboration of what I had already been told by Suanne, only more detailed, and about as encouraging as it could be given the circumstances.

The doctor's central theme and thesis: in cases like Suanne's, early detection of breast cancer tumors is the key to successful treatment and cure, at least in the vast majority of cases. And yes, she pointedly used the word "cure." Hearing it from Dr. Mahoney however, was like having the seal of the highest authority put on the best news I could possibly imagine.

In the course of my conversation with this extraordinary woman, who, without exaggeration, probably saved Suanne's life, I couldn't help but thinking what might have played out and the turn this conversation might have taken had Suanne not received the call from our neighbor Nancy, or just dutifully accepted the clinical judgments that had been given to her and blithely gone along with scheduling her next mammogram and doctor visit twelve months hence.

I wondered what it must be like for a doctor to call a husband, a mother, father, or a patient and disclose that the pathology report showed that cancer was highly aggressive and at an advanced stage; that it had spread to distant sites and that the prognosis was guarded or poor?

Instead of listening to the buoyant voice and prognosis I was hearing, I knew there were tens of thousands of breast cancer patients and husbands were consigned to face just such a grim fate. I realized that Suanne and I could have been among them. I wondered how I would have felt and how I would have reacted to such a report. Sadly, I would soon learn the answer through the experience of two colleagues of mine whose wives were diagnosed with breast cancer a few months after we learned of Suanne's illness. (More on this later.)

"Your wife does have cancer," Dr. Mahoney concluded, "but I think we got it all. The tumor was only about eight-tenths of a centimeter and appeared very self-contained. It also appears to have been one of the slow growing varieties. We will need to follow up with a second surgery to excise the margins and remove some lymph nodes to check them for cancer cells, but if nothing further is found, there is a 95 percent chance that she will have a full life expectancy. The chances are good that Suanne is cured."

"You're saying that the cancer is gone?" I asked, still skeptical of the unbridled confidence with which Dr. Mahoney gave her prognosis.

"Yes and no." She responded. "If there has been no migration of the cancer cells outside the primary tumor in the breast, and assuming there aren't other malignant tumors that we are unaware of, then yes, by taking out the tumor, we have, in fact, removed the cancer.

"On the other hand, you have to remember that microscopic cancer cells could have been carried to a distant site where a new tumor is growing as we speak. That's called distant metastasis. If that has occurred, then obviously the cancer isn't fully cured.[24] We'll learn a lot more when we excise the margins and check out her lymph nodes."

"Is there any way to determine if there are distant microscopic tumors?" I asked.

"At the present time we do not have the technology to accomplish that. But Suanne will go through a series of tests to rule out a gross metastasis in a variety of locations. She'll have a bone scan to rule out cancer in her bones, a chest x-ray to rule out lung cancers, blood tests for cancer in her liver, and so on.[25]"

"What will the treatment consist of, assuming all those tests are negative?" I pressed.

"I don't medically treat cancer patients," [26] she answered, emphasizing the

---

24 - If that more distant site is in the breast it can still be cured but would require a mastectomy .If the cells are outside the breast, cure is much less likely. **EM**

25 - These tests are not always done any more for very small tumors like this one. I would do them if I were contemplating a mastectomy – if there were a 1% chance of a bone metastasis, I'd want to know before I did a potentially mutilating operation. **EM**

26 - I do try to stay up to date on the medical aspects of cancer treatment and frequently opine about it - something the oncologists in many rural counties are not used to! **EM**

word, "treat." "I just do the surgery and at this point I don't think Suanne is a candidate for a mastectomy, provided that her margins are clear and there is no other tumor in her breast."

"What about the lymph nodes?"

"The condition of the nodes has no bearing on the decision for a mastectomy. If the tumor is elsewhere in the breast, then the breast has to be removed. If the nodes are involved, then more systemic therapy is needed, such as more aggressive chemo."

"I will order additional testing before the next surgery and she will see a radiation oncologist and probably a medical oncologist for continued follow-up. Almost certainly there will be radiation treatment for a few weeks. Too, I think it likely that Suanne will be prescribed an estrogen blocker called tamoxifen for a period of three to five years. The radiation therapy can be unpleasant and can cause certain side effects, but most of the side effects are transitory. All of that will be explained to you and Suanne by the radiologist."

"Where will she have to go for the treatments?"

"You have an outstanding radiation oncology group in Santa Cruz County." She said. "Do you know Steven Mann or Ed Sacks?"

"Yes, I do. Steven and Honey Mann are neighbors of ours. We've known them for many years and consider them friends. I don't know Dr. Sacks except by reputation, which is excellent."

"Well, you're fortunate to have such high quality medical care available to you. It's not the same everywhere. In many rural areas radiation therapy still isn't available."

I assumed as we spoke that Dr. Mahoney probably had other calls to make this evening and that some of them might be of a distinctly different variety than mine, so I thanked her for her call and hung up.

I sat there in complete awe. Suanne's doctor, this renown breast surgeon and breast cancer advocate, had just told me, with unalloyed confidence, that she thought Suanne's cancer might be completely gone. Cut out like a shard of glass.

Although I had not seen it at the time, Dr. Mahoney had documented her confidence in her prognosis in a note she wrote to Suanne on the day of her pathology report appointment. I repeat it here verbatim and in its entirety, as penned by Dr. Mahoney:

"Suanne:

Path is not final, but they are

acting like they think

it is suspicious for a

very small invasive cancer

This is ideal for breast conservation -

You would need the biopsy site

Re-excised for bigger margins

The lymph nodes

Sampled, and radiation therapy (1/2 hr. Appt/ weekday)

For 4-6 wks.

Mastectomy with/without reconstruction is the alternative.

I doubt you will need chemotherapy,

based on the tiny size, but we

Will have to wait for the final pathology.

Your job -

Do more reading about small

Stage I tumors

Susan Love's Breast Book

And/or consult the Community Breast Health Project upstairs in Suite 370

If this is cancer (and we'll know later today),

Based on information we have now, it should be

Totally curable (95% chance of normal survival)

Poetry, I thought, pure poetry. But how can that be, I wondered? I was still having a hard time letting go of both my professional fears and my paranoia. My perception of cancer up until the time that its ugly specter rudely entered our lives, was that it was much like being told you were HIV positive five or ten years ago; you were going to die, period; and sooner more likely than later.

But what I was learning from Dr. Mahoney, from my own research and during the subsequent course of dealing with the disease, is that the verdict of a malignant breast tumor is no longer the equivalent of a death warrant.

In fact, assessing and treating many cancers is now something like the triage system in emergency medicine, where when confronted with the application of scarce medical resources to competing interests, the victims are graded ("staged") according to their chances of survival. Some are deemed too far gone, some can wait for treatment, and others will die if they are not treated immediately.

Victims in shock, such as those with massive bleeding or not breathing, are examples of trauma patients that have only a very short time before they die without treatment. By getting to these patients quickly and stopping the bleeding, starting breathing or relieving the shock, their chances of survival are greatly increased.

In breast cancer there is a very well-defined staging system that doctors use to plan long-term treatment and forecast odds of survival. It is called TNM Staging. T for tumor size; N for axillary lymph node involvement, and M for metastasis.[27]

The TNM staging system occurs in two phases. The first is based on the physical examination and screening tests done by the primary care physician. A tumor that feels and/or appears on the mammogram to be less than two centimeters is a Stage I tumor, or a T-1 tumor; between two and five centimeter is a T-2 tumor; and greater than five centimeters is a T-3 tumor.

If the examination of the axillary lymph nodes shows negative it's an N-0 node. If the physician can feel ("palpate" in clinicalese), a suspicious node but concludes that it is negative, it is declared to be an N-1a node stage. If, on the other hand, the nodes "feel" positive for breast cancer involvement, they're classified N-1b. If the lymph nodes feel enlarged and connected together it is an N-2 stage. If an N-2 node is found near the collarbone, it's an N-3. Metastasis is classified either M-0 (no gross distant tumors),[28] or M-1 (distant tumor discovered on gross tests).

The second phase of the staging process commences when the tissue sample from the tumor and (as necessary), the axillary lymph nodes are studied and tested by a pathologist in a laboratory. This information is then all put together to identify the stage of the breast cancer.

In Stage I breast cancer the primary tumor (T) is no greater than 2 centimeters (about 1 inch in diameter); there is no axillary lymph node involvement (N), and it has not spread beyond the breast.

Stage II breast cancer includes any of the following: The tumor is 2 centimeters or less, but has spread to the axillary lymph nodes. The tumor is between 2 and 5 centimeters with or without lymph node involvement. The tumor is greater than 5 centimeters without lymph node involvement.

Stage III breast cancer is divided into states IIIA and IIIB. Stage IIIA is identified by either of the following: The tumor is less than five centimeters, has spread to the axillary lymph nodes and the nodes are fusing together and/or attached to an adjacent structure such as the chest wall. The tumor is in excess of five centimeters and has spread to the axillary lymph nodes. In Stage IIIB the cancer has either spread to adjacent structures (skin, chest wall, ribs, muscles) or spread to lymph nodes inside the chest wall along the breastbone.

---

27 - Actually, staging was developed to be sure that roughly equivalent patients were included in the various arms of a research study – nowadays we have lost sight of that and patients especially tend to use them as a form of fortune-telling, looking at survival rates from those studies... that often isn't valid, but since we can't tell for sure who is cured, it is understandable. **EM**

28 - There is a difference between "clinical stage" which is what the doctor feels, and "pathological stage" which is what the pathologist tells us. The latter is obviously the one that is most valid and which "sticks."

Stage IV breast cancer is when the cancer has spread from the primary tumor site in the breast to form gross secondary tumors in other organs of the body such as the bones, lungs, liver or brain. Stage IV carries with it a very poor prognosis.

According to what we were being told by Dr. Mahoney and from what I was learning from my research, getting to the victim in the early stage of the disease with a definitive diagnosis and treatment is the key to survival. Without early diagnosis and treatment, the tumor has the opportunity to grow and spread, and the prognosis becomes progressively bleak.

But being told the disease was caught early and that everything is "probably" going to be okay is an entirely different matter from being convinced, especially when your mind has been conditioned your whole life to believe that having cancer is the equivalent of a death sentence.

For Suanne and me, it would take a lot more time and a lot more information before the bold and ruddy predictions made by Dr. Mahoney would truly sink in, and even then our fears would prove agonizingly persistent.

Heeding Mahoney's advice, Suanne had already bought *Dr. Susan Love's Breast Book.* She read it and re-read it until it had the appearance of a refugee from a flea market book seller's cardboard box.

I too read it, and after doing so, I believed, and continute to believe to this day, that Dr. Love's book is unquestionably one of the most comprehensive, understandable, and sensitive treatments available, dealing with almost every medical issue imaginable related to female breasts, and particularly breast cancer. It has been hailed by some as, "the Bible for women with breast cancer."

Another extremely valuable source of information for those seeking to gain a deeper understanding of what cancer is, how it develops and spreads, and diagnosis and treatment is the September 1996 issue of Scientific American, a reprint of which can be obtained from the American Cancer Society. There are a number of Internet sites that provide a wealth of information to anyone interested in breast cancer issues.[29]

29 - See *Appendix 1* for a list of web sites, organizations and publications.

• 90 •

CHAPTER 13
Some Other Case Histories

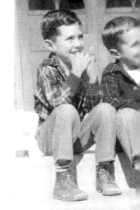

I mentioned earlier that I have two colleagues whose wives were diagnosed with breast cancer at about the same time as Suanne. While the wife of a very close physician friend had been diagnosed with breast cancer a couple of years prior. Then there are Rob and Mendy, son and daughter-in-law respectively, of our neighbor Nancy. The gamut of experiences of these four breast cancer husbands ranged up and down the life expectancy scale from good to terminal. Sad to say, none of these couples were as fortunate as we were in benefiting from an early disease detection.

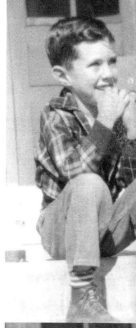

In each of these case histories, the wives were intelligent, educated and sensitive to health issues, yet none discovered their tumor until they had progressed well beyond the early stage.

So as not to skew the picture in favor of the supremely positive prognosis I am relating in the instance of my own wife, I thought it would be valuable - in the interest of balance - to summarize these other case histories. Together, they serve to put our experience with breast cancer into perspective.

Case One

Richard is a successful lawyer from Sacramento. He has been married to Karen, a primary school teacher with a post-graduate degree, for over twenty-five years. Karen works, not out of economic necessity, but because of her love of teaching. They have four children ranging in age from 14 to 22.

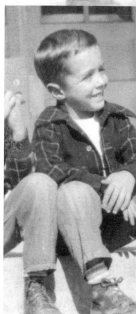

In September of 1997, at the age of 44, Karen found a lump in her right breast while showering. That all of the women cited in this story discovered lumps in their breasts while bathing is by no means anomalous. Indeed, soaping off in the shower is a perfect time to feel changes in the

219243

body and it is commonplace for women to find lumps in their breasts while showering.

Karen did not seem to be a likely candidate for breast cancer. Like Suanne, she evidenced few of the known risk factors.

She entered menarche late (15.7), had an early first childbirth (21), breast fed all four of her offspring, never smoked or drank; enjoyed a healthy diet, and never took contraceptive pills.

Karen exercised regularly and, at 5'6" and 130 pounds, was in excellent physical condition, and had never been overweight. About the only thing they could think of that might be a contributing ingredient was the ground water, which in many Central California communities is subject to a regular diet of agricultural chemicals. To this day, however, a positive link between the groundwater in question has not been established.

Karen had regular mammograms, all of which were negative, including the most recent one, two years prior. Her last Ob/Gyn appointment and physician breast examination was just months before and was negative as well.

In November of 1997, only two months after the self discovery, Karen had a lumpectomy and was diagnosed with a 1.9 cm. (approximately .80 inch) malignant tumor (by comparison, Suanne's tumor was .8 cm or over one cm. smaller).

Karen's margins (the tissue immediately surrounding the tumor) showed some infiltration of cancer cells (Suanne's were "clean"). Like Suanne's, Karen's tumor was hormone receptor positive, which means that estrogen and progesterone promoted its growth. As with Suanne's case, following the lumpectomy diagnosis, a second surgery was scheduled to remove some lymph nodes and expand the margins around the tumor for further study.

The tumor was classified a high Stage I and would have been classified a Stage II if it had been one tenth of a centimeter larger (2 cm.). The life expectancy prognosis for a tumor the size of Karen's usually is given as "poor" in clinical terminology. In layman's language this oftentimes translates to "terminal," accompanied by an 80 percent chance of a five-year life expectancy and a 70 percent chance of surviving for ten years.

Immediately after receiving the pathology report from the lumpectomy, Richard and Karen, a doting, loving couple, embarked on an intense, hurry-up course of study to research for themselves what treatment option they would select. Every option was looked at solely from the perspective of increasing Karen's statistical probability for long term survival.

Richard tells me that no consideration was given to cosmetic or even conservation matters, only survival. In the thirteen days between the first surgery (the lumpectomy) and the second surgery to expand the margin and remove lymph nodes, the couple concluded, based on their inquiry and discussions with doctors, that the mastectomy procedure supplemented with chemotherapy might add between four and six percent to her 70 percent chance of ten year survival. They elected to go with the mastectomy (as opposed to a follow-up exploratory procedure (excising the margins), such as was performed on Suanne.

Following the lumpectomy, the first news Richard and Karen heard was that, statistically, the prognosis for a Stage II tumor is "poor." Richard's initial reaction to this, as would be expected, was one of complete devastation. His second reaction was to commit himself, with every fiber of his being, to his wife and anything he could possibly do to contribute to her survival.

Karen's own reaction to the prognosis, Richard relates, was very deliberate and calm. Richard, meanwhile, experienced classic so-called "sympathetic reaction," in the form of nightmares, insomnia and phantom pain. In his own words, he felt like "a duck whose mate had been shot and wounded." He spent hours and days unable to function, crying uncontrollably, and engaging in the same kind of self-examination and guilt that I have, only correspondingly worse. Richard took it very, very hard; he was an emotional wreck.

The reaction from their children ranged from one similar to Richard's (the 22 year old boy), to initial self-pity from their daughter who resented the intrusion of breast cancer into her life just as she was turning Sweet Sixteen. After the initial shock - and varying emotions - all four of the kids closed ranks with their dad in a total commitment to help their mom beat the grim odds she was facing.

For Richard, the ordeal meant leaving no stone unturned in determining what, if anything, might be done to increase Karen's prospects for long term survival. Besides doing his own medical research (as I did, and continue to do), he consulted with several medical oncologists (cancer specialist), to get as many opinions as possible.

Thirteen days after she detected the tumor on her own, Karen's left breast was removed in a modified radical mastectomy procedure.

As this is written, Karen is undergoing her second round of chemotherapy. Richard, always a contributor and hands on participant around the house, willingly assumed most of the household chores while striving mightily to keep up his law practice.

Following the surgery, Karen came to suffer a variety of complications, including lower extremity numbness, insomnia, chronic constipation (bowel impaction), and severe nausea. All of these are common side effects of chemotherapy.

Richard has become almost obsessed with the possible - albeit unproven - role of stress in general and stress imposed on wives by husbands in particular in the medical and social factors that he is convinced contribute to the breast cancer epidemic. Among the social factors Richard believes contribute to breast cancer are dead beat dads, drug and/or alcohol addicted husbands and fathers, child and/or spousal abuse, and those who simply fail to contribute to the home and fulfill the role of primary provider and breadwinner for their families.

Asked for specifics, Richard notes that historically, women have fulfilled the traditional roles of wife and mother, primary caregiver to children, homemaker/maid, cook, teacher's aid/tutor, resident chauffeur, and household manager/comptroller, plus others. Today, in addition to the aforementioned roles, Richard opines, women are expected to work fulltime, pay the mortgage, and look like Pamela Lee Anderson while serving dinner when the husband gets home at night, assuming that the woman is lucky enough to have an intact "nuclear" family.

It is inevitable, Richard theorizes, that at some point the increasing demands placed on women will manifest in health problems such as heart disease and breast cancer.

Karen was off work for a year after the mastectomy. Coping with the chemotherapy proved extremely hard on her physically and emotionally, and made it virtually impossible to work. During the more difficult phases of the chemotherapy treatment, Karen's primary concern - characteristic of today's put-upon wife/mother - was the impact the illness and its complications was having on her family.

Once the side effects subsided, Karen dove back into the classroom, teaching with a renewed commitment that Richard described as bordering on obsession. But he also felt that the personal and psychic rewards Karen derived from her teaching amounted to perhaps the best therapy she could have.

"She seems to have completely accepted her life as a cancer patient," Richard relates, "both in terms of the opportunities that remain and those that may not remain." At this writing Karen's breast cancer remains in remission. Statistically, she has only several more years to live.

Case Two

Dr. Marcus Stone is a family practice physician in Santa Cruz County now in his late forties. At the age of 48, his wife Sandy found a lump in her left breast, here again, while showering. They have a son, who was 10 at the time.

Sandy was a moderate smoker and had a strong history of breast cancer in her maternal blood line. (Her maternal grandmother died of breast cancer at the age of 70. A maternal aunt was diagnosed with breast cancer in her forties, had a mastectomy, and is alive and well today, a septuagenarian.)

Sandy gave birth to her first (and only) child relatively late (37), had started menarche early (12.1), and took birth control pills for a period of more than ten years in her 30s and early 40s. She did not enter menopause until after the breast cancer diagnosis and chemotherapy treatment.

Sandy was cognizant of and very sensitive to her risk factors for breast cancer when she discovered her lump in the shower. She had been getting annual mammograms since she turned 40.

Immediately upon finding the suspicious lump she told her physician husband she felt certain it was malignant, although she wasn't sure why.

A mammogram, performed two days later, was read as "suspicious for a tumor." A fine needle biopsy aspiration (FNA), done a day later, was inconclusive. Accordingly, a lumpectomy was then scheduled for the following week.

Meanwhile, in the short interval between the inconclusive FNA and the lumpectomy, Sandy and her breast cancer surgeon concluded that in view of all the risk factors, if there was in fact a malignancy, she was going to have a mastectomy immediately.

High on the consideration scale was the experience of her aunt, who was cancer free thirty years after her mastectomy. Sandy did not even want to wait for a pathology report on the suspicious lump. She did not want to have a second surgery to expand the margins and sample her lymph nodes and then wait for a second pathology report before deciding what to do next. Thus, Sandy and her surgeon decided, based primarily on the strong family history, that if "frozen sections" of the tumor analyzed during the lumpectomy procedure showed a malignancy, she would undergo a modified mastectomy without further ado...or delay.

With the full assent and support of her husband, Sandy signed a consent form providing that if a malignancy was found, she wanted the breast removed. Sandy was a strong advocate for herself and believed that she had the greatest chance of long term survival by opting for the mastectomy and chemotherapy instead of the alternatives then available.

The lump removed from Sandy's left breast was almost exactly one centimeter in diameter. The frozen section showed that the tumor was malignant; and as agreed, the surgeon proceeded with the mastectomy; immediately.

In the course of the surgery, eight to ten lymph nodes were removed and biopsied. Three of them turned out positive for breast cancer metastasis, affirming uncannily, Sandy's initial suspicion (and prediction) that the lump she detected while showering would prove to be bad news.

The combination of the strong family history, the size of the lump and the metastasis into the lymph nodes strongly argued for the decision arrived at jointly by Sandy and the surgeon. Meanwhile, her husband, the medical doctor, fully supported his wife's decision to undergo the mastectomy once the lumpectomy results were known.

The role Dr. Stone played in his wife's care and treatment for breast cancer was strictly non-clinical; rather, it was exclusively that of a deeply concerned and caring mate. By agreement, Sandy never looked to her physician husband for any medical opinions or judgments. Nor did Dr. Stone fall prey to proffering any after-the-fact second-guessing. He kept his medical mouth shut, and left the decision making in the hands where it belonged.

Like Richard's, his reaction to the decision to go forward with the mastectomy was unhindered by reservations or demurrals. When I asked Dr. Stone what his initial response was to the cancer diagnosis, the answer was simple and straightforward: fear of losing Sandy and her not seeing their young son grow up.

His take on the mastectomy decision I found interesting...and 180 degree from my own sentiments. He said, "Sexually speaking, for me Sandy's having a mastectomy was certainly distressing, but it wasn't something that I couldn't get over and cope with. I've never really been a breast man. Not that I didn't enjoy Sandy's breasts, it just that I've always been more of a butt man than a breast man.

"Some men are leg men, some are butt men and others are breast men. But in reality, as a physician, I happen to know that the primary organ that controls sexual stimulation and activity is the brain. When the brain is stimulated by the hormones that cause us to seek out or desire sexual activity, the role of our response to visual stimulation or even tactile stimulation is secondary to the brain's own sexual chemistry. In addition, there's the emotional component that also goes into the making of a good sexual relationship. What I'm talking about here is a deep love that we had felt for many years."

He continued: "I love Sandy and I recognized that losing a breast is a very, very traumatic experience for any woman. There just simply is no way around the feeling that any woman would have about her femininity, her connubial desirability, and so forth. I wanted to give Sandy as much time as she needed to work through those feelings. As she was doing so, I made a conscious decision to communicate with her, in every way possible, that I loved and desired her as much without one of her breasts as I did when she had both breasts.

"Once that decision was made, I was able to act on it and I became the person - and mate - that I wanted to be for my wife. And I can tell you that once Sandy understood that as far as I was concerned, she was just as full and complete a sexual being as she ever was, it helped her to accept herself. If every breast cancer husband understood and internalized this posture, my feeling is that it would contribute greatly to their wives recovery from the psychological trauma of breast cancer and mastectomies. And I can also tell you truthfully that our sex life is every bit as good today as it ever was."

Dr. Stone says he strongly believes that women can and indeed must be their own best medical advocates. In Sandy's case she was able to sense what the best course of action was for herself. That said, and as Dr. Stone cautions as a doctor, any decision on a matter as grave as selecting one course of breast cancer treatment over another, should be made only after a thorough and complete discussion of the risks and benefits of all options with the best medical resources available.

Dr. Stone further maintains that the strength and commitment of a cancer patient to her own health can be a crucial element in the odds for long term survival. Sandy's "sense" of her tumor turned out to be medically justified. Seven years after the surgery, Sandy has had no recurrences or signs of breast cancer. She is considered "clean" and her prognosis for long term survival is excellent.

Also of significance here, I believe, is the involvement of Dr. Stone, both before and after Sandy's surgery, as husband and as helpmate. As was true before the surgery, in terms of helping around the house, he continued to be one of the most contributing, supportive, helpful husbands I have ever met. In all respects, he pulls more than his own weight.

Case Three
The two aforementioned cases are both eloquent testimony to the capacity of breast cancer husbands to provide the kind of loving support that a breast cancer victim needs during this time of incredible physical and emotional challenge. As suggested by Dr. Mann at the outset, however, this is not always so. The following is a case in point.

Carol and Doug had been married for only 18 years when she was diagnosed with breast cancer. She was 38 at the time, and an upper level manager for a large insurance company. Doug was 40 and an executive with a major chemical corporation in S.F. Carol had just started with a program of annual mammograms due to the fact that her mother had died of breast cancer at 55 years old. The tumor found in her left breast was not particularly large, only 1.2 centimeters in diameter.

Like Suanne's, it was an invasive ductal carcinoma with poor tubule formation and showed a positive response to both estrogen and progesterone staining. Unlike Suanne's, it had moderately high cytologic atypia, and a moderately high miotic rate. In lay terms, Carol's breast cancer was the same common variety as Suanne's, only more aggressive, more virulent. The treatment regimen elected by Carol was a lumpectomy with radiation. Tamoxafen therapy was not offered.

Nine years later, during an annual check-up, a mass was detected in the breast opposite (right) to where the earlier tumor had been found. The pathology report, after a core biopsy, identified the lump as malignant. This time, after taking into consideration all of the risk factors, Carol's physician raised the possible desirability of a modified double mastectomy.

However, because the newfound tumor in the right breast did not appear to be related to the previous one (in other words, it was not a metastasis from the earlier tumor), the decision was made by Carol and Doug to perform another lumpectomy and treat the area with radiation. This decision was mutually agreed on after much discussion between the couple. This time tamoxafin therapy was prescribed, but after a short time, Carol discontinued it due to the severity of the side effects and Doug's reaction to them. In addition to the side effects from Tamoxafen, both Carol and Doug had a difficult time dealing with the psychological effects of sharing their life, and their bed, with breast cancer.

Approximately six months after the second lumpectomy procedure, Carol noticed that Doug had reverted to a long since discarded habit of working late at the office almost every night of the week. Finally, as a result of finding an unfamiliar article of clothing in their motorhome one weekend, Carol discovered that Doug had begun having an affair with a co-worker at the office. Of course, she was devastated. Upon being confronted, he was contrite and promised to end the affair with his 29 year old secretary. Then disaster struck.

A year and four months after the second lumpectomy procedure, Carol noticed some leakage from her left breast (the site of the original malignancy). Alarmed, she immediately scheduled an appointment with her medical oncologist. This time after an FNA, the pathology report showed positive for a metastasis from the primary tumor in her right breast. A double mastectomy was scheduled and performed within two weeks.

After recovering from the operation, Carol began a long-term course of chemotherapy. At age 50, absent both breasts, with a poor prognosis for long-term survival, and with her hair falling out in clumps, she retired from her job to devote herself to the struggle for survival. Meanwhile, Doug resumed his affair with the co-worker.

Upon her return from a brief vacation to Mexico with a friend between chemotherapy sessions, Carol received an anonymous phone call informing her that during her absence, her husband of almost 30 years had been seen arriving late and leaving early at the home of the secretary.

This time, when confronted with the report of his infidelity, Doug simply responded that he couldn't take it. Soonafter, he packed his bags and left.

Case Four

This case involves Rob and Mendy, who you will recall, are the son and daughter-in-law of Nancy, our neighbor down the street. Due to the ultimate outcome of this "case history" I have included it in its chronological context, at the end of the book.

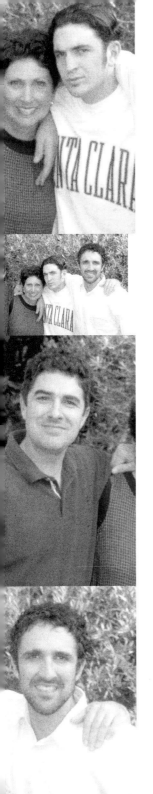

CHAPTER 14
Telling the Boys

May 7, 1996

After the diagnosis, one of the hardest things for me to do was talk about it to others, even our sons. Maybe I should say especially our sons.

Talking about the disease with friends, colleagues and acquaintances seemed to have a magnifying, compounding effect on my own worst fears and what I thought the rest of the world thought about a breast cancer diagnosis. When I was faced with the responsibility of telling the boys about their mother's condition, it felt more like I was getting ready to tell them that their mother was terminally ill, rather than that all the signs pointed toward a complete cure. Finally, when I got my nerve up, I picked up the phone and called Jimmy, who was in his late twenties working in San Francisco.

Of the two older boys, Jimmy was always the more emotional and sensitive. Not that Jerry, our eldest, doesn't have a soft side, it just was not as much in evidence as it is with Jimmy.

When I conveyed the news, all Jimmy could muster, before he started crying, was a weak, "Oh no, Dad;" which, of course, started me crying too. But I managed to tell him what Dr. Mahoney had said in her note to his mother, and assured him that everything was going to be fine.

Once we both stopped blubbering, he rotely repeated that he knew everything would turn out okay and, of course, asked me if he could do anything. I told him I'd keep him posted and if anything came up that I needed from him I'd call. I also suggested that any thoughtfulness toward his mom would be very appreciated.

The call to Jerry, who was in graduate school at the University of Arizona at the time, was similar, just less emotional. Both of the older boys took the news in stride and immediately focused their attention, as I had tried to do, on all the positive aspects of the pathology report and Dr. Mahoney's prognosis. They knew their mother was tough and resilient, not one to throw in the towel; or to feel sorry for herself.

They both had their own families, with their own problems and responsibilities and perhaps had a little more faith than I did in the likelihood of a complete cure. The only one I had left to tell was Josh and I had no inkling what his reaction might be.

When I got home from work, I turned on the news. On cue, there was a discussion about when women should start having mammography examinations. It seems like every time I go on the Internet, turn on the TV or read the newspaper there's something about breast cancer. The National Cancer Institute, said the TV report, was considering changing its recommendations on when women should begin having mammograms. At the time, the NCI's recommendation was that women over fifty have a mammogram every one to two years. Now, the organization was considering lowering the age to forty-five or so.

The American Cancer Society, in contrast, suggests that women begin with mammograms at age forty and repeat them every one to two years. The American College of Physicians recommends starting mammograms at age fifty and having an annual mammogram thereafter. From what I could ascertain, the only universal agreement is that mammograms can reduce the mortality rate from breast cancer in women over fifty by up to a third. Of course this discussion reminded me of the need to broach the subject with Josh.

Before dinner, I asked Suanne if she had said anything to Josh about the diagnosis, hoping that she may have at least mentioned it. She said she had not, thinking it might be better if I broke the news to him. This much he already knew: 1) A lump had been found and, 2) a diagnosis of breast cancer was a distinct possibility. Otherwise, he was purposefully left out of most of the conversations Suanne and I had had on the subject. After the diagnosis, however, we both felt it was important that he be clued in and involved in the ongoing in the discussion.

I thought about broaching the topic over dinner, but it didn't feel comfortable doing so with Suanne sitting there, so I waited.

Josh and I watched the first half of the Bulls Knicks game in the first round of the NBA playoffs. Jordan was doing his thing as only Jordan could do. At half time Josh went into his room to finish some homework. He was sitting at his desk working on the computer when I went in.

"Josh," I said, "you know about Mom finding a lump in her breast?" He nodded affirmatively, without looking up from his studies, probably anticipating what was coming next. "Well, we found out last Thursday that the lump was malignant; that Mom has breast cancer."

For several moments he made no response at all other than letting his hands come to rest on his computer's wrist pad.

"So what does that mean?" he finally asked, still not looking up.

"What it means, as I understand it, is that the tumor is the type that can grow and spread to other places in her body. It's invasive - it's made up of cells that can break out of the original site and establish new tumors in other locations in her body. What it means Josh, is that Mom has the type of cancer that had we not caught it when we did, it could and probably would have eventually killed her."

"Does the doctor say she caught it early enough that she's going to be okay?" Josh intoned, still staring down at his keyboard.

"Yes, the doctor gave us a lot of reasons to believe everything will be okay. She says that if the cancer hasn't spread beyond the site where the tumor was taken out, everything should be fine."

"Good." he said. Josh is not the most expressive kid I've ever known and he seemed perfectly accepting of the prognosis. After a polite interval to see if I had anything else to say, he returned to his studies without asking any more questions. I wasn't quite done, however.

"Josh, even though right now the doctor thinks Mom's going to be all right, this whole thing is really very hard on her. Regardless of what anybody says, including the doctor, breast cancer is a disease that makes any woman who has it wonder about how long she might have to live. I'd really like for you to be as thoughtful of Mom as possible, okay? Try to make things as easy on her as you can. You could start by maybe cleaning up your room, okay?"

"Of course, I'll be thoughtful Dad, I understand what you're saying. When will you know for sure about it? You said 'if,' didn't you? If it hasn't spread."

"Yes, I did say if. Your mother is going to have to have another operation to take out more tissue around where the tumor was and remove some lymph nodes to check to see if the cancer has spread. We won't know until after that if everything's really okay. Even then we won't know for sure for a long time. But for now it's very important that Mom not have to worry about things unnecessarily. Worry isn't good for Mom. I'm asking you to help me take care of her as much as you can, okay?"

"Why does she have to have another operation?" he responded, this time looking up from his studies. I decided to answer his question as completely and as thoroughly as I could. I figured that what he didn't understand, I could explain, or at least attempt to.

I began. "Because one of the characteristics of cancer tumors is that they can invade surrounding tissue and get into blood vessels or the lymphatic system and spread. This characteristic is what distinguishes a malignant tumor from a non-malignant or benign tumor. We know that Mom's tumor is malignant. If the tumor has penetrated into the lymph system or a blood vessel, it can shed cells that then are carried to different parts or areas of the body and start new tumors. Its kind of like some awful disease getting into a water well and being spread to distant locations by people carrying the water from the well to their homes. So, to answer your question, Mom's next operation is basically to learn if the tumor that was in the well, so to speak, has spread or been carried by her blood stream or lymph system beyond the original site in her breast. Do you understand what I'm saying?"

Josh nodded affirmatively that yes, he was following my explanation, and turned back to his studies. My impression was that he didn't seem to fully appreciate the position his mom was in. Maybe it's because of the progress that has been made in treating cancer compared to when I was a kid.

My most vivid remembrance of cancer up until the time it came calling on our household was when I heard that the quarterback on Cal's football team back in the Seventies, a guy named Joe Roth, had melanoma, an extremely aggressive and malignant form of skin cancer.

Roth was one of the best quarterbacks in what was the conference and had enjoyed a terrific senior season. After the season ended he was invited to play in the Hula Bowl All-Star game. He played and as I recall, may have even been named the MVP of the game. Three days later, Joe Roth, the kid with the cannon arm and a promising pro career ahead of him, was dead. The melanoma killed him; just like that. It made no sense to me then, and it still doesn't. Why, I wondered, would God take away one so gifted, so undeserving of such an awful fate.

That was a long time ago, but I never forgot about Joe Roth and the Hula Bowl and cancer. Josh probably never heard of him. Maybe that's a good thing. Maybe not.

Months later, Josh would confide in me that he never really got that worried because he believed me when I told him that everything would be okay. (If only he would believe a few other things I tell him!) But how much does any sixteen-year-old kid listen to anyone about anything? Especially a parent.

Despite his initial languid response, I thought it had been a good idea to get him involved early, hoping as I did as a consequence that he would deal with the whole issue as objectively as possible. Whether this theory worked, I'll never know, but I'm glad I told him when I did. It would have only grown more difficult as time passed. The Bulls won the game. Air Jordan rules.

CHAPTER 15
Sisterhood of Arms

May 9, 1996

I had a trial scheduled in San Luis Obispo County Superior Court ten days hence and a settlement conference was set for that day.

Taking Highway 101, it's a little over two hours from my home in La Selva Beach to the San Luis Obispo County courthouse. Notwithstanding the nice blue coverage line on the map they showed me when I bought my cell phone, coverage is lousy most of the way. So it's either news (KCBS until south of Salinas, then KMJ out of Fresno), sports (KNBR) or as a last resort, my cassette stereo.

On this particular early morning drive I went through Van Morrison's "Astral Weeks," Elton John's "Love Songs," Tom Waits (my cousin) and Eric Clapton before exiting onto the Santa Rosa Street off ramp in SLO. The settlement conference was at 9:00 a.m. in front of a pro-tem judge (a lawyer acting as a temporary judge for the limited purpose of the settlement conference).

I didn't have the best relationship with the attorney representing the defendant, largely because over the course of dealing with her on this case, I found her to treat the practice of law and her declared adversaries much as "Big Nurse" Ratchet did the inmates in Ken Kesey's *One Flew Over The Cuckoo's Nest.* She dished out equal measures of spite, a relished malice and an agenda designed as much to implement her animosity as represent her client. Despite her "Big Nurse" attitude, and the absence of any hint of courtesy and collegiality, for some odd reason I found her rather attractive and even engaging in a severe sort of way.

She was youngish, bright and seemed dedicated to her work. There were times I wanted to take her aside and tell her that not having *cajones* didn't, *a fortiori*, constitute a disability in the courtroom and, to the extent she thought it did, a little civility and cooperation would surely overcome

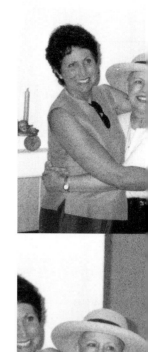

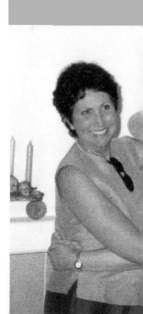

it. I never delivered my little talk, however, opting instead to ignore her antagonistic attitude and parry her legal thrusts as best I could.

As we were waiting in the hallway for our case to be called, I took her aside and told her that I was having a family medical emergency and would in all likelihood have to continue (postpone) the trial. She responded, in her customary caustic manner; that a continuance was out of the question and demanded to know what kind of family emergency would prevent me from attending the trial.

"Thank you for your interest," I said sarcastically, "I appreciate it very much. My wife has recently been diagnosed with breast cancer. She's having her second operation on the 20th. So regardless of what you or the court says, I won't be available for trial." My voice faltered with the words "breast cancer" as it seemed to do with regularity. Even in the course of dealing with a Nurse Ratchet, I could hear the emotion wheedling its way into my voice.

"I'm sorry," she responded. "Truly, I'm very sorry. Don't think a thing about the continuance, Scott." Her tone and demeanor instantly changed, becoming almost intimate and comforting. She appeared to be completely taken aback.

"If there's anything else you need from me, just let me know." Her hand touched my sleeve just below the elbow as she was talking, a gesture I found comforting and sincere. "There won't be any problem. I'll prepare the stipulation and send it to you. I am truly very sorry. I didn't know. I'm sorry for being so curt."

I thanked her again, ingenuously this time, and told her that I'd already notified the court that I would not be available on the scheduled trial date, but that even so, she should let the trial judge know we had talked.

Alas, once into chambers her attitude reverted to the Nurse Ratchet persona. Predictably and lamentably, we failed to settle the case, but on departing she shook my hand firmly and conveyed her best wishes to my wife. On the drive back home I thought about this "anonymous" female attorney's moving response to learning from an adversary of his wife's breast cancer diagnosis. It's as though, in the snap of one's fingers, she changed instantly from a nasty overbearing Nurse Ratchet to a caring, even nurturing Florence Nightingale. Plainly, the abrupt turnabout in her attitude had nothing to do with me or anything I said beyond informing her of Suanne's diagnosis. Rather, I deduced, we now simply share a common language; the common language of BREAST CANCER. Suddenly, she was in the ranks of what might be called, a "sisterhood of arms."

In this so very obvious transformation, I began to appreciate that for every woman, a breast cancer diagnosis, or even the threat of one, encompasses more than a strict anatomic/body image component or even the fear of death. Breast cancer slashes and burns the very essence of feminine identity. The self-same words, "breast cancer," seem toxic and venomous, almost unmentionable, like an infected water well.

Likewise, I began to comprehend, to a degree, that it is the male fixation and obsession with breasts (a phenomenon I frankly have never viewed as particularly loathsome or unfortunate), in no small way suffuses many women with such desperate feelings of terror and loss when confronted with the threat of breast cancer. This obsessive attitude of men toward breasts is as integral and pervasive in contemporary American culture as are violence, television and fast food.

I ask, what other part of the human anatomy serves as such a bright beacon of sexual attraction, allure and neurobiological stimulation between the sexes. Lest there be any confusion or the slightest doubt about this, all one needs to do is go to a checkout stand at any supermarket in our nation and look at what graces the cover of half of the magazines on the rack. From *Cosmopolitan* to *Women's Health*, from *Allure* to *Elle*, breasts are magnets of visual attraction. The well-worn adage that "sex sells," might just as well be stated as "breasts sell."

Fashion designers rack the last ounce of creativity from their brains to come up with new and imaginative ways to display breasts in their latest runway iterations. Moviemakers can't imagine a production anymore without at least a scene or two of bared breasts. (Lord, the first nipple revealed in a Hollywood movie wasn't until 1969 [Sarah Mills in *Ryan's Daughter*).

Far and away, breasts are the most photographed, most commercialized and most fantasized about part of the human anatomy, male or female. Each year, millions upon millions of dollars are spent on elective (cosmetic) breast surgery, with the vast percentage for augmentation (despite the well-documented risks).

Is it a mystery why all this attention and all this money is lavished on breasts? I don't think so! Like it or not, when men in fraternal company use the word "tits" as a superlative to describe everything from clothes to cars to doctoral dissertations, they are expressing a profoundly real, visceral and universal standard of supreme value and carnal appreciation. And it is a characteristic no less intrinsic to men than the natural God-intended nurturing instinct is to women.

But what, I had to ask myself, does this aspect of male carnal appetite do to a woman suffering from breast cancer? What woman does not recoil in horror at the image of a mastectomy?[30] What deep unspoken thoughts run amok in her mind when a woman's chest is threatened with becoming a landscape of scar

---

30 - There are some who don't recoil in horror and some who even see it as relief – they are not always comfortable organs to have – and even their meaning for men is variable. Sexual symbolism is highly variable as is sexual stimulation from breasts – it means little to some people. **EM**

tissue instead of pendulous orbs of alluring, stimulating, come-hither feminine flesh? Indeed, what physiological badge of masculinity (outside of professional sports, that is) accounts for an industry such as is on display in the magazine racks of our supermarkets (not to mention the adult section of our newsstands), an industry in which the models are paid almost as much as the highest paid athletes? The answer, of course, is none, at least not in modern-day society.

The prominence given to breasts in modern American society, where we wear popular culture on our sleeves, is difficult to overstate. From an anthropological to a contemporary cultural perspective, breasts represent everything from a primary source of stimulation of the reproductive/survival instinct, to a marketing tool for products as diverse as cigarettes (no small irony here), to cars, jewelry, laundry detergent and alcohol.

Breasts are a symbol of beauty, allure, eroticism, and the feminine mystique; they are the quintessence of the so-called feminine mystique. Contemporary standards of legal propriety and "political correctness" aside, many men (with the exception of the workplace), can barely look at a woman without first noticing and "sizing up," literally and figuratively, their breasts. Similarly, studies show that many women prominently notice breasts too when first meeting other women.[31]

As I crossed the Salinas River near Soledad, I began to wonder what would my reaction have been if Suanne had been diagnosed with breast cancer and had a mastectomy during my reckless and self-indulgent years "at sea," hunting for the elusive "White Whale." How I would have reacted to the threats posed by breast cancer had I been a young man, say, of twenty-five or thirty years old when confronted by it? Would the bonds of marriage and family have been strong enough at that early stage to fend off the assault that my "instinctual reaction" to the absence of breasts from my life would surely have triggered?

Pushing the envelope back even further, how, I asked myself, would I have reacted as an adolescent male to seeing the picture of the breast cancer patient on the cover of The New Yorker magazine after mastectomy surgery? What crude hurtful remark would have freely parted my lips? The answers to these questions were easier to find than to think about.

I pushed these disquieting thoughts from my mind as I switched on KMJ talk radio out of Fresno. God, I needed some diversion, some relief. Life and all its damned imponderables, was getting to be a heavy burden.

Instead, as fate would have it, I got host Ray Appleton talking to a listener from Visalia about a study done jointly by the National Resources Defense

---

31 - The appreciation of breasts is hardly new. To wit, consider the following very mainstream art: Jacopo Palma il Lecchi (1480-1528), Venus and Cupid; Lucas Cranachi, the Elder (1472-1553) Adam and Eve; Georg Penez (1500-1550), A Sleeping Woman; Jan Metsys (1509-1575) Susanna and the Elders; Pierre Renoir (1841-1919), Nude, 1872; Henri Matisse (1869-1954), Nude On A Sofa, 1923; Pablo Picasso (1881-1973) Woman With A Book and Bust of A Woman, 1923; and virtually all of Edward Degas' bronze statuary.

Council, the American Cancer Society and Harvard Medical School. The study found that the Visalia-Tulare-Porterville area of the San Joaquin Valley (California's "heartland"), leads the nation in deaths per thousand caused by environmental pollution.

The caller was asking about the influence of agricultural pesticides on the study results. I immediately thought about having taken Suanne and the boys out to the ranch in Los Baños that was surrounded by row crops on three sides and a dairy on the forth where we had our own water well. "No place to run; no place to hide."

Even more troubling than these ruminations, as I pulled into our driveway, was the matter of how the mere existence of all the issues surrounding breast cancer was effecting Suanne as the second surgery approached.

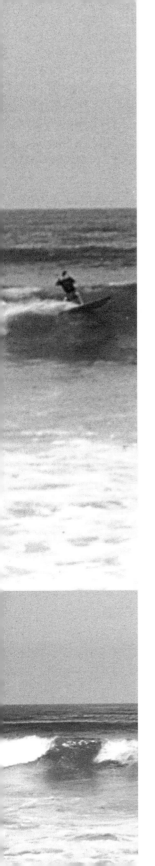

CHAPTER 16
The Second Surgery

May 19, 1996

The day before Suanne's second surgery was a beautiful sun drenched Sunday on the Monterey Bay. I had gotten up early to go surfing with my buddy Howard Gertz (he of California Surfboards fame). After a two-hour session of fairly decent waves at the Hook, thrown up by an early south swell, I was home by 8:45. The three of us sat down to Josh's favorite breakfast of Jackie Cornish's organic barnyard eggs (over easy), thick sliced bacon from the Deluxe Market meat department, Alfaro's Santa Cruz extra sourdough French bread, Ore-Ida hash brown potatoes and my own mother's "famous" homemade fig jam. This repast usually got us all through to Sunday dinner.

After breakfast, I read the Sunday paper. It was replete with speculation on what had caused the horrific crash of ValueJet Flight 592 in the Florida everglades. The evidence was pointing to a fire in the cargo bay. There was an obituary on Thomas Moore. He died from cancer, of course. Tom had been a Peace Corps director in Senegal in the late sixties and early seventies. I knew Tom. He was a really good and decent man and by all accounts, a brilliant lawyer. Our offices were in the same building in Santa Cruz in the mid-eighties.

Suanne and I spent the remainder of the day in the yard where I was engaged in building a new redwood picket fence. Suanne, meanwhile, tended lovingly to her prized rose garden. Neither one of us said so much as a word about the surgery, now less than 20 hours away.

Even though we had been through the drill before and had been given every reason to expect that the cancer had been removed, we were both more than a little apprehensive. As much as Suanne respected Dr. Mahoney, and despite my research, I was still having a difficult time figuring out how she could predict a 95 percent chance that

Suanne would have a full life expectancy, this with no chemotherapy, and no radical surgical treatment and based on nothing more than "tangible" than the size and characteristics of the tumor identified in the pathology report. Old perceptions die hard.

We had also learned about the aforementioned staging formula that included the size of the primary tumor (T), lymph node involvement (N) and distant metastasis (M) used to determine whether mastectomy, chemotherapy, and other treatment options would be necessary. The basic question being addressed after the first surgery was whether the tumor had spread, microscopically or otherwise.

To answer this question, Dr. Mahoney first ordered the battery of tests that were discussed above. These tests are used to rule out "gross" or relatively large identifiable tumors in the blood, bones, brain and lungs. If these "gross" tests prove negative, as thankfully they did in our case, the doctor then surgically removes axillary lymph nodes and more tissue from around the original site (known as re-excising the margins), of the tumor to determine whether they contain any cancer cells.

Dr. Mahoney explained this to me in terms of a target of concentric circles with a bulls-eye (the malignant tumor) in the middle. What the surgeon wants to learn is if there has been any spread from the center to any of the rings outside the bulls-eye.

Particularly in the case of infiltrating ductal carcinoma, medical wisdom holds that the lymph nodes provide a valuable tool in assessing the probability of whether microscopic spread of the breast cancer has, in fact, occurred. The data however, is imprecise. In women with negative nodes, there exists a 25 percent chance that there has been microscopic spread of the cancer, and in approximately 25 percent of the women with positive nodes there has been no further spread. Nevertheless, surgical examination of lymph nodes is considered a useful tool in making a prognosis. Accordingly, it is widely, although not universally employed.

In every human armpit there are thirty to sixty lymph nodes. For the purpose of analysis, the surgeon removes between 7 and 15 modes on the side where the tumor was found. The formula for assessing the lymph nodes goes something like this: If you have one to three lymph nodes that test positive for cancer cells there is a lower probability that the malignant cells have spread. Four to ten positive nodes constitute a medium probability of spread, and ten or more constitute a correspondingly higher probability. Note that the probability range is not low to high in the absolute sense, but rather lower to higher in a relative sense. The reason for this is that any positive finding in the lymph nodes is thought to be a good indication that there has been at least some microscopic spread that requires chemotherapy treatment.

Even with a full day of vigorous physical activity in the yard, Suanne and I both, once again, spent a night of tossing and turning nervously waiting for the next stop and the next news on our breast cancer odyssey.

May 20, 1996

Arriving at Stanford Hospital at 8:00 in the morning, we immediately checked into the surgical suite and waited a few minutes before we heard the woman at the reception desk call Suanne's name. A repeat of the same admittance procedures ensued, except that this time, because the surgery was considerably more invasive than the lumpectomy, Suanne would be spending the night in the hospital.

The operation was scheduled for 10:00 o'clock and would take about an hour and a half to two hours. So, after getting Suanne into the pre-op room, I pulled out my laptop and began working. In addition to the miraculous medical technology and information that has enabled millions of people to live fuller, longer and healthier lives, the advent of the laptop computer has banished all excuses for playing hookey from work. On this particular morning I was reviewing a deposition on an ASCII disk. But try as I might, I found it virtually impossible to concentrate on anything but what I imagined was going on in the surgical suite. No amount of miraculous technology can supplant focus and attention.

It was approaching noon when Dr. Mahoney emerged, informing me that everything went according to plan and that here was nothing untoward to report. She guesstimated that Suanne would be taken from recovery to her room within a couple of hours.

To my disappointment and in spite of my prodding, she declined to offer comment on the appearance of the lymph nodes; indeed, she volunteered nothing other than that there were no complications and that we'd just have to wait for the results of the pathology report on the margins and nodes.

Not fully appreciating that it was only microscopic cells and not a visible tumor they were looking for, I was a little frustrated by her response. I had an image in my mind of lymph nodes matted together or having little tiny growths coming out of them, but by the time the thoughts in my mind were primed for expression, Dr. Mahoney had done an about face and was off to another surgery. With nothing better to do than waddle in my own paranoia, I left the hospital to make my obligatory trip to the Oasis for my L.A. Hot fix. If my head wouldn't cooperate, I figured my stomach would. Bob wasn't there but Mark was, so we shared a small pitcher of Anchor Steam and I lied about what I was doing in Palo Alto. I was in no mood to hear any more of his stories about abandoned erstwhile girlfriends or how luscious their tits were.

At 1:30 I went back up to the recovery room reception desk and was told that it would probably be another hour or so before Suanne was ready to be transferred to her room, so I returned to my laptop and scrolled through more deposition testimony, only half attentive to what I was doing.

At 2:30, a nurse came out and told me I could go to the overnight recovery room which was in a different part of the hospital. About the time I arrived at her room Suanne was wheeled in on a gurney and transferred to the bed. She was still heavily under the effects of the anesthesia. I turned on the TV and watched a special by Bill Kurtiss on mass-killer Richard Spec's life of sex, breast augmentation and drugs in prison. It was quite sickening and I was glad Suanne wasn't able to watch.

After a while, she was able to squeeze my hand and nod in response to my questions but what she really wanted to do was sleep, so I kissed her goodbye and left for home. The clock on the wall over her bed read five o'clock.

I don't know if it was fatigue or relief at the surgery being over, but I went to bed around 8:30 and slept like a baby all night. I returned to the hospital the next morning and drove Suanne home. She was in a little more pain this time, but all things considered, very glad the ordeal was over. We had to wait another three days to get the results of the pathology report, a period of time every bit as agonizing as our first wait.

When the pathology report was issued, it was again a profusion of good news. The margins were completely clean (as opposed to dirty, meaning cancer cells were present), and the axillary lymph nodes likewise showed no signs of cancer. Of the dozen nodes excised and examined, nary a single cancer cell was found in any of them. We were on cloud nine! Somehow, Dr. Mahoney's bold and daring predictions had come true. But we also had become aware that in a large number of cases, even with "clean" margins and nodes, there has still been dispersion of microscopic cancer cells to distant sites through the lymph system and blood vessels. Knowing this, I was still a little troubled by the rosy picture that was being painted.

Dr. Mahoney explained to Suanne that given the previously identified charac-teristics of the tumor (its small size, estrogen receptivity, low miotic rate, etc.), this simply confirmed her original prognosis. Yes, she admitted, there was still the possibility some errant cancer cells could be lurking about somewhere. And yes, there remained the possibility that Suanne did not fit into the statistical categories of women with the same or similar tumors.

It is literally true that no two cancer patients are alike. Each individual displays unique characteristics that together dictate the outcome; among them, genes, environment, hormones and the autoimmune system.

For every ninety-five women with breast cancer fortunate enough to find themselves in Suanne's thumbs-up classification profile, there are five others that aren't so fortunate and accordingly, must come to grips with a less than full life expectancy. And with respect to the identifying traits of those in the five percent category, there simply are none - I repeat, none are identifiable.

Despite all the "qualifiers," Dr. Mahoney remained supremely confident. The next course of medical treatment was as originally predicted by the doctor. Suanne would begin a course of radiation treatment that would last for five to six weeks and was designed to kill any residual cells in her breast. She would also begin tamoxifen therapy that would last for a period of up to five years. The cancer treatment train was about to leave the station, and Suanne was on it. So far, so good.

CHAPTER 17
What Next

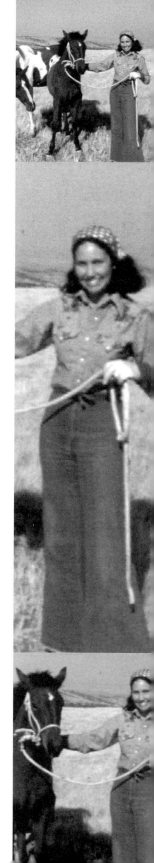

May 24, 1996

I knew that Suanne was going to be seeing Dr. Steven Mann for the radiation therapy, but I hadn't seen Steve since she was diagnosed with breast cancer, other than to wave at him driving through the neighborhood. Although I didn't know for certain, I assumed along the way that Dr. Mahoney had contacted him regarding Suanne's forthcoming treatment. When I did see Steve, the meeting was memorable.

I stopped by Deluxe Market on my way home after work to pick up a few things. As I was going in I saw Steve ambling toward me in the parking lot. Just seeing him headed in my direction started the now familiar emotional response I experienced just thinking about my wife's having breast cancer. How weird, I thought, a sun drenched Friday afternoon in May, neighbors greeting neighbors and friends, and I'm ready to break down in tears over saying hi. But by now, I was carrying this emotional baggage around with me like a bad habit.

"Hi Steve," I greeted him, assuming that he already knew about Suanne's disease, "I guess this is one relationship I was hoping we would never have." Steve is a large, gentle man with a warm smile and the soft hands you might expect of a radiation oncologist. As we shook hands, I could tell that he had no inkling.

"Are you okay?" he asked.

"Yeah Steve, I'm fine. You haven't heard from Dr. Mahoney in Palo Alto?"[32]

"No, I haven't." He responded, "Why, is it Suanne?"

At this point my eyes were starting to well-up and even though I was wearing dark glasses, I knew it would be only moments before little rivulets of tears started running down

---

32 - When a patient first sees me for a consultation, we call the referring MD and request records when the appointment is made, but I don't see the records in advance – just on the day of the appointment. Once the team is established (radiation oncologist, medical oncologist), we get in the habit of sending copies of notes to every other MD automatically every time we see the patient. **EM**

my face. I struggled to maintain my composure as I answered his question.

"Yes, I thought you might have already known. Suanne was diagnosed with breast cancer over a month ago. I believe you're the radiation oncologist she'll be seeing." There was a long pause.

"I'm sorry Scott, I didn't know. Has she had her lymph nodes tested yet?"

"Yes, they are clear; so are the margins around the tumor."

"How big was the tumor?"

"Eight tenths of a centimeter."

"She's lucky. Anytime a tumor measures under a centimeter when discovered, you're very lucky. Early diagnosis is the best thing possible for a breast cancer patient, especially if they're over 50. How is she taking it?"

"Well, she's not back working out yet since her last surgery was just a week ago, but Suannes' very tough and resilient, she's doing okay. Frankly, sometimes I think she's doing better than I am. I'm an off-again, on-again wreck. But if you don't mind I'd like to ask you a question."

"Sure, anything," Steve responded, "what's on your mind?"

"Dr. Mahoney told me on the phone after the first surgery, and before the lymph nodes had even been tested, that she thought Suanne has a 95 percent chance of a full life expectancy. She even used the word cure. It may seem odd, but saying the word "cure" has bothered me. How could she say that even before the expanded margin and lymph node surgery?"

"First, let me tell you that Suanne couldn't have a better surgeon. Ellen is as good a physician and breast surgeon as there is, anywhere. Period. She's seen enough breast cancer tumors and patients that she can tell a lot just from the size of the tumor and the age and history of the patient. She is highly respected in the oncology community. She's very familiar with both the clinical and the research sides of breast cancer. What she told you initially wasn't just based on the size of the tumor. The clinical and demographic characteristics of breast cancer patients with a 95 percent chance of a full life expectancy are very well understood. I'm sure she had the pathology report when she gave that prognosis."

He went on: "At point eight cm. you got to the tumor about as early as you can. The prognosis for a full life expectancy in a woman Suanne's age is excellent when you catch the cancer so early and the pathology report shows it to be a slow grower. The cancer cells were probably not terribly distorted in their appearance. The fact that she didn't have any lymph node involvement is very positive. That's not to say that there couldn't be some microscopic migration but the chances are excellent that she got it all. So the best thing you can do is think positively. Suanne too. Ellen wouldn't have told you what she did if she wasn't very certain in her mind about it."

To say the least, Steve's comments were both reassuring and comforting. But I still didn't feel confident on the "cure" matter.

Before parting, we chatted a few more minutes about the prevalence of breast cancer in our area and about when Suanne would start her radiation therapy. The parking lot seemed to be teaming with people, scurrying this way and that. A box girl with long dark tresses came by pushing a train of grocery carts, babbling on to a friend about something. I fetched what I was after in the market and returned to my car. Steve was just driving away. As I loaded my groceries a couple drove by in one of those rakish Mercedes 500 series convertibles with the top down.

She was a thirty-something comely blond (seems as though every woman I see driving one of those rakish Mercedes convertibles is blonde and beautiful). Her partner looked like he probably owned one of those megabuck high tech firms in Silicon Valley. They were laughing uproariously over something, seemingly without a care in the world.

"Cure, cure, sure. Sure, cure, cure." The words flipped flopped in my head almost in a taunting manner.

After I started the car I sat there for a minute slumped back in my seat and wondered when, if ever again, Suanne and I would laugh so hard as the couple in the Mercedes or feel so free as all those people in the parking lot. I was probably feeling sorry for myself, but at that moment, I wasn't sure it would ever happen.

Ordinarily, I'm a regular news junkie, particularly news of politics. That morning I had read a piece by Maureen Dowd, a syndicated New York Times columnist, castigating Clinton and his lawyers for attempting to clothe the commander-in-chief in the protection provided by the Soldier's and Sailor's Civil Relief Act of 1940 in the Paula Jones sexual harassment case. "Jesus Christ," I thought to myself in disgust. "Does this man have no shame whatsoever?" The turn of affairs (no pun intended) was especially disheartening to me because at one time I identified with the President as a contemporary. A fellow traveler in the Sixties generation, one might say.

Then back home, on the evening news Clinton was quoted as saying, "I am always a little skeptical when politicians piously proclaim their morality." He was talking about Senator Bob Dole's stand on abortion and some pointed criticism Dole had made about his vetoing the so-called live-birth abortion bill. Normally I would have sat down and written an opinion piece or a letter to the editor or something. As things were, I dismissed it as just another news report about a manipulative, self-absorbed President who has no concept of piety, conscience or morality. But for the present, and for who could say how much longer, my world and our world, revolved around breast cancer and we were being held tight in its dispiriting grip.

CHAPTER 18
'Thar She Blows

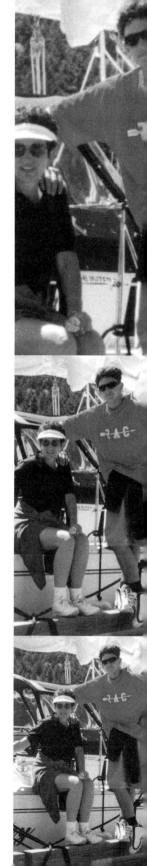

June 5, 1996

In the fall of 1995 we had penciled-in an early-summer sailing vacation in Washington's San Juan Islands. After the diagnosis, of course, things like vacations, recreation, and relaxation just sort of fell off the table. But since I had been planning my trial calendar around the vacation, when the time slot came up on the calendar we left it open, just in case everything fell into place with Suanne and her treatment. Of course, we did not foresee the proximity of the second surgery to our scheduled departure date and had all but given up on being able to go because of Suanne's convalescence. When I got a phone call confirming our reservations, I decided on the spot that it would be a good idea to go if we could manage it. And, to our joyous surprise, Dr. Mahoney gave the trip her blessing.

Literally a day or two before our reservations for the flight up to Seattle and Friday Harbor, word came from Dr. Mahoney that so long as Suanne didn't overdue it there was no medical reason to scuttle the trip. I was at the office when Suanne called.

"Guess what, Honey?"

"You're having a good day?"

"Better. What would you like to do right now more than anything else in the world?"

"I'd like you to tell me that we're going sailing in the San Juans."

"Well, go out and buy yourself a new pair of sailing gloves - that's exactly why I called."

It was like the fog lifting before noon on a long anticipated day at the beach. We were all ready for some diversion and a sailing vacation in the San Juans sounded like the perfect way to find it. I even detected a little twinge of anticipation in Suanne's voice.

Getting ready was almost a celebration in itself. Suanne

busied herself packing clothes for hiking, sailing, swimming, and dinning. Josh was out in the garage gathering his fishing gear and I was pouring over charts planning our sailing itinerary and provisioning. The whole process of just getting ready for a vacation had the immediate and much needed effect of distracting all of us from the doom and gloom of breast cancer that had consumed our household for so long.

To be frank, even with all the positive results from the pathology reports on the lumpectomy and the expanded margin and node surgery, Suanne still had cancer and we knew for a certainty that there was no magic bullet for ridding it; nothing like penicillin for bacterial infections. It's one thing for a physician to tell you that a positive attitude about a cure can help achieve that end, but quite another task to actually develop such an attitude. I had not yet achieved that plateau. But Suanne and I agreed that a change of scenery to the San Juans would be good therapy.

On Wednesday we flew up to Seattle's SeaTac Airport where we caught a Harbor Air puddle-jumper to take us up to the San Juan Islands. The trip from SeaTac to Friday Harbor is an adventure in itself, akin to an aeronautical time warp. Even though you're in this gigantic modern airport, you check in at a tiny little freestanding counter (actually a dais) where an agent asks you your body weight and then weighs your luggage. For safety reasons (the plane can't lift off the ground if there's too much aggregate weight?), you're limited in the amount of poundage you can take on the small nine-passenger, single engine aircraft that serves the Friday Harbor and Oak Harbor airports.

After the weigh-in the pilot comes and gets the passengers and takes us all down a flight of stairs out to the tarmac where he issues parachutes and cold water survival gear and ...(just kidding here), we board the aircraft. I suggested to Josh that he ask if he could sit in the co-pilot's seat up front, which he did and was invited forward by the pilot. Then comes the fun part.

The flight from SeaTac up to the San Juan Islands has to be one of the most breathtaking aeronautical tours one can imagine; spectacular enough to take one's mind off just about anything.

Taking off, you immediately see Mount Rainier off to the southeast, rising 14,410 feet up into the sky, like a huge snowy white sovereign exercising silent dominion over the great Northwest. Once aloft, we bank out over the sparkling azure waters of the South Sound; over Vashon and Blake Islands, until finally we level off on a northerly bearing and fly past Seattle, the fabled Emerald City, off the right wing. Our course took us over Bambridge Island, were my law partner Pete Mair and his wife Mudge live on beautiful Fletcher Bay; the Kitsap

Peninsula, and the southern reaches of Whidbey Island.

To the west are the craggy, alpine peaks and rain forests of the Olympic mountain range; to the east the dryer and more evenly contoured Cascades.

The day was crystal clear with only straggling clumps of cirrus clouds drifting here and there in a turquoise sky, as if they had no place to go. Off to the northeast, the ice-capped peak of Mount Baker, Rainier's little sister, rises up through a soft gray choker of lenticular cloud cover to meet the afternoon sky. To the west, the Hood Canal snakes its way along the foot of the Olympics. As we pass over Admiralty Inlet and head out over the broad blue stretch of the Strait of Juan de Fuca, our pilot points out the narrow isthmus of Whidbey Island at Point Partridge off to our right and Port Townsend to our left.

Down below, out of the strait, you can see white billowy sails here and power boat wakes there, surrounded by an infinite array of golden glitter dancing on the water, heralding the coming of the high tourist season in the islands.

I looked over at Suanne for a sign of how she was feeling. For the entire flight she had sat pensively looking out the window. Was there a message here? I thought there might be. She's never really comfortable on small aircraft, even on our flights up to the islands. Later, once back on terra firma, she allowed that she was feeling "pensive," but still enraptured by the overpowering panoramas of the Northwest.

We've taken this trip over a dozen times and I've found that people seldom talk, as they didn't on this flight; no doubt because they are awestruck at the artistry of Mother Nature's canvas we pass over, where earth, sky and water mingle in such a dazzling profusion of shapes and colors that words become almost irreverent.

At last we crossed over Cattle Pass, made a U-turn over the harbor, touched down and taxied to a stop in front of the "air terminal" at Friday Harbor.

Steve Perser, the owner of Charters Northwest, was waiting outside the terminal to deliver us to the new slips at the foot of Spring Street where our sloop, Odyssey, was waiting, all excited and exuberant over our arrival and the TLC that she knew was in store. With the clean clear air of the islands and 70 degree weather invigorating us, we threw our bags in the back of Steve's pick-up and began to settle in to our vacation in the islands as a celebration of our great good fortune in catching Suanne's disease early and her excellent prognosis. And what a place to celebrate!

The San Juans are an archipelago of 172 named islands in the Puget Sound on the north side of the Strait of Juan de Fuca, east of Vancouver Island and west of Anacortes and Bellingham, Washington. The main islands of the archipelago are San Juan, Orcas, Lopez, Blakley, Decatur and Shaw. These and the lesser islands make up San Juan County, Washington, with Friday Harbor as the county seat. They are nothing short of a pine, birch, and cedar covered paradise hewn from the Olympic Mountain range by the migration of ancient glaciers during some past ice age eons ago.

Suanne and I started coming to the San Juan Islands in the summer of 1992 after a medical malpractice trial I had in Everett, Washington and had returned several times on our first boat, a little Chrysler 26 trailer sailor. Three years later, having fallen in love with the place, we bought a Hunter 35.5 and put it into service with Charters Northwest in Friday Harbor to defray part of the costs. Our plan was to spend as much time as possible exploring the waters of the Puget Sound, the San Juan and Gulf Islands.

After greeting the office staff at Charters Northwest, stowing all of our gear on board and provisioning at King's Market, we sat around the salon table in Odyssey's main cabin debating what to do where to go first.

I cast my vote was for bringing out the cleaning supplies and polishing the bright work. Josh would hear none of that, casting a "dissenting vote," voting instead for an early dinner at the San Juan Brewery Café and a movie afterward. Suanne seconded our son's vote, surprise surprise, so off the three of us went for an evening in town. The silver screen offering was *Twister*, a movie about people who chase hurricanes. During the movie I suspected that Suanne was thinking about the rigors of sailing and sure enough, while walking back to the boat she reminded me that she wasn't up for going out in any high winds. I assured her that we wouldn't be running into any hurricanes here in the San Juan Islands.

The next morning, after checking the tide chart, fuel and water levels, and the NOAA VHF radio channel, we were ready to cast off. That's when the first socio-political-marine problem of our trip began.

Ever since we acquired our first sailboat, Rose (the Chrysler 26), Suanne had always been my best and most dependable crew member. It was not that she enjoyed sailing in the open ocean conditions of the Monterey Bay so much as she just did a damn good job of crewing whenever I needed her; her very real fears notwithstanding. She is extremely strong, agile on deck, and was willing to put up with most of the rigors of sailing so long as I didn't ask her to go too far offshore or out into heavy weather. I think it was probably the physical challenges of sailing that she enjoyed more than anything else. She also was more available than most of my buddies, few of whom shared my passion for spending weekends away from their families on Rose.

After we bought Odyssey, with her roller-furling jib, Dutchman flaking system and all lines led aft to the cockpit, and began sailing in the sheltered waters of San Juans, Suanne's appreciation (toleration) of sailing improved considerably. Odyssey also has a comfortable master stateroom with a queen-sized bed, an actual head with a shower, and a serviceable galley with Corian counter tops, all of which contributed immeasurably to her willingness to participate in my passion for sailing. Josh actually found my love of sailing to be a burden and never showed any interest at all in learning port from starboard, much less how to help get under way, hoisting sails or docking. Hence, the problem of which I speak.

In deference to Suanne being barely two weeks post-op, my choice was to either summon her for help, (which for many things I simply couldn't do), or press Josh into service (a risky proposition, at best with any teenager). Situations like this can and will cause problems on sailboats if they're not thought out beforehand, particularly when you're sailing in 42-degree water.

Fortunately, as we were about to cast off (and before I had to make a decision), Aaron Hayes, the charter boat manager for Charters Northwest, came along and gave Josh a hand and a hands-on lesson in casting off. It goes without saying that any nervousness I show on the boat is amplified many times over in Suanne, so I was very grateful for Aaron's timely and fortuitous appearance.

When we finally were under way and motoring out past Brown Island, I asked Josh to take the wheel so I could go get the deck cushions. I didn't think a thing about it beforehand, but the moment I surrendered the wheel, I sensed that Suanne was not entirely comfortable with Josh driving. No big deal; I assumed it was just the fact of her surgery, our first day on the boat and hopefully, nothing more. Time would tell. Our first destination was Reid Harbor on Stuart Island. I chose Reid Harbor because it's a very quiet anchorage, only about a three to four hour motor sail from Friday Harbor, and the tides were with us most of the way. No use pushing the envelope at this stage.

After getting the life-lines up, fenders put away and the dock lines all stowed, I took off the winch covers and then went forward to remove the sail cover from the main. I was ready to sail. Before hoisting the main, I checked the wind speed. It was very light out in San Juan Channel so I decided to motor for a while and give Suanne and Josh a chance to get their sea legs before heeling over under sail. I knew that Suanne would be more comfortable with motoring since she usually was.

When we turned west in Spiden Channel the breeze picked up to ten knots and I suggested to Josh that we raise the main. But again, I could sense immediately from the way Suanne adjusted her seating and placed her arm around the winch, that the thought of heeling over was still not agreeing with her. Although I did think that perhaps she might have made at least a gesture, I understood where she was coming from. Uncharacteristically, she just wasn't up to it, physically or mentally.

"Never mind Josh." I said, "We'd better motor if we want to beat the tide into Reid." Suanne knew full well it was thereby making a concession, though she said nothing to dissuade me from continuing to motor instead of raising the sails.

At Reid Harbor we picked up a buoy on about the fifth pass with Josh at the helm and me manning the boat hook (which I won't go into), and settled into the first day of our holiday afloat. It was a warm beautiful June day in the islands. There was nary a hint of fog or wind at the anchorage, the water was perfectly flat, and, as we had expected, there were only a few boats moored in Reid Harbor. Perfect conditions for relaxing on the boat.

After lunch, I started on the bright work and, Suanne stretched out in the cockpit with a John Grisham thriller. Josh set out to learn how to row the dingy, the doing of which soon turned into an unexpected (and educational) adventure for him and wonderful (albeit not unexpected) entertainment for us.

Later in the afternoon, after I had finished polishing the pulpit, pushpit and stantions, we dingied into shore for our traditional hike to the Turn Point Lighthouse. On the way in we dropped ourcrab net, which Josh had baited with chicken entrails.

Determined to make the hike, Suanne had specifically asked Dr. Mahoney if a two to three mile hike on fairly flat ground would be okay for her to do, which it was.

Unless I am mistaken, the Turn Point Lighthouse marks the north-westernmost point of land in the continental United States. The name "Turn Point" comes from the fact that just out in Haro Strait from the lighthouse is where the border between Canada and the United States turns from 348 degrees north to 55 degrees east.

Our hike was considerably more leisurely than usual, and Suanne made it without voicing a single complaint. We even caught a glimpse of some orcas (killer whales), out in the strait on the return hike. No luck with the crab net; not even a nibble on the entrails.

That night we feasted on barbecued lamb chops, steamed asparagus, and baked potato. After dinner we started a game of Monopoly that was to last until we left the islands. All in all, Day One of the vacation proved to be excellent therapy for all of us, and the subject of breast cancer never came up once.

On the second morning, we rose to cloudless skies and an awesome sunrise coming up over Orcas Island. So far the notoriously quirky northwest June weather was treating us like honored guests. After coffee and breakfast, Josh dingied back out to bring up the crab net. On this effort he was considerably more successful—on both counts. No wounded duck course in the dingy, and the crab net was filled with three large Dungeness crabs surfeited on the chicken entrails. At 8:45 we motored out of Reid Harbor and headed southeast on a course of 90 degrees past Spiden Island.

Once past Flattop Island we turned north in President's Channel on a course of 15 degrees and headed for our next destination, Sucia Island; depending on tide wind and current, a sail of anywhere between two and four hours. We sailed around the southern edge of Sucia and into Fossil Bay where we dropped anchor and boiled our three crustacean captives for lunch. Tasty, tasty, tasty! And fresher you just can't eat.

Again, in deference to Suanne, I motored all the way from Reid Harbor to Sucia, even though the wind out in President Channel picked up to twelve knots and would have provided some fine sailing. I was privately hoping that Suanne would suggest that we raise the sails, but she didn't. She remained bundled up under the dodger obviously lost in her own meditations, which I had no difficulty imagining.

While we were cleaning up after lunch I asked Josh if he was ready to learn how to sail Odyssey. By now he was beginning to take a shine to her and responded with an almost spirited yes, which ensured at least a modicum of cooperation from Suanne. Clever ploy on my part, I thought. We weighed anchor at around two and motored out past Mantia Island into Rosario Strait.

Out in Rosario Strait we picked up a southeasterly breeze blowing at between ten and twelve knots and I decided it was time for Suanne to bite the bullet.

"Josh," I commanded in good Ahabian tone, "come take the wheel. We're going to do some sailing."

Miraculously, he hopped to with what seemed genuine enthusiasm. After attaching the main halyard (the cable with which the mainsail is raised to the head of the mast), to the sail and taking off the sail ties I got Josh to follow the windvane on the masthead and point up directly into the wind so I could raise the main. He did as he was told and I soon had the main luffing in the wind.

"Fall off, fall off, Josh," I yelled after I winched up the mainsail the last few feet to the masthead. Again, Josh quickly followed my instructions and moments later I cut the engine and winched down the mainsheet. Finally! We were finally sailing.

Suanne was watching Josh at the wheel of Odyssey for the first time under sail and I could tell that just seeing him driving the boat was a thrill for her. I unfurled and sheeted in the jib, put on a tape of Pavarotti, and took a seat on the stern rail, as Odyssey heeled over to 15 degrees and sliced smoothly through the deep blue waters of Rosario Strait. This is what I had been waiting for. No internal combustion engine noise, no smell of fossil fuel burning; just pure sailing in one of the most beautiful spots on earth! I had an overwhelming sense of thanksgiving and well-being.

From Sucia we sailed on a southerly course down Rosario Strait to Obstruction Pass and into East Sound. Josh was in a particular hurry because he wanted to see at least part of game one between the Seattle SuperSonics and the Chicago Bulls. Our destination was Rosario Resort on Orcas Island, the largest and most populated on the San Juan Islands.

We had barely pulled into the slip at Rosario when Josh leaped onto the dock and sprinted up to the Orcas Café where the game was in progress and where he joined a small group of avid northwest fans cheering on their Sonics.

Rosario Resort and Marina is located on a sheltered cove about half-way up East Sound. The hotel, a one-time private mansion, was built in the early 1900s by Robert Moran, a Seattle ship builder, with money he raked in constructing battleships for the United States Navy during World War I. No doubt, due to the fact that Moran and William Randolph Hearst were contemporaries and built comparable fortunes, Rosario is often referred to as the Hearst Castle of the Northwest (the Hearst Castle, of course, is located on the Central Coast of California).

For us the main attractions of Rosario have always been the Friday night seafood buffet in the Cascade Room, climbing Mount Constitution, (at 2410 feet, the tallest peak in the San Juans), and a romantic swim in the indoor pool after dinner. On this trip I knew there was no way Suanne could make the arduous trek up Mount Constitution, nor was she likely in the mood to don the racy bikini I ever-so-thoughtfully kept on the boat for the titillating after dinner swim. So, as could be predicted, she stayed on the boat, relaxed and read while Josh and I did the hike, went swimming and rented bicycles for a ride up to East Sound. During our two evenings in Rosario, we settled for the ongoing game of Monopoly, the seafood buffet and attending an organ concert in the Mansion featuring Rosario's gifted resident composer and pianist, Christopher Peacock.

On Sunday morning we slipped out of Rosario and headed for the west side of the islands, Roche Harbor and the elegant Canadian city of Victoria on Vancouver Island. NOAA (National Oceanic and Atmospheric Administration) weather radio reported an earthquake with a Richter-scale magnitude of 7.7 near the island of Adak in Alaska. After a uneasy discussion of its tidal effects, I assured my apprehensive crew we had no need to worry about a tsunami, being, as we were, ensconced in the protected waters of the Puget Sound. It did strike me, nevertheless, after seeing the *Twister* movie, that my out-of-hand dismissal of a hurricane in the San Juans may not have been as fully warranted as I proclaimed, but I didn't mention anything about it.

The weather was sunny, the winds light and the water flat; marine conditions that I call "Suanne sailing." After our uneventful sail from Sucia and two days of relaxation hangin out at Rosario, Suanne was finally beginning to really relax. The trip from Rosario to Roche Harbor took us through Harney Channel between Orcas and Shaw Island (almost a due westerly course), and back out into the San Juan Channel and Spiden Channel. In San Juan Channel the wind picked up a little and I had Josh man the wheel while I unfurled the sails. There was no hesitation on his part; indeed, it appeared he was really taking to it.

Once on course, Odyssey immediately heeled over to 15 degrees, but this time Suanne didn't seem to hardly notice. Oh yeah, this was a very good sign! She even took the wheel for a few minutes and looked very comfortable, just like she used to. Finally, our vacation on the boat seemed to be taking the edge off of Suanne's anxieties. No discussion of breast cancer. No newspaper reports. Nothing untoward, save for the 7.7 earthquake hundreds of miles away in Alaska.

By late afternoon we made radio contact with the Roche Harbor Harbormaster on VHF channel 16. "This is Odyssey calling the Roche Harbor Harbormaster, come in please."

"This is the Roach Harbor Harbormaster Odyssey. Over."

"What is your availability of slips? Over."

"What is your length overall and beam, Odyssey? Over."

"Length is thirty-five, five and beam is eleven, nine. Over."

"We've got plenty of open slips, Odyssey. Come into the guest dock and check in and we'll assign you a slip. Are you familiar with the Roche Harbor Marina? Over.

"Yes, I am familiar with the marina. I'll be arriving at the guest dock in approximately fifteen minutes. Thank you harbormaster. Odyssey, over and out."

We checked in with the Harbormaster and were assigned a slip on D-Dock.

This time, when we pulled into the slip, Josh handled the docklines like an old salt. We replenished our water supply, hooked up the AC power, and I fixed a delicious taco dinner that was enjoyed by all, including the chef. After cleaning up the galley we went up to the bar at the Haro Hotel and listened to music for a while before retiring to the boat, and of course, continuing our game of Monopoly, which is another story in itself.

Suanne was monopolizing the game (no pun intended), and we had many good laughs over Josh's unique approach (or shall I say "dexterity") to rolling the dice and shuffling the chance cards, which somehow always seemed to come out in his favor. When we went to bed that night I could sense the cumulative tension and stress of the past few months being lifted from Suanne's body, not unlike awakening from a bad dream.

On Monday morning, after a sumptuous breakfast at the Lime Kiln Café and some fresh provisioning at the Roche Harbor Lime and Cement Company General Store, we motored out of Roche Harbor around 10:15. We timed our departure on an ebbing tide, passed in the lee (protected side) of Battleship Island and headed down past Henry Island and the west side of San Juan Island toward the Straits of Juan de Fuca. Our destination was the port city of Victoria on Vancouver Island, the ever-enchanting picturesque capital of British Columbia.

A half-hour out of Roche we picked up a light northwesterly and hoisted our mainsail and jib. This time there wasn't the slightest sign of anxiousness from Suanne. As the sails billowed in the breeze, I asked her to cut the engine and take the helm while I went below to get my camera and binoculars. We were headed for prime whale watching waters. Josh nominated himself chief whale watcher and stationed himself on the bow pulpit seat, binoculars in hand, looking out for whales.

After a half-hour or so on a heading of 140 degrees, I asked Suanne to take the wheel again and went forward to join Josh at the pulpit to search the water ahead for orcas. Even before I reached the shrouds, Josh cried out, "Whales! Whales straight ahead and coming right for us! Mom, Dad, do you see them? Wow, there must be two dozen!"

The wind suddenly picked up to around twelve knots and Odyssey was beginning to heel past 15 degrees as I saw off in the distance the dorsal fins of a pod of orcas bearing directly toward us. Worried that Suanne might be getting nervous with the wind picking up, I looked back toward the cockpit to see what she was going to do.

What greeted my eyes was a scene so wonderful and so enchanting that it will be etched in my mind until the day I die. Here was the most beautiful girl in the world, now of middle age and struggling against breast cancer, wearing this come-hither navy-blue bathing suit top, shorts, black sailing gloves, and a white sun hat, with one hand on the wheel, her right knee propped against the starboard gunnel and binoculars to her eyes scanning the sea ahead for the approaching pod of whales.

"God," she exclaimed, "this is one of the most incredible sights I have ever seen." Indeed, I thought to myself, indeed! She took the words right out of my mouth, only we had different subjects in mind. Wanting in the worst way to preserve this image for posterity (and my enduring visual benefit), I scampered back to the companionway and, seconds later snapped the picture that graces the cover of this book. That's "my" Suanne, as delicious, as delectable and as enchanting as she was to me when we were both in our teens; a long, long time ago.

At the magical moment I turned to look back at Suanne driving Odyssey, running before the wind down Haro Strait, I could swear my heart skipped a beat in utter awe of what I was seeing and feeling. I may never in my life know a more pure feeling of transcendent joy and true boundless love. For in that enchanting moment, in the coalescing of wind and sail, sun and sea; with breaching orcas playing in the water ahead and bald eagles flying above, with our son in the bow of the boat whooping with delight, the most beautiful sight I had ever seen - or could ever hope to see - was my wife at the helm of our boat, alive and vibrant, lacking only a harpoon held high above her head, to bury in the heart of the demon cells that had invaded and attacked her body. My lungs filled with the clean salty air of hope, my eyes brimmed with sweet tears of joy, and my heart billowed as a soft sea breeze blew away the dark clouds of fear that had settled into our lives. I wish for every man and woman, every husband and wife, the profound joy of such a feeling of love and that it would never leave them.

After snapping pictures of Suanne, Josh and the orcas, I finally made my way back to the cockpit and took over the helm in order that Suanne could go forward to be with Josh and commune with the frolicking whales. With both of them holding fast to the pulpit, and Josh with his arm around his mother's waist, the distance steadily closed between the pod and Odyssey.

Soon we were surrounded by the magnificent black and white creatures. We counted 26 in all, ranging in size from young adolescents to great bulls that must have exceeded 22 feet in length and weighed four to five tons. The entire pod seemed to be putting on a show; breaching, splashing, and generally looking like they were having as much fun entertaining us as we were having watching them.

Josh and Suanne were laughing and shrieking with excitement as one of the great creatures came almost completely out of the water not 25 yards off our port bow and sent a sheet of sparkling sea water over the both of them. Then, as quickly as they appeared, the pod was past us, heading north up Haro Strait and entertaining perhaps a dozen whale watching boats out of Friday Harbor, Roche, Sydney and Victoria. It was like a traveling road show. When the excitement of the whales wore down we returned to the tasks at hand of sailing Odyssey out into the Straits of Juan de Fuca on a heading of 210 degrees toward Victoria.

The rest of our stay in the islands was imbued with the enchantment and joy of our encounter with the orcas and the contentment we all felt that night in Victoria as we said our goodnights in the warm glow of the main cabin's hurricane lantern.

"What do you think about the day Josh?" Suanne asked.

"I'll never forget it," he responded, "It was like being touched by God."

We returned to Friday Harbor on the 15th and caught our flight home on Sunday morning. The time invested - eight days in all - proved the perfect elixir for the three of us. A great time, a great timeout - just what the doctor ordered...or at least okayed. We were all the better for it.

In dealing with a disease like breast cancer, there is, I believe, a natural and perhaps inevitable tendency to allow it to overwhelm, to overtake our lives - to intrude into every waking moment, to infect our sensibilities and sensitivities, and to compromise the integrity of all joy and optimism. Without a conscious and dedicated effort to prevent this from happening, it can blot out the importance and countervailing influences of pleasure, recreation and intimacy. The trip to the San Juan Islands was our made to order antidote. Sure, the reality of what we were facing when we returned home was never far from our thoughts no matter what we were doing at any given moment, but it didn't mean that we couldn't laugh and smile, hike out to the Turn Point Lighthouse, make love and eat, drink and be merry. And that's what we did on our vacation, for eight fun filled glorious days we were able to leave the world of breast cancer in our wake and set sail on a course to find beauty and joy in our lives. Now that the holiday had ended, we would be able to re-engage the world of breast cancer and its treatment regimens with renewed spirits, a newly replenished reservoir of hope and optimism, and with visions of cavorting orcas dancing in our heads.

CHAPTER 19
Reveries and Radiation Therapy

June 17, 1996

The first workday after returning from our San Juan Islands vacation, Suanne came into my office a little after noon and asked if I wanted to go get a bite to eat before her medical appointment. From the outset, I tried to attend as many of her informational medical appointments as possible, even though I missed a couple of very important ones that I should have attended. To be sure, never did I consider breast cancer to be solely Suanne's problem. To my mind (and heart), it was our problem and Suanne treated it that way too.

I saved the computer document I was working on and closed the file. We stopped by our favorite deli in the world called Carried Away (which conveniently is located in Aptos, a couple of miles from our office), and got a curried eggplant sandwich, Arizona Ice Tea, and a fruit salad, (Yes, very California!), all to be shared, as is our habit. We then drove to a scenic cliff overlooking the ocean near Seabright State Beach.

It's a place we often go to be alone and discuss family and/or office matters over lunch. By the time we parked, a low covering of clouds was being driven across the water by the prevailing westerlies that sweeps across the Monterey Bay every afternoon in the spring and early summer. From our vantage point on the cliff we could see all the way down to the PG&E stacks at Moss Landing and across to Pleasure Point and Steamer Lane; all spots where I had hung out and surfed since my undergraduate days at Stanford in the late 60s. A young couple were wrapped around each other in the car parked just ahead of us, oblivious to our presence, or anyone else's. The wind scoured surface of the bay had the restless look of a Winslow watercolor.

Neither of us spoke for what seemed like a long time. Suanne carefully unwrapped the buldging eggplant sandwich

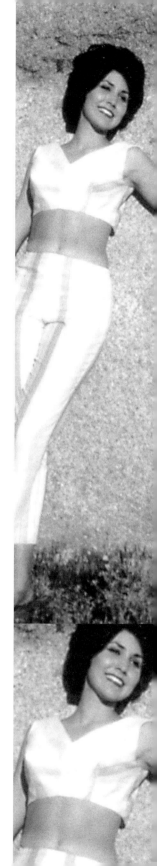

and handed me half. We ate in silence as my thoughts wandered out over the sea change that was taking place in our lives.

It is truly remarkable, I thought in silence, how the past looks through the prism of life's transformations - the relativity over time of what is important and what is not; the immutability of the past. We dance across life's stage, embracing this partner, then that, struggling to make sense of the music, the steps, and ourselves, most of us eventually wishing that we knew then what we know now, thinking how much easier things could have been. IF. That damn little word!

Across the bay near Pleasure Point I could make out a small sailboat beating up toward the Santa Cruz Yacht Harbor. The skipper, I mused, probably didn't have a care in the world other than sailing his boat. I remembered a day sail out of the yacht harbor that Suanne and I gone on two years before.

I had provisioned the galley on our little vessel named Rose (Suanne's childhood nickname), with fruit and cheese and a bottle of Santa Cruz Mountain Chardonnay. Very contrived; very purposeful. In the gear hammock in the forward v-berth was one of Suanne's old bikinis I had retrieved from the Goodwill sack and left it on the boat for just such an occasion (the same one I later transferred to Odyssey).

It was probably my most favorite bikini Suanne had ever worn because it was so threadbare, her breasts fairly spilled out with just about any movement, which also probably explains why I found it in the Goodwill donation sack. She didn't even know that I had salvaged it, much less secreted it on the boat.

This particular afternoon was one of those rare hot August days on the Monterey Bay, with a light breeze and flat water. The Chardonnay was icing down in the galley sink.

We sailed from the yacht harbor down around Pleasure Point and over to Capitola in the early afternoon and anchored far enough away from the wharf so that we had some privacy from the tourists, fishermen and the other boats moored in the anchorage.

After playing out the anchor rode and setting the hook, I laid out our lunch of sliced apple, pear, and peaches and French Brie, and then put a tape of Bob Dylan's greatest hits. The lyrics of one of his songs go: "Lay lady lay/ Lay across my big brass bed..." It was one of Suanne's favorites.

Like almost every other special occasion we'd ever shared alone, eroticism and allure played an important, perhaps crucial role in our relationship. Even after more than thirty years of marriage, observance of our sexual rituals remained subtle and mysterious, even a bit intimidating for me. Although now in her fifties and by most men's (or women's) judgment, "no spring chicken,"

Suanne had remained my greatest sexual fantasy. She was a visual and tactile feast for my carnal appetite, and occasions like this on Rose remained as exciting to me as they did when we were first married, particularly in the planning and anticipation.

"Would you like to sun for a while, Honey?" I asked, confident that the weather was to her liking. After quaffing a half-bottle of the iced Chardonnay she was already recumbent on the port cockpit seat and snuggling up to the bed of beach towels I had spread out for her. An afternoon snooze in the sun was in the offing.

"Sure," she responded demurely, "but I didn't bring a bathing suit to put on. I can't just take my shirt off, can I?" The "can I?" resonated strongly with my now-welling-up fantasies du jour. "Do you have anything onboard I can wear?"

"You know, Honey, I just might." I then went below and returned with the salvaged bikini. "How about this?"

Suanne looked at me with a sultry, knowing smile. "Been shopping at Goodwill?" she asked.

"Here," I said, handing her the flimsy little top, "take your shirt off and turn over and I'll put some sun block on you." Suanne sat up and slowly looked around at the neighboring boats, the wharf, and the beach maybe 150 yards away, then with her eyes fixed on me, she began slowly unbuttoning her blouse.

Once fully unbuttoned, she unhooked the catch on her bra and let it dangle for a few moments underneath her blouse, all the while keeping her gaze fixed on me. She then lifted her arms up with her hands clinched into fists behind her head, closed her eyes and stretched like a cat preening in the sun before removing her shirt and bra at the same time.

She sat there for a moment or two, with an inviting smile on her face, seemingly oblivious to - or better, indifferent to - the surrounding boats and tourists, before reclining on the towels. I gazed at her, feeling the power of her magnetism overwhelming me. God, did I love it whenever she put her feminine charms on display for my erotic pleasure and excitement, as she did in spades on Rose that day. Make no mistake, it wasn't just Helen's face that launched a thousand ships!

"What are you thinking about?" Suanne asked, jolting me back to reality from my reverie.

"Oh nothing. Nothing. I was just thinking about the Yancy case. The trial is only a month away; I've got a lot of work to do. Are you ready to go?"

"Sure Honey, I'm ready. Are you ready?"

When we pulled into the lot at the radiation oncology center and parked, I had one of those strange sensations sometimes referred to as out-of-body experiences. I could see myself getting out of the car in slow motion, locking it and then walking to the back of the car and taking Suanne's hand, then walking across the parking lot toward the double doors that had "Radiation Therapy" and the doctor's names inscribed on them.

The first thing I noticed about the couple I was watching was how healthy and vigorous they both looked. They could have just as easily been walking into a movie theater, a restaurant or a gym. Their stride and carriage were robust and brisk; their aspect determined and sure; their posture erect. Then they passed through the radiation portals as if entering a foreboding Gothic temple and descended down a set of stairs to a reception area that had a distinctly, and appropriately, sepulchral ambiance about it.

In the waiting area there were rows of chairs geometrically laid out with an assorted collection of cancer patients scattered about quietly waiting to have the lethal beams of high energy radiation shot into the nasty little tumors or cells that were growing in one part or another of their bodies. There were the usual congeries of dog-eared magazines strewn about, along with a passel of pamphlets dealing with the many forms of cancer and radiation therapy.

Most of the people looked old and decrepit, but there were a couple of younger people too. The couple I was watching looked too young and far too healthy to be there as patients; they struck me more like visitors in a nursing home. I wondered to myself what their situation could be to have brought them to a place like this.

I took a seat picking up the newspaper and began thumbing through the pages while Suanne went to the reception desk. I read that ValueJet had been grounded by the FAA for "several serious deficiencies." It was reported that the airline had a history of deficiencies. I thought about what the families of the one hundred and ten people that perished in the crash and wondered how they might be reacting to the report. Here today, gone tomorrow.

After checking in Suanne returned and sat down beside me. By then I was scanning the table of contents of a publication entitled "Radiation Therapy and You," a pamphlet put out by the National Cancer Institute. I turned to the section on what cancer patients need to do to take care of themselves during radiation therapy: Get plenty of rest, eat a balanced diet that will prevent weight loss, keep the sun off the area that is being radiated, avoid using any type of foreign material on the treated area (such as soaps, deodorants, lotions, perfumes, etc.) Reading it brought me back to the reality of what we were there for and how cancer knows no boundaries of age, physical condition or body image. Before long, the young woman at the reception desk called Suanne's name and directed us to Dr. Mann's office. This was the first time I'd seen Steven since that day in the parking lot at Deluxe Market. I hoped I wouldn't break down like a blubbering wimp.

The doctor walked in, greeting us with a delicate combination of neighborly intimacy and clinical detachment.

"Hi Scott. And Suanne, how are you? I'm sorry we have to be meeting like this, but if for any reason you're uncomfortable with me treating you, I'll be happy to have one of my partners handle your case." It was a conversation I expected.

"No, Steve," Suanne responded, "if you're concerned that either one of us might be uncomfortable in social settings because of your professional intimacy with my breasts, perish the thought. I've shown my breasts to so many doctors over the past three or four months that I don't look at it as any different than opening my mouth for my dentist. If it doesn't bother you, it doesn't bother me or us. In fact, we're very pleased that it is you who will be treating me." She was direct and right. I nodded my agreement.

Steve then launched into an explanation of the role of the radiation oncologist in the treatment of cancer patients. The radiation oncologist is usually the next member of the breast cancer treatment team that comes on board following surgery, if he or she hasn't been involved from the beginning.

Typically, the radiation oncologist is the first physician that is specially trained (and often "board certified") in the treatment of cancer. This is in contrast to a woman's primary care Ob/Gyn that performs physical examinations and orders the mammograms (and is specially trained in obstetrics and gynecology), the diagnostic radiologist who reads the mammogram films, and the surgeon (who is specially trained in particular areas of surgery) who performs the needle biopsy, lumpectomy, mastectomy, and so on. At this stage, the radiation oncologist essentially takes over the role as the "captain of the ship" in the care and treatment of the breast cancer patient, even though this role is usually temporary.

Steve said that since it was highly likely Suanne would be having tamoxifen therapy, it would also be a good idea for her to be followed by a medical oncologist, whose role he went on to explain.

Medical oncologists are physicians who are trained in internal medicine with a sub-speciality in oncology. Oncology is defined as involving the treatment of cancer patients with drug therapy or with chemicals (commonly known as "chemotherapy"). Depending on a variety of yet-to-be-determined factors, Steve suggested it might be possible that Suanne would need a course of chemotherapy. He recommended a young medical oncologist named Richard Shapiro who had recently completed his fellowship at Stanford.

Steve had already consulted with Dr. Mahoney, reviewed Suanne's entire medical chart and had concluded that she was a good candidate for radiation therapy. He explained that sometimes when a patient is referred to him, he and his group will decline to offer treatment for any number of a variety of reasons, including medical history (for example, a woman with a history of chronic lung disease may be at a peculiar risk with radiation therapy), equipment (some women may be of a bust size that is incompatible with particular equipment), or any other reason that suggests to the radiation oncologist that the risk of radiation is greater than the potential benefits of radiation therapy.

Having determined that Suanne was a good candidate for radiation therapy, Dr. Mann explained that radiation therapy had made great technological advances in recent years. Whereas in the early years of radiation therapy the machines used bore a closer resemblance to a meat clever than a scalpel, today the radiation therapy is extremely precise in terms of both the energy used and the focus of the radiation beam. Because of the precision and focus of the radiation on the site of the tumor, much less energy is required. As a direct consequence, there are fewer risks and side effects, although some remain.[33]

The side effects of modern radiation therapy include what the doctor called the "sunburn effect," a condition of the skin similar to a rash or sunburn. The skin in the areas of radiation in some patients may thicken and change colors. The nipple can show changes ranging from a darkening or lightening, to a scaliness.

Many patients experience fatigue, thus the need for plenty of sleep and rest. Others experience pain, swelling and tenderness in the breasts. Loss of appetite is a common side effect. Some patients develop a dry cough and the feeling of a lump in the throat. Nausea is not uncommon. Some women's breasts change in size and shape. Most, if not all of the side effects, in the majority of patients go away within six months to a year. Some patients suffer from chronic lymphedema, which is a swelling caused by fluid retention that typically manifests itself in the patient's arm on the side treated.

The doctor next explained what the radiation therapy would consist of. First,

---

[33] - The first widely used machines for the treatment of cancer in radiation therapy were Cobalt therapy machines. They consisted of a radioactive piece of Cobalt 60 housed in a lead container to which the patient was exposed when the door of the container opened by remote control. They were inexpensive and reliable (there were few parts that could fail), but had the disadvantage of the edge of the beam of radiation on the patient's body being very broad. In other words, if you were to measure the amount of radiation just inside the radiation field (the target) to a point just outside the field where it fell to zero, the distance would be in centimeters. this was because the source of radiation in the Cobalt machine, the piece of Cobalt, was about the size of a quarter. Newer machines called linear accelerators have a radiation source only a few millimeters across and the transition area in the patient from full radiation to zero is measured in millimeters. This results in a more delineated beam of radiation and less exposure to the patient. Linear accelerators for medical use were developed at Stanford by Dr. Henry Kaplan and came into common usage in the 1970s. **SM**

the area of treatment is carefully identified. This is done at a planning session prior to the initiation of radiation therapy. Permanent marks in the form of tiny tattoo dots are placed on the skin to provide landmarks for the area to be radiated.

There are a couple of reasons for the permanent markings. One, the marks allow the radiation therapist to focus the radiation machine during each treatment session on the precise area needed. Two, it is important to have the radiated area permanently marked in the event there is a recurrence of the disease. In this manner the future radiation oncologist will know what area has received prior treatment.

For a period that typically last six weeks, the tumorous breast is blasted with a high energy beam of electron radiation from a device called a linear accelerator. Suanne's sessions, we were advised, would take place five days a week and last about fifteen minutes, start to finish. The blast from the radiation beam lasts between three and five minutes. At the end will come a one-week "booster session" in which the radiation would be focused more narrowly on the lumpectomy site. After painstakingly reviewing this entire "preamble," Dr. Mann directed us to an examining room where Suanne changed into a paper blouse.

As I watched Suanne remove her blouse and bra I began contemplating how I would respond to watching my neighbor, and a man to boot, looking at and feeling my wife's breasts. Until now, I hadn't actually thought about this aspect of her treatment. It was minimally disconcerting, but before I could even organize my thoughts, Steve knocked on the door, entered and walked over in front of Suanne and said, "Let's take a look." Suanne was sitting on the examining table.

He carefully undid the bow on the paper blouse and pushed one side away, revealing Suanne's right breast. I watched as he poked here and pushed there, first on the outside of her breast then around the bottom and then up the cleavage side. He grasped the nipple firmly between his thumb and index finger as if he were lightly threading a nut on a small bolt. After completing his examination of the right breast, he repeated it on the left.

As I watched Steve perform this very "hands-on" examination, I wondered if he could see beyond the clinical aspects of the breasts that he was examining. I wondered if he could see the lovely mounds of pendulous flesh, the tan lines, the areolas and the sweet nipples that had given so much carnal sustenance to me for more than three decades. More likely, I decided, examining breasts for a male radiation oncologist is more like visiting a nudist colony. After a while the sexual attributes of the naked bodies just fade into the whole of the human animal and are regarded little differently from, say, a thumb, or a molar, or the inside of the lower colon - perhaps not unlike the manner in which I suspect that Louis Leakey, the famous anthropologist, might view Lucy if he were to see her scampering naked around the Olduvai Gorge. The key word here, I satisfied myself, is context. Yes, context. After Steve completed his examination he asked us if we had any other questions.

I asked him how the radiation can kill the cancer cells without also killing the healthy cells that surround it. It was one of the few questions I had that I had not yet researched and was more than a little confusing to me.

His answer: Normal (i.e., healthy) cells are very resilient and can literally repair/regenerate themselves when they are damaged. The process is similar to the way healthy soft tissue repairs itself by scarring over when cut. But if the cut becomes infected, it has a much more difficult time healing because of the near-liquid consistency of the purulent tissue. The same general principle likewise applies to the mutated cancer cells. Because of the defects that make a cell cancerous in the first place, they cannot repair themselves as healthy cells can when shot with the beams of radiation. Instead the cancer cells die and therefore stop dividing and multiplying. In contrast, the healthy cells simply roll up their sleeve and go to work repairing themselves.

"That's it? I asked, feeling considerable relief. "Three minutes of radiation therapy five days a week for six weeks, and nothing other than self-limitations on activities?"

"That's it." said the doc. "See you on Monday." With that, the appointment with Dr. Steve Mann, radiation oncologist and neighbor, was over. Suanne got dressed and we left with instructions for Suanne's planning session.

On the way out to the car, I asked Suanne if it made her uncomfortable having me there while Steve was examining her breasts. She said that it was no biggie, and turning the tables, wondered how I felt watching Steve "fondle" her breasts. Her question sounded serious, but I though perhaps she was trifling with me a bit. Quite honestly, I was feeling pretty good about everything. Radiation therapy didn't sound to me as though it was going to be anything to onerous or unbearable. Nonetheless, I took the bait.

"Well, it really wasn't like he was fondling your breasts," I responded as we got in the car and drove away, "it was more like he was palpating them. Palpating, you know, is different from fondling or feeling breasts. It's not like he was feeling you up or anything. No, frankly the palpating didn't bother me a bit. But, since we're on the subject, I was wondering, have any of the doctors you've seen, ever just sort of leaned over while they were fondling your tits and started sucking on them?" I tried to suppress a smile, but couldn't.

"Yeah, Scott, now that you mention it, every one of them in the past has. Steve is the lone exception and I'm sure he'll get around to it sooner or later. My understanding is that's part of the standard therapy performed, and at no extra charge. They do it to prevent the cancer from recurring. Honest, it's the God's truth."

I countered, doing all I could to stifle a guffaw: "Have they said anything to you in that regard about home remedies?" I gave her a friendly little pat on her right inner thigh.

"Yes, I'm told home remedies work amazingly well. Would like to go home right now and administer some?"

"I love you, Honey," I said, "I love you more right this minute than I did the day I asked you to marry me." As I uttered those words, I suddenly found myself trying to suppress not a laugh, but the tears that were forming in my eyes. God, I love this woman. I am such a lucky man.

We zipped right past the office and went home. We engaged in sweet, sweet love for what seemed like hours. But I didn't look at the clock and made no entries in my Daytimer. Instead,

I kissed her misty tears,
like rain upon the land,
In a black all consuming void and beyond,
And the songs she sang to me
Were of beauty and sorrow,
Of dawn and springtime

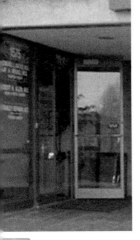

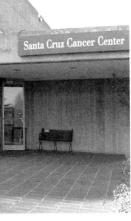

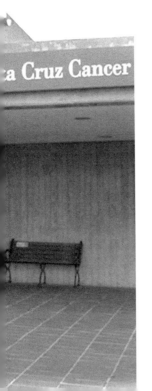

CHAPTER 20
The Planning Session

June 18, 1996

After a morning at the hospital undergoing various tests, Suanne went to the radiation therapy center to have her planning session with Dr. Mann and his team.

The first test at the hospital is a CT (computerized tomography) scan that takes a cross-sectional image of the chest, showing the breast, chest wall, lung and heart. The CT scan is done with the patient in a position that is intended to mimic the exact same position in which she will be in during her therapy sessions. The images from the CT scan are then fed into a computer allowing the radiation oncologist to view the distribution of radiation in the patient's breast and adjacent tissues by virtue of the fields being targeted from slightly different angles. The angles selected are those that give what is clinically termed "a homogeneous distribution of radiation" to the breast and with a minimum of unwanted "overspray" (my term) to heart and lungs.

The simulation procedure sets up the treatment as though it were to be delivered using the plan (angles) from the computer. But, instead of treatment x-rays, diagnostic x-rays are employed so as to allow the area through which the x-rays will pass to be seen. This procedure permits the radiation oncologist to confirm the accuracy of the computer generated treatment plan and to modify it if it should be deemed there is too much lung or heart tissue in the treatment field.

By the time of the planning session the tenderness from Suanne's lymphnode surgery was fully healed and she had unrestricted range of motion with her arms. This is important because while setting up and undergoing radiation therapy she would have to have one or both of her arms raised up and over her head to accommodate the requisite positioning for the therapy. Sometimes a so-called cradle is used to ensure that the elevated arm remains in the exact same position throughout each session.

In addition to all of the technical preparation it entails, the planning session also affords the patient time in which to acquaint herself with the people and the procedures she will encounter.

The *radiation oncologist* [34] typically works with a group of highly trained specialist that function as a close knit team in administering the radiation therapy.

The *radiation therapists* (sometimes called radiation technicians) assists the patient in the radiation therapy room and operate the hi-tech "zap" machines that deliver the radiation. Radiation therapists are required to have at least two years of college and pass a rigorous written examination administered by the state.

The *radiation therapy nurse* assists the patient on an ad hoc basis in dealing with such matters as side-effects, diet, nutrition, and various medical issues. Their training is similar to that of the therapists.

The *dosimetrist* calculates the radiation energy used and the duration of treatments to be administered according to each individual patient's particular needs. Dosimetrists undergo the same requirements as a therapist plus an additional year of formal schooling.

The *radiation physicist* calibrates and maintains the radiation machines. This specialist has a masters degree (meaning two to three years of post graduate work and must undergo an oral and written examination) or Ph.D.(four to six years of post-graduate work and written and oral examination) in physics.

And, of course, there are the *office personnel* (front office and back office), who together run the business end of radiation therapy practice.

When Suanne got home from the planning session, she showed me the mapping all over her right breast and the tiny little tattoos that denoted the area of treatment. She then described for me in detail what the planning session entailed.

"The first thing I did was change into the johnny vest (the paper blouse), with the tie strings and opening in front. Steve then introduced me to his team, which consisted of the radiation technologist or therapist, the dosimetrist and a radiation physicist. The therapist then escorted me into a room where there was a treatment table and this very menacing looking machine above it.

"This room is where the "set up" is done prior to actually undergoing the radiation therapy. The set up, or planning session, consists of "mapping" the area to be radiated to ensure that the radiation beams are directed to the precise areas where they want to eradicate any cancer cells that may remain after the tumor was removed. The mapping is also to avoid radiating lung, heart and

34 - Until the 1980's the physician was called the *Radiation Therapist* and the person carrying out the treatment was called the *Radiation Therapy Technologist* (RTT); today the physician is called a *Radiation Oncologist* and the RTT is now the *Radiation Therapist*. **SM**

other adjacent tissue.

To accomplish this the device used to simulate the actual radiation therapy machine (called a "simulator"), takes actual diagnostic X-rays to precisely define the anatomical structures under the breast.[35]

"I lay on my back on the radiation table with my head in a cradle and my arms extended over my head while all this is being accomplished. After the x-rays were taken and read the information was fed into a computer that confirms the precise angles of the radiation therapy."

Pointing to her chest, she added: "When this was finished they made all these marks on my breast with a purple marking pen. These marks will then be utilized by the radiation technicians in administering the radiation therapy. If it were someone other than myself going through this, Scott, I'd find it all very interesting. After Steve reviewed everything and was completely satisfied that the area to be radiated was precisely identified, the permanent tattoo marks were made."

"You and Cher now have something in common." I jested. My off-hand (and admittedly not at all funny) remark was in response to an article we had read in the paper that morning that Cher was having her "menagerie" of tattoos removed, including the "rose garden" on her butt.

"Let me see the marks." I politely insisted. What she showed me could hardly even be called a tattoo. They were little tiny dots on her chest, above, below and medial to her right breast and barely visible or distinguishable from her normal skin.

"I'm not to wash off any of the purple lines you see on my skin until the treatment is over. My first session is on Monday." [36]

The planning session on the treatment table, described by Suanne, lasted a total of about an hour and a half. Hearing her describe the process, even with

---

35 - The patient lies on the "treatment" table and the machine is aimed at the patient's body at the angle and field size specified by the treatment plan generated by the computer. When the machine is turned on instead of a treatment beam, diagnostic x-rays come out which expose x-ray film mounted in a film holder perpendicular to the beam on the other side of the patient. When this film is developed it gives a picture of what the x-ray beam "sees" as it passes through the patient. This film is reviewed by the radiation oncologist to ensure that the computerized treatment plan is faithfully being carried out and really works, as is modified as necessary. As a final check to the accuracy of the treatment plan, once the simulation films are passed, the patient has her first treatment. However, the first day of treatment is frequently a repeat of the simulation process, but this time on the actual treatment table using the treatment machine. Here the x-ray film is different, being less sensitive to radiation, because the exposure is so much longer. The film is arranged the same way as in simulation, perpendicular to the x-rays. If the x-rays are coming from above or below, at a 90 degree angle to the patient, there is a slot in the table under the patient to slide the film holder into. **SM**

36 - The dose of radiation is measured in a unit called a rad (acronym for "radiation absorbed dose"). The rad is a measure of energy the radiation deposits in a gram of tissue. One rad is equal to 100 egs/gm. The rad has been around for a long time and has allowed doctors to compare doses with one another. Over a long time, experience has taught us that a safe and fairly standard dose for breast cancer treatment was 180-200 rads/day, up to a total of 4500-6000 rads. Although the dose inside the treatment field is known, it is not the same dose entering the patient's body and some radiation is absorbed before it reaches the target volume. The factors that influence how much is absorbed are the type of tissue, the energy of the x-rays, and the distance of the machine from the patient's body. Taking all these into account, one can calculate the dose the machine needs to give in order to get the desired dose to the target. Knowing the rate at which the radiation is emitted from the machine allows one to calculate the time the machine stays on. Today these calculations are all done by a computer program. **SM**

the uncomfortable hard surface of the treatment table, seemed fairly perfunctory and tolerable to me. I didn't regard it as being that big a deal. Heck, she'd be in and out in fifteen minutes and whatever side-effects incurred would be transitory and manageable. Or so I told myself. In truth, however, I needed more education.[37]

37 - A week or two later, after Suanne had began her radiation treatments, it became clear to me that going through radiation therapy was taking a much greater psychological toll on her than I had anticipated. I called Steve and asked him if Suanne's response was to be expected.

Steve told me that radiation therapy affects different people in different ways, and that it's a lot more difficult than one might imagine. He told me he thought Suanne was handling it very well from what he was observing."

By this time I had told Steve that I was seriously considering writing a book about my experience as a breast cancer husband and he was very supportive and enthusiastic about the project. Out of the blue, he asked me if I would like to go through the whole radiation therapy process myself. I thought he was kidding but I was intrigued by the prospect of learning first hand what a radiation therapy patient goes through.

Steve explained that, of course, I wouldn't actually be radiated but I could go through everything else. He told me to give it some thought.

A few days later I arrived at the radiation therapy clinic for my planning session along with one session of radiation therapy. Steve had made all the arrangements and wanted to make it as realistic as possible. I walked down the stairs into the sepulcher and gave the receptionist my name. She looked at me a little funny, I thought, but asked me to take a seat and a nurse would be with me shortly. I took a seat towards the back of the room and picked up the same brochure had before put out by the National Cancer Institute and started thumbing through it again. There were several other patients in the waiting area waiting for the real thing, and I began to feel a tinge of self-consciousness about my experiment. Here I was doing a mockup of a process that they were depending on to perhaps save their lives. In a few minutes a nurse came out and called my name. I followed her back to the cubby hole area where she instructed me to change into the little green vest and to then take a seat just outside, just like Suanne had described.

Soon a different young woman came up, introduced herself as a radiation therapist and asked if I was there for my planning session. I indicated in perfect patient-speak that I was and she took me into the simulator room. Once inside the room where I would be prepped I began to get a sense of how the process might affect a patient psychologically. The simulator room is very stark and the simulator machine menacing looking. Then I was given the he whole business including the mapping of my chest with the purple lines, but no tattoos. The table was every bit as hard and uncomfortable as Suanne had described it. Next, I was taken into the radiation therapy room where I was strapped on to the treatment table. While being positioned the therapist explained each step that would take place. She raised and leveled the table until the laser beams coming from the he walls and ceiling were in perfect alignment. Then I was left alone. At this point the intimidation factor became very clear even knowing that I wouldn't be showered with electron beams from a high energy linear accelerator. Soon a voice came on over the intercom and told me that the therapy was about to begin. Next I heard a sound that was a combination of a low hum and a soft grinding. This went on for about three minutes. Finally, after the sound stopped, the voice over the intercom came back on and said the treatment was over. The same therapist came back into the room and released me from the table. JSL

Dr. Mann comments: For a variety of reasons that the reader can guess, it is highly unusual for a non-patient to be subjected to the treatment planning process or simulation session. Yet to experience something is always better than listening to a description or watching; it is much more profound. It's like the difference between watching and participating in an athletic event. The author's "planning session" was the first time for me (and obviously for him), and in fact the first time I had even heard about a family member undergoing an exemplar planning session. There was certainly no danger involved, but it did take away from valuable staff time. However, I was impressed with the potential value of the project Scott had embarked on and I wanted to give him the opportunity to understand in more depth the experience and fears that a breast cancer patient faces while undergoing radiation therapy.

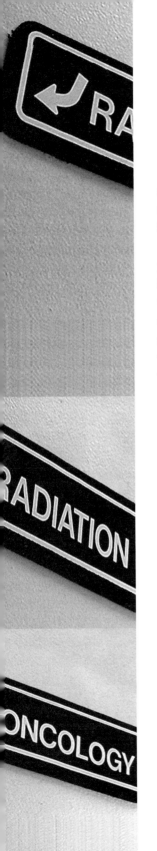

CHAPTER 21
Medical Oncology

June 19, 1996

At the initial appointment , Dr. Mann had given us a summary explanation of the field of medical oncology in the context of Suanne's continuing care, and the chance that Suanne would need a course of chemotherapy.

Beforehand we had not given any thought to the prospect (in my mind, "specter") of chemotherapy, but after Steven's clear reference, it was a topic of discussion. Even the possibility, much less the probability of chemotherapy, came as somewhat of a surprise to both of us. As early as after the first surgery back in April we had been told that it was unlikely Suanne would need chemotherapy, and after the second surgery produced no evidence of dirty margins or lymph node involvement, we assumed that the tumor had not spread beyond the primary site and she would not need chemo.

Our thinking went along the lines of: If, a) the surgeon had completely removed the cancerous tumor; b) there was no evidence of any spread; and c), the radiation therapy would kill all remaining rogue cells in the immediate vicinity of the tumor, then why were we now talking about the possibility of chemotherapy? Then I recalled that Dr. Mann had said any decision on chemo would be left to the judgment of the medical oncologist.

Before the first appointment with Dr. Shapiro, we tried to bring ourselves up to speed on the role of the medical oncologist as a member of the breast cancer treatment team. Medical oncologist, we learned, are physicians with a high degree of specialized training; first in the field of internal medicine (the diagnosis and nonsurgical treatment of adult diseases) and then in the treatment of malignant tumors (oncology).

The standard training for a medical oncologist is often done in a combined residency (a period of four to six years following their internship during which time they are trained in hospitals in their specialized areas of medicine), and sometimes they complete independent residencies in both specialties. There are board certifications (certifications of competency by a board of medical examiners in specialized areas of medicine) in both internal medicine and medical oncology.

Medical oncologists provide cancer patients with a type of treatment called chemotherapy (the introduction into the body through the blood stream of cytotoxic chemicals that are designed to zero in on and destroy cancer cells).

Another treatment used by medical oncologist is the hormonal therapy that had been described to us by Dr. Mahoney in conjunction with the drug tamoxifen. Hormonal therapy differs radically from chemotherapy in the way it works.

Chemotherapy performs in much the same manner as radiation therapy. Cells that are dividing and multiplying go through several steps. These steps are called, in the sequence they occur, interphase, prophase, metaphase, anaphase, telophase and back to the beginning, interphase. The whole process of cell division, as everyone who took high school biology may remember, is called mitosis. While the names of the various phases of cell division may serve only to conjure up some vague recollection of high school biology, the important thing about these terms is that they describe each of the necessary steps for cell division or replication to occur. The "cytotoxic" drugs used in chemotherapy are designed to interfere with one or more of the phases of metosis resulting in the death or inability of the cell to replicate. Different drugs are needed to interfere with different phases or processes in cell division.[38]

The problem herein, of course, is that any drug that interferes with cell division in cancer cells, also will interfere with the same mechanisms in healthy cells that are dividing normally. This explains why cancer patients who are undergoing chemotherapy suffer side effects such as hair loss and the reduced inability of the healing process to close wounds (scarring). The hair cells are constantly dividing and multiplying (resulting in hair growing), and bone marrow is constantly "growing" new red and white blood cells and platelets, which together promote healing of damaged tissue. This is in contrast to tissue and organs that are not constantly growing, such as the heart, lungs, liver, brain and skin. Where no cell division is taking place the chemotherapy has little or no effect.

Chemotherapy is almost always administered in "cycles" (installments) to

38 - Chemotherapy means the use of drugs against cancer at any vulnerable point. There are several dozen drugs used both by themselves and in combination with one another. In breast cancer, the most common combination of drugs consists of Cytoxan (trade name, aka cyclophosphamide, which is the generic name), methotrexate and 5-flourouracil or 5-FU. It is also know as CMF. In a typical regimen C is given orally and M and F are given intravenously. The pills may be given for two weeks and the injections as a single injection repeated around two weeks later. This "cycle" is then repeated after the blood count recovers and is continued for around six months. **JSL**

enable the bone marrow factory that is producing the good stuff we need for a healthy body and to fight disease and infection, to take time off to rebuild itself.

Hormonal therapy on the other hand, works not by interfering with the phases of mitosis or cell division, but rather by shielding and protecting the cell from what are believed to be external growth stimulating influences. In Suanne's case, the pathology report showed that her tumor was positive for estrogen and progesterone, two female hormones produced mainly in the ovaries but also in the adrenal glands and elsewhere in the body. It is these hormones that produce the female sexual characteristics that begin to manifest during puberty such as the growth of pubic hair, development of breasts and "rounding" of hips. The operative word here is growth.

Most contraceptive (birth control) and HRT (hormone replacement therapy) therapies incorporate use of synthetic estrogen. Since Suanne's tumor was positive for estrogen and progesterone, tamoxifen therapy was prescribed to protect her from the influence of these growth producing hormones on the cells in her breast.[39]

We arrived for our first appointment with Dr. Shapiro carrying considerable apprehension over the possibility of having chemotherapy, or alternatively, that without it the chance remained that some cancer cells might escape and begin replicating elsewhere in Suanne's body. There were three other people in the waiting room; a couple and an elderly and visibly anxious gentleman that alternated between pacing around the room and peering blankly at the pages of magazines from the end-table beside the chair he occupied. The couple actually seemed relaxed as they discussed the news that Richard Allen Davis, the defiant, deranged abductor and slayer of young Polly Klass, had been found guilty of first degree murder with special circumstances by the Santa Clara County jury, which under California law, entitled him to the death penalty. From my perspective, a well-deserved criminal sanction, if ever there was one. After a few minutes a nurse came out, announced Suanne's name, and motioned for us to follow her back to an examining room.

Suanne perched on the examining table while I helped myself to the only chair in the room. I noted that from the diplomas on the wall that Dr. Shapiro was board certified in both internal medicine and in medical oncology. Good, I told myself. He had done his residency at Stanford. Double good. I always find Stanford credentials comforting, but when the person I presumed to be Dr. Shapiro walked into the examining room, I wasn't sure if he was the doctor or a

---

39 - Actually, no one knows how tamoxifen works – there is a school of thought that it works by direct effect on the replication of DNA, but that it needs the estrogen receptor to hoist itself into the cell in the first place... It is not simply an estrogen blocker though... Where the tumor has these receptors, the opportunity exists to use this medicine which is easier to tolerate. But in dangerous tumors, even with estrogen receptors, we will often do regular cytotoxic chime first... this one had all the good features, so even if you had wanted chemo we would have been hard-pressed to show any advantage of the chemo over tamoxifen based on research results. **EM**

student intern. He looked all of maybe thirty years old at best, certainly younger than my older sons and was quite handsome. His boyish appearance notwithstanding, he immediately won us over with a broad smile, a strong handshake and the kind of caring demeanor that immediately relaxes and inspires confidence in patients. After introducing himself (yes, it was Dr. Shapiro), he launched into a veritable exegesis of the role of the medical oncologist in the treatment of cancer.

He began by explaining that he would be assuming responsibility for the primary care of Suanne's cancer treatment. Once the surgeon and the radiation oncologist were finished with their care and treatment, Suanne would need regular follow-up visits to monitor her condition, particularly with respect to any chemotherapy or tamoxifen therapy that might be needed. At this point I interrupted.

"Doctor, we have been under the impression, perhaps mistakenly, that once the tumor was removed, in all likelihood there would be no need for chemotherapy. Our understanding is that there is a 95 percent chance that Suanne has been cured of her cancer without chemotherapy. Do you have any reason to disagree with that?"

Without saying so explicitly, what I was really asking was, is there reason to believe that metastasis had taken place despite everything we had been told to the contrary?

"No," he replied, "not at all. I have reviewed Suanne's entire chart beginning with the mammograms back in January and going through Dr. Mahoney's surgeries and I concur with her prognosis. As I'm sure you've been told many times, the tumor was very small and discovered very early. But even when you discover a malignant tumor as early as you did, there is always the statistical possibility, however remote, that some cancer cells managed to wrest loose and travel to another location in the body. Unfortunately, there is not test, at least not yet, to ascertain whether this has, in fact, occurred. As I said, in your case, the statistical possibility is small and typically we don't want to use chemotherapy to medicate the entire body after surgery and radiation therapy unless we feel it's absolutely necessary."

Dr. Shapiro went on with his medical oncology lecture, confirming much of what I had learned from my own research. He concluded by telling us that the decision on whether to use chemo or hormonal therapy, is ordinarily left to the medical oncologist. While indicating that he did not foresee the need for chemo in Suanne's case, he was careful to point out that there are exceptions to every rule and his job is to determine what the best course of treatment is for each individual patient.

Dr. Shapiro next said that while Suanne would probably not be receiving chemotherapy, it is important that she be monitored closely while taking the estrogen blocking drug, tamoxifen. She would require regular blood tests and doctor visits. He explained that tamoxifen can cause a variety of side effects including weight gain, vision problems, depression, and hot flashes, on the milder side, to increased risk of uterine cancer. Although in Suanne's case, having had a partial hysterectomy years earlier, the issue of uterine cancer was not a statistically serious threat. The tamoxifen therapy, he said, usually lasts from three to five years. While Suanne was aware of the phenomenon of hot flashes, she was certainly not aware of the severity of the tamoxifen hot flashes that awaited her.

The doctor next handed Suanne the obligatory little green vest with the string ties in front, then demurely excused himself from the room for her to change. After reappearing, Dr. Shapiro performed a physical examination of her breasts similar to, and no less thorough than the one by Dr. Mann. By this time I was beginning to feel like I too was opening my mouth for the dentist, but we left hugely relieved to have learned that chemotherapy was not in our future.

CHAPTER 22
Radiation Therapy

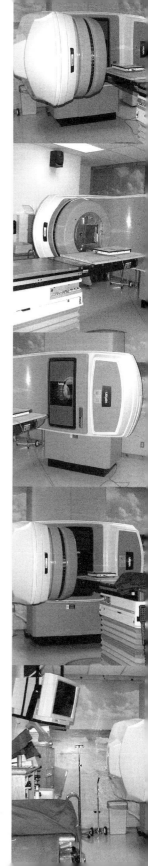

June 24, 1996

Early summer mornings in the "fog belt" of Santa Cruz County, hard against the Pacific, can be very reminiscent of the dead of winter. Once the fog wanders in from the ocean, depending on the prevailing temperature in the inland valleys, it can settle in for most of the day. On cool dreary summer days, such as this, when the fog hasn't lifted, sitting in a warm office in front of a computer screen isn't the worst place to be.

Suanne's first day of radiation therapy wasn't such a hang-dog day weatherwise, however. Indeed, as if flaunting the arrival of summer, the day of Suanne's first radiation treatment was nothing but blue skies, windless and warm; the kind of day that stirs the imagination to ponder wishfully all manner of things you might be doing other than sitting in an office, or more to the point, undergoing radiation therapy treatments.

At about 11:45 I heard Suanne's car door close outside my office. As is her habit, she came into my office before going upstairs to her office. I could read on her face some of the inaugural effects of being blasted with a beam of high energy radiation that is meant to kill or disable any mutated cancer cells that remain near the site of her tumor. Pushing myself away emotionally a tad, I opted for some diver- sionary small talk.

"Did you hear about O.J.'s fund raiser?" I asked. No, she hadn't, so I told her about Simpson's plan to put on a benefit for an organization dedicated to stopping domestic violence in the African-American community. He had also announced, the news report said, that he'd be "totally vindicated" at his upcoming civil trial in Santa Monica. I made some lame comment about Simpson's being a clinical psychopath, but it was obvious that the conversation was vacant and meandering, so I finally asked how her visit went. She was ready to sit for a while and give me a blow by blow account.

"After arriving," she began, " I changed into the same cute little vest that I wore during the first examination with Steve. I put my clothes in a cubby hole assigned to me in the changing room. Then I went to a separate waiting area until being called by the radiation therapist.

"There were two other women waiting for their turn in the spotlight. They'd both been going for a while and knew each other. We introduced ourselves though there wasn't any chit-chat.

"When the therapist called me, I went into a stark large room with a treatment table and a space age looking radiation therapy machine at one end. The whole scene is very "Star Wars" looking. The part of the machine that shoots the beams of radiation is on a rotating arm that pivots around the patient while you're lying on the table. This enables the therapist to deliver the radiation from 180 degree opposite positions.

"I lay down on the table with my head in a cradle and with my arms raised up over my head. The therapist moved me around to get me into the proper position and unfastened the vest exposing my breasts. There are laser beams coming from the wall and ceiling that enable the therapist to position me on the table in precisely the same position at each session using the markings and tattoos applied at the planning session. The table moves back and forth and up and down to achieve the exact correct angle of attack for the radiation beam.

"Once the technician got the table into the correct placement, she then re-positioned my body until the laser beam markers intersect perfectly with the mapping on my breast. Then the therapist left the room.

"During the positioning, another radiation therapist sits at a control panel outside the room observing everything on monitors and communicates with the therapist in the room through an intercom. There's a little window up high on the far wall where the technician who operates the machine sits.

"Then the therapist left the room and the person up in the booth asked me over the intercom if I was comfortable and explained to me what would happen next. He said that the machine would be rotated into the position and it would make some noise during the movement. Moments later the machine rotated into position while emitting a high-pitched whirling noise. Then the same faceless voice over the intercom said that the therapy would start in 15 seconds and I would hear a buzzing sound.

"The actual delivery time of the radiation, I was now advised, would be between three and a half minutes. From the time the buzzing sound started until it ended seemed like a lot more than three or three and a half minutes, but I didn't time it. I didn't feel a thing, except the macabre image I had of being a cadaver on a slab in a morgue.

"When the buzzing noise ended the voice from the control panel told me I was done and that I could go back to the dressing room and leave. The only thing she said other than that was to leave my gown in the cubby hole. From start to finish the whole appointment took about fifteen minutes. Everyone was very nice. That's it."

"Did you see Steve?" I asked. She didn't.

With little change, this was "the drill" Suanne would be going through five days a week for the next six weeks. It all sounded dreary to me and I knew that the whole exercise would be mentally and emotionally draining on Suanne, as it doubtlessly would be for most people. But at this juncture I had no idea what her psychological and physiological response would be to the treatments and neither did she. We would find out over the summer of her radiation therapy.[40]

---

40 - A Patients psychological response to radiation therapy is as varied as the patients themselves. The best predictor of how a patient will respond is how the patient has responded to illness or stress in the past. There's nothing particularly unique about the type of stress caused by radiation therapy, other perhaps than the duration of the daily treatments

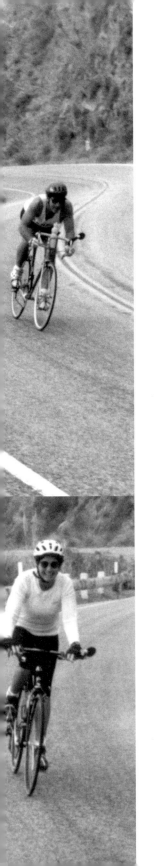

CHAPTER 23
Radiation Therapy: Week One

June 28, 1996

When Suanne came into my office at the end of her first week of radiation therapy, I could see that she was feeling pretty down. For my part, I still was trying to relegate the treatment sessions to a minor intrusion into the daily routine of our lives so I tried to focus the conversation on current events for a few minutes.

There was the horrific blast at an Air Force base in Saudi Arabia where 19 Americans were killed and 105 others wounded. The attack was carried out by a terrorist group led by a Saudi millionaire named Osama bin Laden. Simpson's gala black-tie "Stop the Violence" affair the night before at his Bundy estate, was also in the news. There were protesters outside to remind the media audience of the heights of clinical hypocrisy Simpson is capable of. Meanwhile, Ted Krczynski, the so called "Unabomber," had been booked in Sacramento and charged with capital murder.

Suanne warmed slightly to the conversation, but I could tell she needed to talk about how she was feeling. "How'd it go today?" I finally asked.

She had been leaning on my stand-up desk during the conversation thus far, but then crumpled into one of my client chairs when the conversation turned to the suffocating topic of breast cancer. She allowed that today was no different than the other days, but that she knew the whole treatment regimen was going to make for a rather depressing summer. I had been tinkering with my computer while we were talking but then turned to give my full and undivided attention to whatever it was she wanted to talk about. (From time to time I needed to remind myself that we were dealing with "our cancer-treatment" program, not just Suanne's. I did not want to come across to her, anyone else, and most importantly, myself, as sitting on the sidelines or being nothing more than a cheerleader.)

"There was a young man who was brought in in a wheelchair. He appeared to be in his late teens or early twenties. Maybe a little older, but he looked so frail that he had a very child-like appearance. Most of his hair had fallen out and he looked pale and gaunt yet he somehow managed a smile and a cheerful greeting to everyone there. It was his mom who had wheeled him in.

"I don't know what kind of cancer he has or how long he's been going to radiation therapy, but he didn't look good. There was an older woman with breast cancer who had had a double mastectomy fifteen years ago. Two months ago they found out that she has a tumor in her lung. While we were sitting in the waiting area in our leaf green radiation vests, she told me that we are all sisters; all women with breast cancer, she said, are sisters in a war for survival.

"She talked about how lucky we are because of the great strides being made in the detection and treatment of breast cancer. She laced her commentary with a lot of military terms like 'battle,' 'frontlines,' 'conquer,' and 'victory.' Her words and her tone were very inspiring. She has so much fighting spirit. Yet, I told her I feel more like a draftee into an unpopular war than a sister engaged in a holy crusade. I still find myself asking the question, 'why me?'

It was hard to imagine Suanne in such grim circumstances; surrounded by frail, sick, and "last leg" cancer patients. Outwardly, she retained her hard athletic appearance. I wondered too about the "why me" question. But the answer is actually easy. It is that there is no answer.

Suanne was (and remains) an athlete, a picture of strength and health, and possessed of more energy, strength and stamina per pound than almost anyone I know, male or female. She was an inspiration and role model for everyone at her gym, including high school, college and professional athletes. In high school Suanne had been an all-around athlete, a cheerleader, and a class officer. At Stanford, in the late sixties, well before physical fitness became a popular obsession, she took up serious weight lifting, bicycling and running and pursued them with a vengeance. When we moved out to the ranch after law school she began playing tennis and racket ball, constantly moving up the competition ladder until she was the number one payer in both sports at our club. She was the quintessential jock.

And, at fifty-one, to me she was no less beautiful than she was at the age of thirty-one. Yet here she was walking in the company of death and disease, being showered with lethal beams of radiation on a daily basis and, like every other cancer patient, not knowing what the future held in store, or if she even has a future.

As she was telling me about her fellow patients her voice began to crack. She looked down at her lap. I could tell she was fighting back tears. She finally broke down and began to cry, which instantly brings tears to my eyes. "Jesus Christ," I said to myself, "this really sucks."

I walked around behind her, gently and lovingly rubbing her shoulders and neck, wishing and hoping that by laying my hands upon her I could simply rub away the pain, like an oldtime faith healer. But I knew that the power of my hands upon her was nothing but a mere palliative and it would take all the love, consideration and affection I could muster just to blunt the emotional challenges the summer would thrust upon is. As for the physical challenges presented by radiation therapy, I was again nothing but a bystander.

Powerlessness is a mighty incentive to believe in the paranormal, the occult, and blind faith. Few among us are so rigid and fatalistic that we can't bend our knees in prayer when we're feeling vulnerable and helpless, and, believe me, pray I did. Often and in earnest. And I'm not, nor have I ever been a particularly religious person. But I do believe in an infinite divine source of creation. And I do believe that communication is possible with the Infinite Divine One.

With cancer, there is no place for smoke and mirrors, there are no magic formulas, no silver bullets, and, to be certain, no simple or easy answers, notwithstanding the avalanche of unsupported claims for such homeopathic remedies as eating apricot or papaya seeds and drinking unwashed aloe vera mixed with honey and tequila. There is only the ever increasing bona fide power of medical science to take the battle ever farther and ever deeper into the cellular world of genetics, DNA, molecular mutations, and advancing medical technology. This is not to say that the power of prayer, faith, and Carnegieesque-positive thinking are without their salutary effects in the fight against cancer. Who am I to say such modalities of thought and belief don't work? Who is anyone to say?

Indeed, I believe that good humor, a smile on one's face, benevolence and faith can and do work to achieve positive ends. Studies are coming out one after the other, that serve to confirm the benefits of everything from laughter and prayer to compassion and charity (along with a reduced-stress lifestyle) on all manner of not only industrial strength-maladies, but personal goals as well. But the fact remains, I am convinced, that the battle to find a cure or prevention for cancer won't be won on "a wing and a prayer" alone.

At the end of her first week of radiation therapy Suanne's mood, while not noticeably down or depressed nor even melancholy, had changed. Since February she had seen nine or ten different physicians and a raft of medical technicians, assistants, and nurses. The doctors ranged from her Ob/Gyn, radiologist and surgeon, all actual warm-blooded bodies that she knew by sight, sound and name, to anonymous name-badge anesthesiologists, pathologists, and internists, who, one and all, hovered about at the periphery of her ever-evolving, ever-dynamic care and treatment making arcane decisions and recommendations to their lords and masters.

She had been stuck, poked, probed, radiated, incised, excised, photographed, medicated, discussed, contemplated, charted, and analyzed, like a common, university-issued rat undergoing clinical trials. Her tests ranged from chemistry panels, urinalyses, and MRIs to bone scans, needle biopsies, C-T scans and x-rays. It was like she was in training for the Olympics and was spending almost every minute of every day in pursuit of the gold, except the reward here neither fame nor glory, but simply to return to her previous normal, healthy, vital self. This became the elusive prize, in and of itself.

But in pursuit of that prize, Suanne displayed the same obsession, the same dedication, the same passion, that she had throughout her life for every goal she had ever set for herself, if not with an even greater sense of dedication and motivation. All of this because of a wanton, miserable, virulent disease in the most photographed, most prominent, and to many, the most alluring aspect of the female anatomy. If anyone could beat The Big C, Suanne could. I told myself this over and over and over.

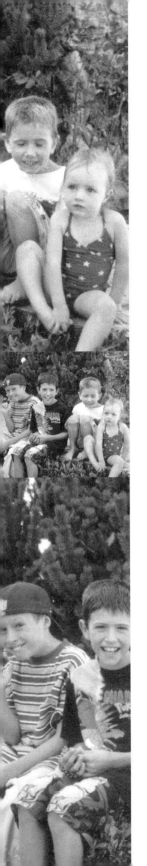

CHAPTER 24
Radiation Therapy: Week Two

July 5, 1996

I heard the sound of Suanne's car door slam and the whistle of the remote locking at the usual time after her appointment. It would take but a second or two before my door opened and she walked in. The second week of having a beam of electrons fired into her breast was over, but I was not expecting a TGIF celebration.

When I rose to greet her, however, I was surprised by the radiant smile on her face and her upbeat demeanor. A day earlier, on the fourth, we had been to the La Selva Beach parade and had our two older boys and their families over for hamburgers and hotdogs in the afternoon. The day was warm, relaxing and upbeat. After the evening fireworks down at the beach she seemed to be in good spirits . Being around family was always like a balm for her. This morning over coffee we got a good laugh from a column by Maureen Dowd in which she excoriated some Clinton-basher for being unduly concerned about whether the young women in the White House were wearing underwear or thongs or nothing. God forbid, nothing. Tongue firmly in cheek. Suanne offered she'd definitely be concerned if she had a daughter working in the White House who paraded around sans underwear or wearing thongs!

The Supreme Court has just recently ruled that Paula Jones suit against the Commander-in-Chief could continue. What, for heaven's sake, will come next?

"What happened?" I asked, as I took the mail out of her hand and placed it on my stand-up desk, "Did Steve do a particularly good job with his digital examination today?" I figured a little humor here might not hurt, although male (read chauvinistic) levity at this point was probably a little out-of-place.

"That's disgusting." she snapped back. "No, I had the most incredible conversation with Mrs. Johannes today. You remember, she's the lady with the double mastectomy; sisterhood, the war on cancer and all that?"

"Sure, I remember." I responded as I put my arms around her waist and began massaging her rock hard gluts, "What did she tell you, that they can transplant tits?" Although probably deserved, she refrained from hitting or kicking me. Her cheerful attitude was a welcome change.

"No," she said, "and would you like to hear what I have to say or do you want to continue being gross and crude? You know, you're not funny."

"Yes, I know I'm not funny, Honey. But when I see you looking like you do right now, my heart sings like a rock. Is that okay? And of course, I want to know about your friend. What happened?"

"It's SOARS like a hawk, stupid, not sings like a rock." She managed with a slight smile, but went on.

"While we were waiting together for our treatments Mrs. Johannes told me a lot about herself when she was a young girl. Now I know where she got all of her war metaphors. She grew up in Holland and was a member of the Dutch underground in World War II when she was a young girl. She actually fought against the Nazis in Amsterdam. She was only fourteen when the war ended. You could feel and hear so much pride and character in her voice while she was telling me about the war and the underground fighters.

"The way she talks about fighting cancer is no different than the way she talks about fighting the Nazis. She made me take pride in being a soldier in the war on breast cancer. She talked more about the sisterhood of women with breast cancer and how important it is for us to support each other and to contribute to the total war effort. It was almost patriotic."

I started to interrupt, but was overridden by Suanne's exuberance.

"I was very moved by her spirit and commitment," she continued. "She has so much strength and gumption and there are so many women like her. Here she is retired, getting old, living alone, and fighting a new war toward the end of her life, just like she did in the beginning. I didn't really relate to what she was telling me the first time I met her in the waiting area, but I do now. We are all sisters fighting a war, not only for our own lives, but for all women. Scott, I think I want you to write the book you've talked about. We need to do our part." **41**

By the time Suanne finished telling me about Mrs. Johannes I had tears in my eyes. The book part didn't escape me, but I have to admit that I felt pretty crude

---

41 - The writing this book has been an issue with Suanne from the beginning. For my part I would be less than candid if I did not admit that simple act of writing hit has been a great challenge and even enjoyable. I enjoy writing. But for Suanne it has been a long drawn out reminder of her disease, an unwelcome invasion of her privacy and drain on my time. The one thing that has sustained her though the whole process and allowed me to finish the project is our shared hope and belief that we will have made a positive contribution to the war on breast cancer.

and stupid saying the thing I did. I apologized for my remarks, to which she replied, with a smile, "Apology accepted, you insensitive cretin! After all, you are a man.

"So I don't really have a choice; do I?" I asked, as Suanne walked out the door.

CHAPTER 25
Radiation Therapy: Week Three

July 12, 1996

On the way to work I listened to a report on KCBS describing the security efforts taking place in Hotlanta for the Olympics. Between the local, state and federal agencies involved in the security operation, there are going to be three times as many people protecting the athletes as there are athletes. Domestic and foreign terrorists like homegrown Timothy McVeigh (Oklahoma City) and Saudi millionaire Osama Bin Laden, among others, are the focus of all this attention. The sarin gas attack in the Tokyo subway in March 1985 by a Japanese cult known as "Aum Shinrikyo" (translation: Aum Supreme Truth Cult), was prominently mentioned in the report.

As the world comes together under the banner of sport and athletic competition, it seems as though there is a parallel world awash with evangelical zealots of one stripe or another, all seeking venues great and small to wreak vengeance on their heretical foes. To such zealots words like peace, hope, friendship, respect and fair play are nothing more than epistemological aberrations to be sacrificed on the anvil of their own bitterness, hatred, despair and self-loathing. But in truth, they are nothing new, they are the flotsam and jetsam of the human condition.

In the arena of the Great World, it's not surprising that the vast number of these zealots and their venal minions of true believers are young males blinded by rage and convulsing with a need to express their manhood. In my own obviously less sensational way, I traveled down the same obsessive path in my youth. As a young man I viewed Ahab and his hunt for the White Whale as the quintessential hero and the quintessential quest of the philosopher-warrior in search of the true meaning of the nature of good and evil, man's highest calling:

"The path to my fixed purpose is laid with iron rails, whereon my soul is grooved to run. Over unsounded gorges,

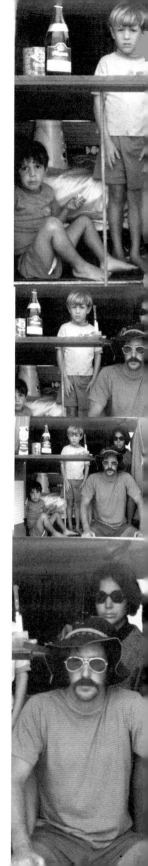

*through the rifled hearts of mountains, under torrents' beds, unerringly I rush.
Naught's an obstacle, naught's an angle to the iron way." (Ch. 37, Sunset)*

When I first read these words (and others like them), it transported me to a
place that could almost be compared to the spiritual notion of raptureña, a
hidden place where zealotry and obsession mingle in splendid isolation from all
competing values and interests of the visible world. The competing view of
Ahab, as a madman, consumed by bitter rage and willing to sacrifice all to feed
that rage, has certainly occurred to me in my middle life. What great fortune for
our species that the hormonal rails upon which we travel decline as we age.

When Suanne arrived at the office from the sepulcher she told that the young
boy in the wheel chair was brought to radiation therapy this week on a gurney.
The spring in his voice, she said, was noticeably weakening and even his pallid
translucent skin is washing out. His mother was with him all week, still painting
scenes of sun filled days with words of encouragement, faith, hope and love.
Some mothers can be such strong, heroic figures when life tests us with insults
and injuries to our children. While men go about their work, wrestle with their
testosterone, and hunt and gather, these women heal, mend, nourish and nurture.
And now, in addition to all this, they pay the mortgage, attend parent child
conferences, and sometimes even struggle to allure us back to the hearth.

How, I wondered, could I have been so blind, so long to the heroism of my
very own combination of Aphrodite, Diana, and Venus all rolled into one
incredible woman? How, would I have ever managed my life without her? The
fact of the matter is that I probably wouldn't have managed, at least not as well
as I did. Of all the challenges I managed to meet, of all the bullets I have
dodged - and they were mostly the same bullets and challenges that cut down so
many of our cohorts in the sixties and seventies - being able to still share a bottle
of vintage wine from old glasses with the queen of my adolescent dreams is now
unquestionably, the greatest source of pride and thanksgiving in my life.

Yet now, in the waning summer of our middle life, my queen marches in the
ranks of the foot soldiers in the war against breast cancer. What changes, I
wonder, might I have made, what maladies and pitfalls might have been avoided
had I half the appreciation of this woman in my younger years I now have.

CHAPTER 26
Radiation Therapy: Week Four

July 19, 1996

This was a week of major ups and downs. On Wednesday TWA flight 800 from New York to Paris plunged out of the sky from 13,500 feet killing all 230 people on board. There was a lot of unconfirmed speculation about a terrorist act, including a report of something that looked like a missile striking the plane. On Friday the Summer Olympics in Atlanta were opening at Centennial Olympic Stadium amid much pomp and circumstance. While the world continued spinning on its customary axis, Suanne and I were looking for the light at the end of the tunnel.

Radiation therapy itself is a silent painless form of treatment that takes only a short amount of time each visit to complete. For most patients, the side effects are transitory and manageable. But after four weeks of radiation and tamoxifen therapy, I could see that the cumulative side-effects were beginning to exact a mounting psychological toll on Suanne.

Item: The determined upbeat young man in the wheelchair, maybe just slightly older than Josh, died from a brain cancer that had metastasized in his body like the hydra-headed monster that it is. For him, the radiation was nothing more than palliative. He was checking out, no matter what they did. Suanne couldn't even think about the boy's mother without tearing up.

Item: Mrs. Johannes had to stop radiation therapy because of severe nausea and weight loss.

Item: One of the new patients this week was a twenty year old young woman with some form of bone cancer.

In all, not what would be described as leavening news out of the radiation oncology unit.

In addition to the daily psychological trauma of being immersed in the society of cancer patients, the tamoxifen therapy was creating a veritable maelstrom of hot flashes,

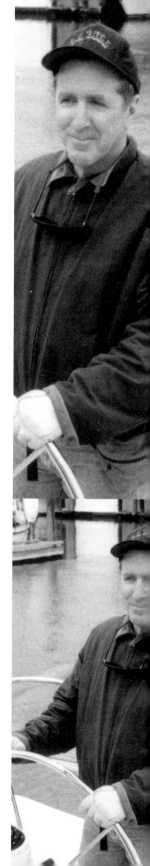

and for Suanne, an unusual degree of emotional vulnerability.

To the extent that Dr. Shapiro had described the hot flashes as one of the "manageable and transitory" side effects of the tamoxifen therapy (I think he used the word, "minor"), he had made it clear that the adjective "minor" was qualified by the standard bell shaped curve of each individual patient's reaction to it. Some women get mild and occasional hot flashes that barely wake them up at night. Others experience huge swings in body temperature caused by the confusing and dramatic change in their hormonal equilibrium.

In Suanne's case, she was waking up several times a night in a profuse sweat that would literally soak her side of the bed. The surface temperature of her body would suddenly rise to over a hundred degrees causing her skin to become clammy like a fish. She would have to get out of bed and go outside in an attempt to cool off in the cool moist air coming up from the beach. Then, once cooled down, she would then get severe chills and goose bumps all over her body and ward them off by covering up with extra blankets or even turning up her electric blanket. These chills often get so bad that she shivers violently. Then the whole cycle would start over again. Within the statistical bell shaped curve, Suanne probably was up near the peak. Then, there was the issue of sex.

From the onset, the cancer had a profoundly depressing effect on Suanne's libido, and therefore, my own. At first it was simply the shock of my wife being diagnosed with breast cancer. Then it was the pain from the surgeries. Even giving her a little hug was at times intolerable. Then came the radiation therapy, which meant a prolonged uninterrupted period of daily magnified focus on her breast cancer.

Not only were the hot flashes a nightly disruption, but were adding to Suanne's deepening fatigue during the day. Sex not only disappeared from the landscape, it dropped off the edge of the earth. For weeks on end, when we would go to bed my mind would run wild with every dark image it could conjure up to torture me with, and every option to the torture my fantasies could summon.

"What," I asked myself, "if the termination of Suanne's estrogen therapy, combined with the cancer and menopause dried up her libido, literally and figuratively? What if a few malignant cells had already escaped and the cancer was spreading and we didn't even know it? What if the cancer reappeared in the opposite breast and she had to have a double mastectomy? What would I do if I could never again touch her breasts for sensual gratification and pleasure? What would this do to her self-esteem; her femininity? What if the doctors were wrong about her chances of survival? What will I do every time I see a woman with beautiful breasts? What will Suanne be thinking I'm thinking every time she sees me looking at a woman with beautiful breasts? What if, what if, what if?" Don't try to tell me that fatigue and anxiety aren't contagious. I know for a fact that they are.

Assuming that the doctors are right about her survival, maybe, I thought, I should consider comfortably sliding into middle age without the pressures and distractions of sex. I read a Scott Turow novel once about a middle-aged lawyer with a wife who didn't care much for sex. He was accepting of this and turned his attention to developing other interests; work, golf, gardening, reading, puttering, and the like. He allowed the fantasies and activities that had fed his carnal appetite to be sliced, diced, chopped up, wrapped up and put in the freezer. But then his wife died and he met this sexy young tart that defrosted his fantasies and reacquainted him with his pre-morbid sexual self.

Then, with the help of the beguiling young seductress , the ashes of yesterday were reconstituted into a veritable conflagration of carnal appetite and erotic pleasure. I thought a lot about this character's "rebirth." But none of the answers to my questions, literary or otherwise, were any more satisfactory or palatable than most of the questions. I finally attributed my own disturbed thinking to the weather. It was the long dry spell that was turning my mind into freeze dried mush, or so I told myself.

At about the time I was reduced to wondering what I might find for diversion on the Internet or in the personal classified ads in *Good Times,* Suanne would wake me up in the middle of the night, snuggle up next to me and ask me how I was holding up. She would run her fingers through my hair and whisper in a sultry voice that the summer would pass and that we would once again reacquaint ourselves with each other, physically and otherwise.

"Before you know it," she said, " we'll be back aboard Odyssey, sailing up East Sound to Rosario for their Friday night buffet. Maybe we'll anchor out like we did the first time we visited there on Rose. In the evening we'll take the water taxi in to the mansion and go for a swim in the indoor pool before dinner. I'll wear the bikini you left on the boat and after dinner we'll go back to Odyssey and make love for hours. You can wait for me can't you, Honey? I just have to get through this."

When Suanne would talk to me like that, my eyes would fill with tears of anguish and joy, and I would wish that I could take all of her pain, all of her fears, every malignant cell that had ever been in her body and every form of medical treatment she had received and substitute myself in her place. I would also remember and revisit every violation of her trust and her love that I had ever engaged in, and want to again, beg for forgiveness and absolution.

The gift of true love is so sweet, so rare. And when accompanied by such commitment and devotion as Suanne showed unremittingly and unstintingly throughout our marriage, it is a treasure beyond compare. She was so patient for so long; seeing me through my poet years, my warrior years, my cowboy years; suffering through an immaturity that dogged me well into adulthood. How could I even think the thoughts that plagued my nocturnal mind? But these thoughts, I knew, were only the prattling of idle neurons and synapses basted perhaps with the residual testosterone of a middle age man, suffering through the conjugal absence of his mate. Her midnight voice on these occasions was like a welcome summer breeze - mollifying, soothing, and consoling:

Welcome sweet sweet magic,

Summer breeze,

Moonlight and afterglo,

From a star, reflecting reflecting,

From so far yet so near, my pulse,

Deliberate and halting,

From wrinkled time,

To stand alone and give,

In truth together,

From me to you, this only moment.

"Yes, honey. I can wait. I can wait as long as it takes and longer still. I love you so."

CHAPTER 27
Radiation Therapy: Week Five

July 26, 1996

Five down, one to go - the end was in sight. I almost felt as if it had been I and not Suanne who was racing against time and now the finish-line was coming into view. Howard had called me Thursday night with a surf report of eight to ten-foot waves from a south swell hitting the coast. Enough said; we had an epic two hour session at the Hook. But notwithstanding the great surf, the day didn't start out well.

When we awoke on Friday morning huge headlines in the morning papers screamed "HORROR IN ATLANTA." A massive explosion rocked Centennial Olympic Park at 1:15 a.m., the work of a terrorist. Four people were reported killed, scores injured. One witness reported that "There were rivers of blood."

At the end of week five, when Suanne came into my office, I could see once again that she was feeling the pain and stress of the radiation therapy. "Rough day?" I asked.

"Yes," she responded drearily, "today when I was getting my blood work done at Dr. Shapiro's office before the radiation appointment, there was a young woman and her husband there for her chemotherapy. I hadn't seen them before. Even in her condition, with no make-up on, she was so beautiful. She had pale blue eyes, beautiful high cheekbones and a strong chin. She was wearing a baseball cap, but I could see that she had almost no hair. Her husband sat very close to her, almost as if he was propping her up. The whole time they were in the waiting room, she sat motionless with her head leaning against his chest staring off into space.

He had a look on his face that reminded me of the way Jerry (our eldest son) looked after his dog got run over when he was a little boy. I think, she's John's client; you know the one that had the mammogram that was placed in

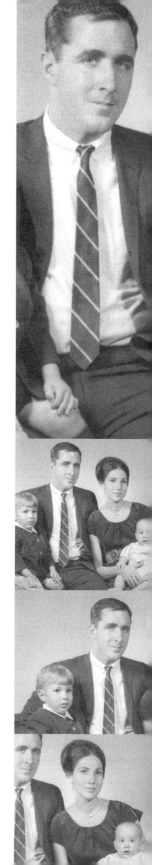

the wrong file and not read and they didn't find the cancer until over a year later." Suanne's voice began trailing off, then stopped. She leaned over, her elbows resting on her knees and buried her face in hands and sobbed. "Give me some Kleenex, please," she finally said. Tears rained down her cheeks.

I knew exactly whom Suanne was talking about. She was a neighbor and client of a lawyer who is a good friend of ours. About two and a half years ago this young woman had gone to her Ob/Gyn for her annual check-up, and because there was a strong family history of breast cancer, she had begun having mammograms, even though she was still in her thirties.

On the occasion of this mammogram, mistakes were made. Mistakes are a fact of life and can happen for reasons as simple as the violation of an office procedure or as complicated as failing to distinguish between shades of gray on the film, but the results of the mistakes can be catastrophic either way, as they were in this tragic case. I learned that the mammogram of this young woman somehow ended up in the wrong file and didn't get read.

Shortly after the misfiled mammogram incident she had become pregnant with their second child. After the deliverery she had a routine post-partum checkup including a mammogram. This time the mammogram was suspicious for malignant lumps in both breasts. Follow-up surgical exploration confirmed the malignancies and her lymph nodes showed extensive invasion on both sides by the breast cancer and distant metastasis in her brain and bones. When the doctor sought to retrieve the earlier mammograms for comparison, they were not in her chart. It was then that they discovered the earlier mammograms had either been misfiled or misplaced without having been read at all.

Upon review, the earlier mammograms showed a suspicious lump of approx-imately one centimeter in the left breast. The right breast was clear in those films. Even at her young age, assuming no lymph node involvement, on the TNM scale this would have been a Stage I tumor with an excellent prognosis for long term disease free survival. When it was found it was a stage IV, meaning virtually no chance of long term survival. Although errors of this nature are rare, they do occur, and in this woman's case, the price was the death of a young mother, a wife, a daughter and a sibling.

While the most common forms of breast cancer are very slow growing, sometimes taking decades before they can be detected, some forms are highly virulent and aggressive, and can multiply rapidly and metastasize within a few short months. As I alluded to at the outset (regarding Mendy, our neighbor's daughter-in-law), breast cancer in younger women can be much worse and much more difficult to treat than in older women.

To begin with, tumors in young breasts are more difficult to diagnose both by mammogram and physical examination. This is due mainly to the density of the breast tissue in young women. Left undiagnosed and untreated for even a short period of time, metastatic breast cancer in young women can be a death knell, as it proved to be for John's young client who was dead within eighteen months of her diagnosis. Her youngest child was still nursing when she was scheduled for her bilateral mastectomy.

When Suanne regained her composure, I knelt in front of her chair and let her rest her head on my shoulder. She whispered, almost as if talking to herself, "If we had not gone to see Ellen after the radiologist said my mammogram was negative, I would be in the same condition that young woman is in. I would never see Joshua throw a baseball again, I wouldn't be there to see him and graduate from high school and college. I wouldn't be able watch our grandchildren grow up. We wouldn't grow old together. I would've left you alone in our home."

"I know, I know," I said, "but you did go to see Ellen and we caught it in time. Everything is going to be fine. Everything is going to be fine. I promise, Honey; I promise. Let's go to a movie tonight, okay?" God, I hoped and prayed and willed it to be so with every ounce and fiber of my being.

The fact is that mistakes are made all the time by medical professionals. Lawyers in the business of suing doctors, hospitals and other health care providers, are a remedy of last resort when these mistakes are made.

It is equally true that the remedies provided by the legal system for medical mistakes are a very poor substitute for proper care. In June I went to trial on Doug Yancy's quadriplegia lawsuit which serves as a case-in-point. As noted earlier, Doug was partially disabled prior to his auto accident by a condition in his neck known as ankylosing spondylitis, a condition wherein the disks in the neck degenerate, calcify and the vertebral bodies get very brittle and fuse together.

Despite the handicap, Doug was able to function well as a small engine mechanic earning enough money to support his very modest lifestyle. Of course, after becoming a C-7 quad, he couldn't do anything; not even sit beside a lake and hold a fishing rod. The popular perception is that such an injury would be compensated handsomely by a jury. Not so.

In California (and 35 other states), we have tort reform laws to shield and protect health care providers from the consequences of their negligence. California's law is known as MICRA, the Medical Injury Compensation Recovery Act. The act was passed in the aftermath of the so called "medical malpractice insurance crisis" of the mid-seventies. During this period the medical establishment, aided and abetted by its confederates (I'll refrain from the use of the term "partners-in-crime"), was able to persuade the California legislature that if they did not implement measures to protect health care providers from trial lawyers, the medical malpractice insurance carriers would all leave California and there would be no medical care to speak of.**42** In other words, no insurance or unaffordable insurance, no doctors. Swayed by powerful lobbying (and a larding of politicians' warchests), the legislature obliged by passing a whole package of very brilliantly crafted measures to protect the doctors and other health care providers from their own negligent acts.

First, to reduce the incentives for lawyers representing injured patients they restricted the attorney fees down to an amount that would make it unprofitable to take serious cases like Doug Yancy's. Then they restricted the amount of damages that could be recovered by the client to further discourage representation.

In Doug's case, as in all medical injury cases in California, the maximum he could recover for his quadriplegia was the $250,000 cap put on non-economic damages in 1975. And because the $250,000 cap was the amount that was set in 1975 and because it still obtains in 1996, the real amount Doug could recover in terms of purchasing power of 1975 dollars was more like $92,000. What isn't restricted is loss of earnings and future medical care which obviously goes right back to the doctors and hospitals that Doug and others like him require due the malpractice committed on him in the first place. Then, to top things off, the defendant in a medical malpractice case can elect to have his or her insurer pay out any award in periodic payments over the life expectancy of the plaintiff. This enables the insurance carriers to keep the money invested in their portfolios and pay the plaintiff out of their dividends or interest. Nothing short of a legislative tour de force. You really have to tip your cap to the success of their Machiavellian, self-serving machinations. Few do a better job of it than they do.

We showed up for trial in Doug's case, and as often times happens in a case of clear negligence on the part of the defendant, a settlement was reached at the eleventh hour, just prior to picking a jury. Of course, by that time we had spent tens of thousands of dollars on expert witness testimony and the defense attorneys had milked the case for all it was worth.

What Doug received in the settlement was just about enough to enable him to pay for his own medical care and the necessities of life without going on the

---

42 - In reality what was actually happening was that the medical malpractice premiums paid by doctors to their insurance carriers had been invested in the stock market and between 1971 and 1975 we had been in a very strong bear market. Millions, if not billions of dollars in stock portfolios had been lost. Compared to these losses, the payouts for jury verdicts were hardly even a drop in the bucket. But scapegoating trial lawyers was a clever way to scare both the Califronia legislature and the public into carving out special treatment for some of the most privileged member of society. And, of course, at the expense of some of the weakest and most needy member of society, they were successful.

public dole. A much simpler solution would have been for the health care providers to follow their own protocols and keep Doug in C-spine precautions as an inpatient in the hospital instead of sending him home with instructions to stay off work for a week. Whatever rationalizing supports such a system is difficult to fathom, particularly for the poor victims of such negligence like Doug Yancy.

That night we went to see the movie, *A Time To Kill,* based on the novel by John Grisham.

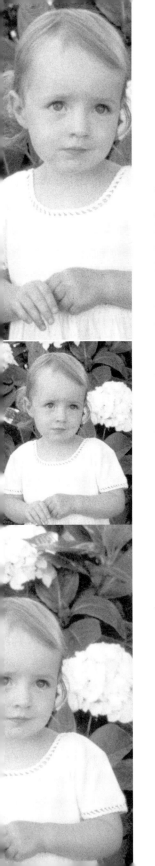

CHAPTER 28
Week Six of Radiation Therapy

Friday August 9, 1996

In the last week of Suanne's regular radiation treatments the Atlanta Olympic games ended with the United States garnering 110 metals and the jury, in the penalty phase of Richard Allen Davis' murder trial, ignored pleas of a troubled childhood and sentenced Davis to death for the killing of Polly Klass. Dr. Mann had said that she would be getting a "booster" for five days next week, and then our summer of radiation oncology treatment would be over. As the cliché says: All good things come to those that wait.

Booster treatments differ from regular radiation therapy in two ways. First, a different type of radiation beam is used. In Suanne's case her regular radiation therapy was done by a machine called a linear accelerator that produced a beam of electron radiation directed at the general area where the cancer had been. This beam is deep penetrating and passes through the area of treatment. The booster consists of higher energy radiation treatments aimed at the precise area where the lump was removed (including the scar tissue) and usually uses a different type of beam that has only shallow penetration.[43] We were counting the days. It was appropriate that the battle, if not the war, would be ending in August.

Jerry, our first-born, was delivered on August 6th. Jimmy came two years later on August 9th. We called them our atom bomb babies. Joshua, our youngest was born seventeen years and twenty days after our oldest, delaying our empty nest for an additional sixteen years or so. Both

43 - When breast irradiation first started, no one knew how much radiation was needed to kill any remaining tumor cells after the original lump was removed. It was known, however, that the entire breast could not well tolerate more than about 5000 rads, and that microscopic deposits of tumor in other areas of the body were destroyed at a higher rate with 6000 rads than 5000 rads. Moreover, the breast location that had the highest chance of tumor recurrence was at the site of the original tumor. Therefore it made sense to give an extra or "boost" dose of an additional 1000 to 1500 rads to the area of the scar after the entire breast received 4500-5000 rads. this was originally delivered inserting radioactive material into the breast a the site of the original tumor. Subsequently this was replaced by external beam radiation in the form of electrons or x-rays. It has never been determined for sure if the boost is really needed, and the most recent consensus from experts from all over the country gathered at the National Cancer Institute is that the boost may or may not be given. **SM**

our older boys were married in August. My mother and our first grandson and granddaughter were born in August. So as a matter of course, we do a lot of celebrating in August; but in August of this year, the celebrations were the best we had ever known.

Every blessed event, every troth of love, faith and hope, every smile, every peel of laughter, every tear of joy, was like a magnificent celebration in itself. My mom and dad were there, still in love after 58 years of marriage, and presiding over a brood of one son and a daughter-in-law, three grandsons, two granddaughter-in-laws, and three great grandsons. And at the center of all of our celebrating this year was Suanne. She was the rock and mortar, the foundation upon which our family was built, something everybody knew and acknowledged.

My feelings were that not only had we won the battle, but also the war. From the warm spring afternoon back in May when I was rowing upstream against my river of tears on Highway 152, until Suanne's last radiation treatment on August 13th, we had experienced almost every shade and degree of emotion imaginable. We had felt the anxiety and fear of finding her lump; the disappointment and frustration of being left in limbo by her Ob/Gyn and radiologist, and the sheer terror and panic of learning that she had breast cancer. We had felt the rebirth of faith and hope engendered by Dr. Mahoney and the pathology report following her lumpectomy surgery. And, we had felt the thrill of a hard fought victory at the conclusion of the radiation therapy.

With the exceptions as noted, we believed we had been the beneficiaries of the best, most personal and most caring medical treatment possible. By August we believed that the muses of medical fortune had smiled on us at every critical turn.

My metaphorical glass had always been half full, but with the conclusion, no the euphoric apotheosis, of Suanne's treatment and absolutely nothing to impeach Ellen Mahoney's bold and confident prediction of a complete cure, my cup now, truly runneth over. It was as if some whimsical mystical phantom had descended upon our lives to protect and reward Suanne for all her goodness, her caring, her patience, and her love. As our month of celebrations began, it was almost as if the whole breast cancer experience had been a dream:

A dream?
Whimsical mystical phantom,
Drifting to and fro, between eternities,
It was long ago,
Before your life, and mine,

That we met in a dream,
Whimsical mystical phantom that you are,
I touch your hand,
I look into your eyes,
I see you, and you me,
And Spring echoes back, into the mystery,
We are of the oceans and the seas,
The air above, the land below,
Dream on...

CHAPTER 29
Reflections

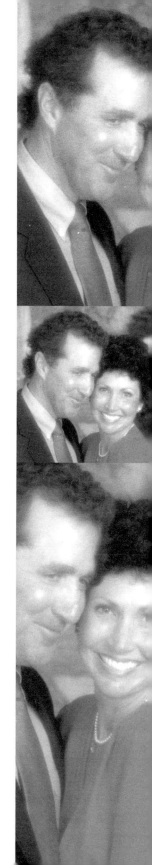

October 10, 1996

With the passage of time, even when counted in the days and weeks following the end of radiation therapy, the all-consuming role of breast cancer slowly began to subside from the high water mark that it had reached in our lives during the daily radiation treatments.

For three seasons, nine months, thirty-nine weeks, 273 days, or 6,552 hours, not a minute had gone by without thinking about what frightful changes the future might hold in store for us. Now, in fewer than 180 days after the confirmed diagnosis of breast cancer, we were left with the challenge of overcoming our still troubling, still persisting fears that the truth of a complete cure - as Dr. Mahoney had predicted so early, might be no more than wishful thinking. Not infrequently did we have to pinch ourselves mentally, while musing "Are we back in Kansas yet?" While the fears are very real and justified, it was not a difficult adjustment.

Not unlike the ease with which any of us can end up at the bottom of the proverbial slippery slope by agreeing to a false premise (or false promise), so too do we all have this wonderful capacity to reach out so far as is necessary in order to embrace that which we want to be true. And when the protocols of peer group validation sprinkled its holy water over the prognosis of a complete cure, we were true believers of the first order.

My birthday afforded a perfect opportunity to celebrate our good fortune. I was excited about the evening. Even getting ready was a smorgasbord of long neglected fantasy delights. For the past nine months, even thinking about eroticism in connection with my wife's breasts seemed unbecoming. I had sorely missed my fantasies.

Suanne was finishing putting on her makeup as I stood in front of the mirror shaving. We talked about the little 12 year old kid that insured Derrick Jeter of a home run in game one of the American League Championship Series between the Yankees and the Orioles. Funny how peculiar little unpredictable acts can dictate the outcome of great events. The Orioles would have won the game and perhaps the World Series if that kid hadn't stuck his glove out over the right fielders glove and snagged the ball. The polls had Clinton leading in 44 states with 339 Electoral College votes, with less than four weeks to go. No surprise (or excitement) there.

I didn't know what Suanne might be planning on wearing, but I was more than a little interested. I allowed my mind to stroll, and perhaps revert, among the unforgotten gardens of my erotic reveries. I wondered if she might be thinking of wearing something to my prurient liking.

Her closet was full of delicate little articles of finery, including very sheer blouses that I had bought her over the years for birthday gifts, anniversary presents and even mother's day tributes. Truth be told however, in reality, they were all as much articles of personal self-indulgence as they were presents for her.

From this collection, my most favorites were the ones that were so revealing that with very little imagination, I could have an almost unobstructed view of her breasts in their most delicious detail. On this evening, however, I suffered from no delusions that she would be putting her breasts on display over dinner for my visual consumption. But no (and alas), I rather expected that she would choose to wear something more appropriate and, shall we say, "decorous." I actually upbraided myself - a little bit - for the salacious thoughts. I looked myself in the eye while finishing shaving and thought about the expectations that I had placed on Suanne for so long and the pronounced role her breasts played in our sexual conventions and protocols.

What I saw in the mirror was a man who allowed his self-indulgence and selfishness in the sexual arena to distort all too many aspects of his relationship with a woman that had demonstrated the greatest commitment and success imaginable in her respective roles as wife, mother, friend and business partner.

Demands of any sort can be oppressive, and sexual demands, stated or not and no matter how they are sugar coated, packaged or presented, can be extraordinarily oppressive. Most of the time we (meaning men in general) recognize it, but manage to ignore the better angels of our nature when they tell us things we don't want to hear. I was now trying to listen.

I saw a man in the mirror that while considering himself sensitive to and even intuitive about other's sensibilities, had too often burdened the relationship with his wife with selfish, sometimes immature, perhaps by some account even abusive sexual expectations. In light of the current circumstances, no matter how much I tried to deny it, what had once seemed natural and even expected, now struck me as crude, vulgar and primitive. Without saying it at the time, I felt embarrassed, maybe even ashamed.

Don't misunderstand me now. I am not recanting my particular sexual fixations, desires or even my consuming appreciation of breasts and the fantasies involving breasts that I (and most men, I dare say) so enjoy. God help me the day I go that far. What I am saying, however, is that as a man, I should be man enough to listen, to hear, and to care about and consider the thoughts and feelings and sensibilities of my wife in dealing with my own sexual desires and fantasies. Perhaps what I'm really addressing is the general tendency of some males (myself included, for certain), to allow the encoded messages from our testosterone to overcome even the most rational and understandable of conventions of dignity and self-respect. I'm not saying that the penetration of male fantasies, however slight, into a woman's sensibilities amounts to psycho-logical rape. In this arena, like most others, it's a two-way street. But in the process of going through my experience as a breast cancer husband, the parallels between my sexual expectations and unwelcome demands were coming ever-sharper into focus. I'm hardly interested in mimicking the dogs on the beach that are totally dominated by the neuronal pathway between their olfactory faculties and their gonads, and I wish I could have recognized that unsavory part of me earlier in my life. Suanne deserved it. The boys deserved it. Maybe even I deserved it.

But recognizing the error of my ways and mending them are two different matters. I finished shaving and got dressed, unable to shake my feeling of self-reproach. This would not do for an evening of celebration. I sat down on the bed and watched in the mirror as Suanne finished dressing. I tried to put myself in her shoes.

Here was a woman who had spent the prior nine months in the maws of a deadly killer. During the entire time, I doubt more than mere moments passed when she did not entertain terrifying thoughts of what fate might hold in store for her. Some might say that because of her age and the remarkably early detection, she shouldn't have really been so distressed. And, of course, the five percent of women who fall into Suanne's profile and die from breast cancer would vehemently disagree.

Suanne had been completely immersed in a massive, coordinated, and multi-faceted medical counterattack on the malignant cells that had invaded her body. And here she was now, barely finished with repulsing the assault, and already returning to her many and demanding roles as business manager, legal assistant, receptionist, bookkeeper, housekeeper, cook, wife, lover, confidant, mother and friend. All this without the benefit of a single night of uninterrupted sleep, a nagging emotional malaise and an unwelcome weight gain that she seemed powerless to do anything about.

Suanne put on an elegant Eileen Fisher dress I had bought her for a birthday present, but one that she had picked out. The distinction being that she had a more shall I say, "holistic" view of how the dress would look than I did. She looked radiant, beautiful and full of her indomitable, indivisible feminine mystique. Usually the word "radiant" is reserved for describing brides on their wedding day, but tonight Suanne looked - and hopefully felt - radiant.

I felt a compelling need to find answers or at least address a whole panoply of questions about my own experience with breast cancer and how it was now affecting me and my relationship with both the real and my very frisky fantasies of my wife. As I pulled out of our driveway for the short drive to the restaurant, instead of diving into my birthday celebration my mind was bestirred by a jumble of questions fairly screaming for answers.

The sweep of male responses to breast cancer in a spouse, no doubt, runs wide and deep, just as does the male psyche's response to gender issues in general. It admits of no doubt that there are many men who see women in terms of being nothing more than objects of sexual gratification. Take away the "tits and ass" and there is nothing left of any perceived intrinsic value to this type of man - not unlike the example I gave earlier of a male dog chasing a bitch in heat down the beach. As soon as the male exhausts himself and/or the female's heat is over, the male goes back to eating, sleeping, belching and channel-surfing, awaiting only the arrival of the next anonymous bitch in heat to come trotting along to plunk his magic twanger.

Lest there be some doubt as to the application of this description to segments of contemporary male society, one need only to listen to the unvarnished talk of men in fraternal societies, hear our complaints about women, or listen to our jokes. One such joke that comes to mind here, which I will quote verbatim by way of example, is the following: "Why did God create tits?" The answer has something to do with auto-eroticism and one of the options men have for what to do with idle hands. This by itself would be convincing enough, even if much of it is only half-serious.

Likewise, it also admits of no doubt that there are men (I like to think that I can honestly now count myself among them), that love and respect their wives for reasons that include a healthy sexual relationship, but extend far beyond the purely physical. I like to think that most men understand and respect their vows when asked: "Do you take this woman to be your lawful wedded wife, for all seasons, for all reasons; for richer, for poorer; in sickness and in health? Do you promise to love, protect, honor and respect her, from this day forward, until death do you part?" However, such belief in and respect for these vows in many men, is but a conscious veneer, camouflaging the capacity of the male human animal to revert to his more primal instincts under the right circumstances. The conditions giving rise to these instincts in even the best of husbands, are not hard to fathom.

I recall having discussions with more than one or two of my close friends when we were young (twenties and thirties), over a hypothetical question that goes something like this: You're out of town on a business trip staying in a hotel in a city where nobody knows you. After dinner you go into the hotel bar and sit down in one of the few seats available to have a drink. As it turns out there is this totally gorgeous babe sitting next to you who is happily married (discrete), a gynecologist (safe), and displays an enthusiastic interest in almost every topic of conversation you come up with, including, you learn after a few drinks, most of your mutually inclusive sexual fantasies. (Hello? Is this heaven?)

In short, this hypothetical circumstance presents the ideal opportunity for the perfect assignation. The question is not whether you'd take Dr. Perfect One-Nighter up to your hotel room and indulge your erotic fantasies, but rather if there are any circumstances you can think of that would prevent you from doing so. Needless to say, short of Dr. Perfect being a transvestite, none of us could come up with any realistic answers why we wouldn't take advantage of this opportunity. Okay, so it references the absurd to prove the obvious, but it doesn't mean that the decision may not come back to bite you. Dealing with your wife's breast cancer or any number of other personal tragedies, is a case in point.

The experience of having your wife suffer through the ordeal of breast cancer challenges a man to ask himself a multitude of very revealing and difficult questions about himself. For example, is the vow of fidelity the same as the vow concerning keeping her, "...in sickness and in health." And if you treat the vows differently, or to use a popular adjective, "situationally," why should you? Can a man or a woman for that matter, choose which vow/ethic to follow and which not to follow? On this occasion I'll heed this vow and on that occasion I won't?

When breast cancer appears on the scene, the distinctions between the vow relating to fidelity and the one on sickness and health can become blurred. Some men react with honor and virtue when their wife becomes sick with breast cancer or other maladies, and others react like barbarians or the dogs on the beach. However, because breast cancer deals with a part of the female anatomy that is intrinsic to the survival instinct and the sexual stimulus-response mechanism, a tangled, even barbaric response to the threat presented by breast cancer cannot simply be dismissed and ridiculed. After all, the encoded messages are exactly that; encoded!

The human male's neuro-biological attributes have evolved (not necessarily refined), over millions of years and cannot be eradicated overnight simply because somebody etches in contemporary stone that such instincts are "politically incorrect."

To believe instinctual sexual responses can be casually manipulated or are limited to some salacious minority of men, I believe, to be plainly and patently mistaken. These instinctual reactions exist in all of us males; at least all of us with a healthy complement of testosterone and normal neural reactions. There is no way that I can recount the multiplicity of complicated, contradictory, unsavory, and primitive thoughts I have entertained on this subject during my own breast cancer experience, particularly during the early waiting periods. All I can say about such meditations is that they came and, thankfully, they went. And I do not intend to offer any judgments on how every man, or any man, should deal with the threats posed by breast cancer, or any other major trauma, in someone you love. Rather, I should like to suggest that every man might want to think about is what certain responses say about who and what we are as individuals, and as men.

What kind of man, for example, would, if he could, trade his wife's breast cancer and the threat of a mastectomy, for, say, bone cancer requiring the amputation of a leg, or spinal cord cancer resulting in quadriplegia, or some other disease resulting in blindness? Few to none of us would admit to such a choice. What kind of man would leave his wife because of breast cancer and/or a mastectomy? Untold thousands have and many more will, but in the abstract, few would like to admit that we might end up in that category. How many men view a woman with breast cancer, or more graphically, a woman that has had a mastectomy, as a freak, a mutant, a pariah, to be shunned or discarded? More than we might think? Finally, how many husbands of wives with breast cancer undertake to walk the proverbial mile in the emotional and psychological moccasins of their stricken partners? Hopefully, many. Whatever the response of the individual might be, a healthy dose of introspection and contemplation of the bonds between husband and wife will help the breast cancer husband get through the ordeal. And I use the word "ordeal" advisedly. Actually, it's more like hell.

One of the first things I observed in Suanne after being diagnosed with breast cancer was a profound feeling of betrayal and failure by her own body. She had done just about everything that could be asked of her to fend off cancer, all seemingly to no avail. The fact that she had a good prognosis at first seemed to have little effect on her mood. With her sense of physiological betrayal came a withdrawal from her enjoyment of her physical and sensual self; an enjoyment that, naturally, had always been to some degree influenced and impacted by her breasts.

After the positive diagnosis was made, it was almost as if every aspect of our past and present sexual relations that involved her breasts, from the way she dressed (or the way I liked her to dress), to our foreplay, was a harsh reminder of the failure of her body to resist cancer and the threat that the mammary organs pose to every woman.

With Suanne's withdrawal from the sensuality and eroticism that had been a mutually exciting lifelong fixture in our sexual relationship, I found my myself falling in step with her. For a time, I believed that showing even the slightest hint of interest in sex might be interpreted by her as a reminder of the deadly disease that was growing in her breast. It is not hard to imagine that in some couples such reciprocating negativity or stress will lead to alienation, antagonism, and hostility. Then comes blame. Thankfully, Suanne and I have the type of relationship that has always permitted us to communicate on just about any topic, including our emotional and intellectual responses to our withdrawal from our normal sexual relationship, and I had little trouble understanding that her feelings of betrayal was a normal response that we both needed to deal with.

Compounding the problem of Suanne's sense of betrayal was the fact that her surgeon had taken her off of the hormone replacement therapy immediately after the breast cancer diagnosis had been made. This occurred at the time of life when menopause was dealing Suanne "Everywoman's" down-and-dirty-middle-age hand (like a cruel double-whammy, breast cancer appears in most women contemporaneously with menopause).

Then there were the surgeries, the attendant scarring, and the side effects of her lymph node surgery, radiation, and the relentless kapow of the tamoxifen therapy. I tried to think of what it would be like to experience such an assault on so many fronts at once. I had only one experience of a sufficiently similar nature to draw upon with any degree of confidence.

At the age of forty-four, during one of the biggest trials of my career and one of the longest civil trials in the history of California, I awoke one morning with a sharp pain in my abdomen. I called a physician friend who came to my house at about 6:30 a.m. and examined me (obviously a close friend). He immediately recommended that Suanne take me to the emergency room for a complete physical examination. I thought about just toughing it out and going to work, but he convinced me that I might be suffering from appendicitis.

Up to that point in my life the only surgeries I had ever had were for various common sports injuries and a couple of minor traumatic amputations of digits that I suffered in my cowboy days from bulldogging and dally roping. I had emergency surgery that morning for a ruptured colon caused by diverticulitis (infection of the lining of the colon that can and often times results in a rupture of the colon). Bowel matter had been leaking into my peritoneal cavity for hours during the night and by the time they opened me up I had peritonitis so bad that I was literally minutes away from full blown septic shock. In more lay terms, what I had was fecal matter leaking from a hole in my gut into my stomach cavity where a massive infection was being spawned. Peritonitis can quickly lead to septicemia (where the infection gets into the blood stream and spreads throughout the body). Needlessly to say, the operation I underwent was much more complicated than the originally contemplated.

The removal of a foot and a half of my colon necessitated the installation of a colostomy bag. A colostomy is the procedure wherein bowel matter is diverted from the colon and rectum (the lower GI track), into a bag that hangs on the left side of the stomach just about at the level of the belly button. The colostomy bag, while not clear, is opaque. Although hermetically sealed, it does not prevent all odor from escaping. Sometimes the colostomy can be reversed by reconnecting the lower part of the colon with the upper part. Sometimes it cannot be reversed and you have to wear the bag for the rest of your life. So for several weeks I didn't know if my colostomy bag was going to be a permanent accessory or not.

After recovering from the colostomy surgery, to the extent that my libido was able to recover, I struggled with all the psychological insecurities that I imagined anyone, including Suanne, would have about having intimate relations with someone who was sporting, literally, a bag of shit on his stomach. The psycho-logical impact was paralyzing. I did not get over that feeling of sexual paralysis until late one night three weeks after I got out of the hospital when Suanne, gently and with great sensitivity, showed me that I was not that colostomy bag, but rather, her companion and partner in life, her best friend, and her emotional and sexual lover, regardless of whether I was wearing that bag or not. It was like being rescued from a pitiless psychological maelstrom in the middle of a dark and frozen sea by some beautiful shining angel - my wife.

My memories of the night that Suanne calmed the psychological torment created by what turned out to be a temporary colostomy bag, came back to me time and time again when I was being plagued with my own frightening thoughts about her breast cancer diagnosis. Suanne was not only the princess of my adolescent dreams and the object of my erotic fantasies, she is the mother of our children, the matron of the hearth upon which we had always placed our hopes and dreams for the future. She is the rock upon which we built our family and our life. In sickness and in health, it was she and she alone who wiped away our tears, exalted in our victories, kept the candle lit in the window during stormy nights, and loved me completely, passionately, and without reservation, in all seasons, in good times and bad, without and with my colostomy bag. What, I wondered over and over again during the darkest hours of my experience as a breast cancer husband, what would life be like without her?

For starters, there would be no one with whom to share all of our memories. Who would I laugh and cry with at Joshua's marriage, our grandchildren's births and birthdays, and our parents' funerals. How could I write my poems to a stranger who had never read a single road sign on the path of my life? How would I ever create another family album like the one Suanne and I created together since our teenage years? Who else could I invest a lifetime of love in? The answer: No one. I knew this was true, because I realized long before Suanne was afflicted with breast cancer that the very air I breathe is permeated with the oneness of who we are as individuals.

From the time I awake until the last image of my day fades away, the sounds, the colors, the smells and the tastes of my life are infused with Suanne. Would I love her less if she changed her hair color? Would my commitment be less if she had a toe or two or a foot amputated? No, of course, not. Do I love her more now than before she was diagnosed with breast cancer. Actually, I believe I do. Not because I understand her any better, mind you, but because I now know and understand myself a little better...as a mate and as a man.

I believe this is true because the experience has given me the opportunity to think about a lot of things that I never really considered before, at least not with the degree of concentration and duration that I have now given. A lot of the things I have thought about, as suggested at the outset, had to do with my selfishness and the stress I had caused in Suanne's life pursuing my own adventures and conquests.

The studies seem to be coming in every day verifying that stress is a major risk factor in how the body's autoimmune system deals with disease in general and the mutations that cause breast cancer. What if I contributed to Suanne's breast cancer? Not a pleasant thought.

Over my birthday dinner that night I reached across the table and took Suanne's hand in mine and drew it to me. I turned her hand palm up and kissed it gently. We then picked up our glasses and I toasted her with the following: "To being together, to feeling love, to our health, and to the anticipation of tomorrow." We softly touched our glasses together and drank long and deep.

CHAPTER 30
Getting Back To Normal

January 15, 1997.

The fall of 1996 turned to winter and suddenly a new year was upon us. Clinton was reelected and the Patriots and Packers are in the Super Bowl. For us, the year of 1996 had brought victory; the war it seems, had been won.

Yes, I was aware, "intellectually," that fifteen to twenty percent of breast cancer patients have recurrences within two to three years, but these statistics are for a much broader range of patients than Suanne and her cohort. They included, for example, larger tumors at the time of detection, patients with positive lymph nodes, and much younger women with more aggressive tumors.

On this, the first anniversary of our breast cancer experience, I totally believed Dr. Mahoney's way-back-when prognosis when she said that Suanne had a 95 percent chance of a full life expectancy.[44] As far as I was concerned, the tumor had been completely self-contained and no cells had escaped outside the primary site. The radiation and the tamoxifen were prudent, precautionary and prophylactic measures to insure our victory.

But, as I have said repeatedly, it was not I that had been diagnosed with a life-threatening disease. Nor was it I who was declared at risk for a local recurrence of the disease in the same breast, the opposite breast, or a distant metastasis in just about any other part of Suanne's body, even if the risk was only five percent. No, I was not the patient. Champion and advocate, yes, but still not the patient. The undeniable truth remains that to this day there is still no cure for cancer in any form.

Breast cancer is "cured," in the sense of the word used by Dr. Mahoney, by way of a) detecting it early, and b) surgically removing it before it spreads. But now, my mind allows me to embrace conclusions consistent with my hopes and the optimistic spin we all like to put on colorably

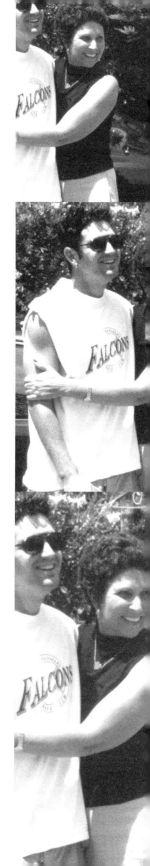

---

44 - In practical terms, what this means is that Suanne will die from a cause other than breast cancer. The life expectancy table for a 51 year old white female in 1996 was approximately 34 years.

favorable but possibly equivocal evidence. I also happen to believe in the theory that optimism is the foundation upon which is built the self-fulfilling prophecy of good fortune.

For Suanne, even though she denies subconsciously massaging the site of her lumpectomy scar whenever sitting in front of the TV without her beloved needlework in her hands, I know that the dark thought of a recurrence of her breast cancer always lurks nearby with only a microscopically thin coat of psychological gloss walling it off from her conscious mind. Regardless of the size of the tumor, early detection, age of discovery or rosy prognosis, the threat of recurrence of breast cancer does not fade quickly away like a bad dream.

The daily obituary columns, news reports of new cancer studies, fund raisers, and the like will likely rekindle some understandable if modest anxiety in Suanne, but nothing that she cannot handle. Of course, contributing to her return to normalcy is the welcome drop in what had been a long parade of doctor appointments, tests, monitoring and therapy.

We estimated that by the time of her last appointment for radiation therapy, Suanne had attended (more accurately, "subjected to") over 80 medical visits in a six month period. That translates into one visit every one and a half work days. Each and every appointment was a stark reminder of the gravity of the threat posed by breast cancer. With the cessation of weekly or even monthly medical appointments, Suanne's mind was turned lose to wander about in greener pastures; pastures in which she could plan on pursuits involving home, family, friends, me, and a future we could look forward to sharing together with confidence. And, a future in which she didn't have to show her breasts to just about every stranger she shook hands with. But some things had not returned to what had been normal for us.

New Year's Eve had not been a particularly big deal for us for a number of years, or since the thrill of self-abusive partying began paying less than cathartic dividends, but we did have a quasi-custom of starting off every new years with an intimate dinner and a rapturous love making session. And no, contrary to what most teenagers and twenty and thirty-somethings think, a regular, fulfilling, even raucous sex life doesn't crash on the rocks and shoals of middle age or grandparenthood. But there is no doubt that one of the active ingredients of a vigorous and active sex life is a positive self image as a sexually attractive and desirable partner who maintains a certain gusto and enjoyment of sex.

As previously suggested, Suanne's self-image had taken a big hit throughout the treatment period. Pain, scarring, swelling, radiation, fatigue, weight gain and the emotional distress attendant with a life-threatening disease are not catalysts for an alluring, sensual self image, and particularly when the situs of the disease was her breasts. But of equal or even greater impact was the termination of the HRT or hormone replacement therapy. It's no accident that my faithful canine companion Rufus, once neutered, barely had the desire to sniff the air when a bitch in estrus came frolicking by. Likewise, it's no head-scratcher, that once spayed, Trinka, the female, once spade can't get a rise from even the most promiscuous of her would be male suitors.

Fact: When the production of human sex hormones declines to a certain point or is "cut off" so to speak, as in the case of the medical necessity of terminating HRT due to an estrogen and progesterone receptive cancerous cell, all of the benefits associated with the HRT therapy are shut down accordingly. The combination of all of these events in Suanne's fifty-first year had the immediate effect of a psychological clear cutting in the sexual area.

Feeling trapped between Scylla and Charybdis, I was at a loss how best to respond, or frankly, whether to respond at all. (Don't even go there," I would tell myself time and time again.).

For eons, men have treated the symptoms of menopause (the period of a woman's life typically beginning in their forties and early fifties when the ovaries commence a steady decline in the production of estrogen and progesterone), as everything from feigned to exaggerated to manufactured. Even today, I suspect, most men have a difficult time understanding and certainly dealing with the mood swings, depression, hot flashes, diminished libido and other emotional and physiological symptoms that are precipitated by the withdrawal of estrogen from a woman's body during menopause. For the most part, I believe men's difficulty in dealing with menopause results not from emotional estrangement from their wives, but rather from ignorance about it cause and effects. Here again, I suspect it's a case of the male choosing not to know, because to know might mean having to change his attitude, his behavior, perhaps even his entire belief system. Many men, perhaps more than any of us think, cannot handle this. Thus, it's a situation of "ignorance is bliss." Only it isn't. Ignorance come at a great price, to the man, to the woman, to the couple and to the family. As all of us learned, or were told, at an early age, sex (and sexiness) lies more in the head than in the loins.

For me, New Year's Eve brought to a head some of my own frustrations in dealing with the complex amalgamation of factors that had been bearing down on both of us for the past year. But, before getting into the events of the occasion, perhaps a little history is in order.

Before breast cancer (fittingly "BC"), Suanne and I enjoyed what would described as a normal, healthy and fulfilling sexual relationship. Our love making was warm and intimate, at times exciting, and if I may say so (please pardon the hyperbole), on occasion, even symphonic (seldom, if ever would I describe it as perfunctory or mechanical). With the onset of breast cancer and the consequent ongoing medical care, our love making – both quantitatively and qualitatively – plummeted to a level just sufficient to keep my eyes from crossing and maintain the semblance of focus required to carry on the activities of daily living. (Granted, I exaggerate, but it had degenerated to a state of borderline extinction.)

Even so, I had little difficulty accommodating this change in our routine during the course of Suanne's care and treatment for breast cancer. I figured this was the least I could do to be a "Good Soldier" in the war on breast cancer. When the treatment ended, however, and with the prognosis was for a complete cure, I expected that our sex life would "eventually" return to the state I had known, and now keenly and increasingly, wanted it to be. And maintaining our tradition on New Year's Eve was not, to my way of thinking, an overly demanding expectation in this regard.

Josh had a few of his friends over in the early evening on New Year's Eve and had plans to attend a lowering-of-the-crystal-ball-in-Times Square party at a friend' house in the neighborhood. The two of us had reservations at the Duck Club Restaurant at the Monterey Plaza Hotel on Cannery Row. We were escorted to our table next to a window where we could almost feel the waves crashing into the shore. Dinner was excellent and Suanne looked stunning in a new Adrianne Vitadini dress I had given her for Christmas. Even if I have mentioned it before (at least once), it bears repeating: Even after the year we had been through, and the ever increasing "tug" of age (literally and figuratively), at 52 years old, Suanne remains one of the most beautiful, elegant, sensuous, and desirable women I have ever laid my eyes on, in the flesh or otherwise, and I have always made a habit of telling her so.

Our conversation over dinner was eclectic, as usual, ranging from the unprecedented flooding in the Central Valley to the mysteriously deafening silence coming from the feminists establishment over the Paula Jones case. Of course we also talked about our good fortune during the past year, Josh's schooling and basketball games, up-coming trials, and office business. All in all, our dinner was a grand prelude to the sensuous dessert I fantasized about as we got back in the car for the thirty-four mile drive back home. Dessert, berserk, smuzerk! No sooner had we fastened our seatbelts than Suanne, my dessert du jour, fast in the clutches of the seat heaters, had nodded off to sleep.

"Suanne," I delicately inquired as we passed Fort Ord, "you're not tired are you?" No audible answer; only some silent squirming.

"Honey, we're almost home." I murmured as we reached Moss Landing, testing the depth of her slumberous response. Still no response.

"Shit," I said to myself, "this is just fucking great. New Years and we're going home to go to sleep. Not to bed, not to make love, but to fucking sleep! God forbid that on New Year's Eve we'd go "to bed" together, and make mad passionate, erotic, sensuous love for an hour or so, and then fall exhausted into one another's arms for the first few hours of the new year. No, that's all part of the past. Now that my wife is a "poster woman" for Susan Komen, I need to start looking at her breasts more as a reminder of what was and could have been rather than a stimulating sine qua non ingredient to our love making. Maybe though, I thought, she'll wake up when we drive into the garage and have a burning desire to rip her clothes off and make love right here in the car. Good luck on that one!"

"Honey, we're home," I said as the garage door opener came to rest, "time for dessert."

I figured that the litmus test would come when she got into bed. NAKED would be a good tip-off. Flannel pajamas? Hell, she might as throw a cooler of iced Gatorade on my nether regions.

Hearing no response, I shook her gently after switching off the ignition and told her we were home. Yawning broadly, she said, "I didn't realize how tired I was." Bad sign! Very bad sign! But hope spring eternal, as they say.

While I'm getting undressed and brushing my teeth, my mind was engaged in an old and familiar, if near pathological pursuit of setting the stage for a tragic ending. " I'll slip into bed before she does, strategically place some conspicuous signal of my erotic intentions in open sight and wait for her response." For me, the signal might be something like a rose colored night light, music, a fire, the sheets turned down suggestively, what have you.

So, there I am. It's fifteen minutes till 1997 and the stage is set. I built a fire. I turned on the music (romantic favorites), and her side of the bed was suggestively turned down. I even placed a Godiva chocolate mint (courtesy of the Monterey Plaza Hotel) on her pillow. "Will she or won't she?" I asked myself.

The moment of truth arrives. She comes out of the bathroom wearing a long nightgown, although not flannel, it was not diaphanous either (anxiety!), and says, with a hand-over-the-mouth preening yawn, "I'm really tired." I started feeling hypertensive, but I am still hoping for the best as she tumbles mechanically into bed. I extinguish the light above our headboard (allowing the pink glow of the night light and the dancing flames of the fire to suffuse the room), and lay motionless waiting for something to happen. I wait and I wait. Nothing. Soon I hear her rhythmic breathing. It's 1997!

"What the hell am I going to do", I wonder, "stoke the fucking fire?"

Here I am, fifty-three years old. I can still surf ten foot waves on the North Shore. I can bench press 245 pounds (55 pounds over my body weight), and I've recently done my first hundred mile bicycle race, the Big Sur century. And, I have a powerful craving for a healthy carnal relationship with my wife, and she's fucking asleep! On New Year's Eve! About 2:30 a.m., January 1, 1997 I can't take it anymore. The fire - in the fireplace that is - is almost completely burnt out.

"Suanne, are you awake?" I asked in a loud whisper. No, response, so I shook her. "Suanne, wake up!" I demanded in a low voice. "Are you awake?"

"What is it?" she asked through the haze of sleep.

What is it? "Honey, look," I said, "I'm just not ready to throw in the towel. I can't sleep. It's New Years, or it was, and we get home from a lovely evening and you put on your armor and plop into bed and go to sleep for Christsake. I lay here awake, wondering if we'll ever have a normal sexual relationship again. Do you have any interest in sex at all? You've got to be square with me about this; I need to be able to stand up and give opening statements and closing arguments without feeling like poking every knothole in the courthouse men's room."

Suanne turned over to face me, reached out and took my hand in hers. It was warm, as in with sweat.

"Scott," she said, "there are times when I feel some of that old desire, but to be honest with you, for the most part, it seems like my desire, at least compared to the way it used to be, has gone the way of my estrogen count.

"The truth is that I don't seem to have the same urge or need for sex I once did. I wish I did. I wish too that I could just sleep through the night once in a while. It's not that I don't enjoy it when we make love, because I do, very much. It's just that I need more help from you than I used to.

"Our sex, for a long time, was based, as you have always said, on my allure, my sensuality. You've said that umpteen times. You usually respond rather than initiate and if I'm not the initiator, you interpret that as a lack of interest on my part. Then you pout. That's the truth. You pout like a little boy that was expecting a particular dessert and didn't get it.

"Well, I'm sorry, it's different now. I don't want to seem cold or indifferent, because I'm not, and you know that. But maybe you just need to get used to it. The fact that I don't produce as much estrogen as before and can't take HRT has made a huge change in the way my body works. Everything is different with my body chemistry. Without enough estrogen in my bloodstream, whether from my own sources or from HRT, my libido just isn't the same. I've talked to my doctors about this.

"But this doesn't mean that all of the pleasure that our love-making has imprinted on my brain has been erased. Once the right neurons and synapses are stimulated in my brain, I enjoy love-making as much now as I ever did. It's just that it has to come from a different source. Instead of coming from my ovaries or a pill or patch, sexual stimulation now comes more from my brain, literally. Maybe we have to work as hard now at love-making as we have in the past at making love in our marriage. Do you understand this, Honey? It's not as though we can simply flip a switch on the wall that's been taped over. When I got into bed, if you hadn't just lay there waiting for me to snuggle up to you, you wouldn't have had to lay there awake until now."

In the shimmer of her eyes I could see the warm glow of old embers burning in her heart. She squeezed my hand and gently pulled me toward her. As we melded into one, my heart soared to heights perhaps I had never known before. Truly, love can conquer all. If I had scripted something for her to say to me that would make things right, to the perfect thing to say at the time, I couldn't have penned anything more appropriate, more beautiful, or more moving. Before drifting off into the land of nod, I mused:

What is love,
An acorn falling to earth,
The touch of another's hand,
Knowledge, experience,
Some or all of these things,
To me love is
Rain upon the land,
a misty spring day,
Motion, growth and time,
Love is recognition of self,
Of who and what and why we are,
Dignity, self-respect and understanding,
It can be seen occasionally,
In a glance.

CHAPTER 31
Déjà Vu

March 4, 1997

As winter eased into spring the rhythm of our lives was settling back into the predictable patterns of a daily routine that had for so long seemed but a distant memory. At the gym, Suanne's levels on the VersaClimber, the Stairmaster and the bicycle were back to her customary levels and better. With two major trials of mine having been completed (and won), the law practice was humming along and we seemed to be coming out of two years of precipitous and unexpected declines in revenue. Josh continued to make his high school honor roll every quarter and as a starting pitcher sported an eye-popping earned-run average of under one on his baseball team. Yet some things I realized, might never return to normal (defined as "The Way Things Were or Are Supposed To Be"), or at least not for the foreseeable future.

The nature of cancer, I had learned over the past year, was so complex and so insidious that no matter how good the prognosis one may be given, there still always exists the very real possibility that a few cells from the original site have managed to migrate or metastasize to a new location elsewhere in the body and set up a colony. Yes, the probability, in cases of early detection, as Suanne's doctors had said over and over, were heavily in favor of a "cure." But even a cure does not ensure that the disease will not reappear.

After all, Suanne did have cells in her body with mutations that had managed to override and defeat the extraordinary Mother Nature given defense mechanisms that our autoimmune system provides us with. What had started out in the Lord-knows-when distant past as a single cell embarking on a course of uncontrolled division, years later (no one can say for sure how many), resulted in a small pea-sized lump and her diagnosis of breast cancer. Our knowledge of the first failure of Suanne's body to prevent this from happening, was eloquent and never to be forgotten evidence to its cursedly wicked ability to do so again.

In addition, there could be other malignant cells, among the thirty trillion or so that make up a healthy human body, at as-yet-unknown locations, that were surreptitiously and methodically establishing new tumors, encroaching upon surrounding tissues, and even sending out new expeditionary forces of their own to stake yet other new colonies of cancer cells. Although the mind-numbing complexity of cell mutation and uncontrolled replication is understood by precious few cancer patients, the insidiousness and mortal peril involved is lost on almost no one. Suanne continued to subconsciously knead and probe her breasts in a prophylactic search for any new sign of changes, but never really expecting to find anything.

On this particular evening Suanne was sitting on the couch needlepointing and listening to a news program that was re-running a video clip of the pitched gun battle on the streets of Los Angeles the previous Friday. (It was actually carried live on TV for several hours as the event unfolded, à la the infamous police chase O.J. Simpson in his white Bronco.) The two fatigue-garbed gunmen with automatic weapons were killed, but six bystanders ended up getting wounded in the fusillade. Before the clip ended I commented to Suanne that it had all the elements of a made-for-TV movie scene.

The phone rang. It was Suanne's sister Bonnie calling from Lawrence, Kansas. Josh was in his room studying and I had just retired to my study to read depositions. During the conversation with her sister, Suanne's fingers found their way to a spot on her right breast - yes, the same breast that had just gone through the metaphorical "wringer" - that she had lived in absolute dread of finding. She quickly ended the conversation and called me into the family room. I found her with her right arm crossed over her chest and her left hand underneath her sweat shirt, obviously feeling her right breast.

"I think I can feel something in my breast." she said in a calm voice, betrayed only by the slight trembling I could see enveloping her body. "Feel right here."

I sat down beside her as she exposed her breast and moved the tips of my index and middle finger over a spot just forward and a little above the incision scar on her right breast. The ritual, by now, was extremely familiar. My heart was pounding so hard as I pressed my fingers into her flesh, that I thought for certain that Suanne could probably feel it.

Recurrence of metastatic breast cancer within the first year is extremely ominous. What it says is that virtually everything that had been done to eradicate the malignant cells has failed. It also says that the proliferation or growth rate of the cancer cells is extremely fast; fast enough to build a new palpable tumor in only a year. It may also say that the new site was colonized by a yet undetected cancer from another primary point of origin.

Treatment options become circumscribed with recurrences of cancer. The down-and-dirty fact is that mastectomy becomes the principal option, with chemotherapy just as likely. Repeat exposure of the original site to a second round of radiation presents new problems with more severe and long-lasting side-effects. Most importantly, the probability rates for long term survival rates plummet! My fingers touched what I was praying they would not, a small, irregular but distinct mass. A mass of something that didn't belong. A mass of renewed horror. Or were we both jumping conclusions?

"It doesn't feel at all like what we felt the first time, does it?" I observed, trying to sound as matter-of-fact and unfazed as I could. "This one feels more like a scar or maybe some swelling, as opposed to a small round object like a pea. I don't think its anything to worry about."

Looking into Suanne's hazel eyes, I knew exactly what she was thinking, and her next words confirmed it.

"Scott, that's what you said last year too, do you remember?"

Yes, of course I remembered. But I had hoped for her sake, my sake, our sake, that it was nothing but a brush-aside false alarm; an illusion perhaps, an imagining. Surely it could not be real. We had escaped the clutches of breast cancer. Our world was returning to normal. Lawyer that I am, I could not repress the thought that now pelted my mind like a shotgun blast against a corrugated-tin wall: "Doesn't this constitute double jeopardy? We were found free once already. They can expect us to be put on trial for the same disease a second time, can they?"

As fate would have it, Suanne's next appointment with Dr. Shapiro, the medical oncologist, was only a week away. All we could do was wait. Waiting a week wouldn't be so bad. We'd been through this before. Bull shit! Double bull shit! Waiting is one of the most hideous, heart-searing burdens of cancer. Predictably, this wait proved to be one of the slowest, most distracted weeks of my life, as I'm sure it was for Suanne. If we spoke "little" during the waiting periods of the first go-round, this time it was as if someone had sewn our lips shut in an effort to prevent even the slightest verbal negativity from becoming a self-fulfilling prophecy.

Another inescapable aspect of dealing with breast cancer, or any other form of cancer I suppose, is that each and every experience you have with the disease, especially the feelings of terror and impotence, are never completely eradicated, regardless of what you're told by others, be they medical professionals, family, friends or other cancer survivors, and regardless of what you may tell yourself. With the threat comes the fear - gripping you upon awakening, sidling up to you during the day and haunting you through the night - it's always there.

In cases like ours, where we felt we had begun to shake off the chronic fear and anxiety, the reality is that they are simply put into a kind of cancer patient's "Pandora's Box," awaiting any opening, any chink in the armamentum of optimism, to return to their keeper with renewed fury and virulence. Everything you have read, everything you have seen, every fragment of fear that has kept you awake at night, every tear you have cried - it all comes galloping back into your mind with the slightest provocation, like the Four Horsemen of the apocalypse wearing frayed hooded habits, pulling behind them a caisson bearing the still-warm corpses of your hopes and dreams.

March 12, 1997

I accompanied Suanne to the appointment with Dr. Shapiro. Being it was a regularly scheduled appointment, the doctor wasn't aware of anything out of the ordinary. The news magazines on the end tables all dealt with the Vice President Gore's fund-raising activity from his office in the White House and the massive flooding in the Midwest. The Pope could have been in town, I wasn't interested.

In a few minutes the doctor greeted us in his usual cheerful manner and walked us back to one of the examining rooms. The standard drill was for the doctor to hand Suanne her white pressed paper johnny vest while asking her a few preliminary questions (any new pains?; changes in your breasts?; etc), absent himself while the patient top garments and bra for the vest, then returning for the examination. On this occasion, Suanne, as fitfully anxious as I was, got to the point immediately. Hearing the obvious distress in her voice, he handed her the vest and proceeded post haste with the examination.

"Show me where you think you feel something new." he instructed. Placing her right index finger on a spot just above and anterior to the still pinkish excision scar, she responded, "Here."

The doctor's expert fingers then glided over the area until he stopped on the mass Suanne had found. "Yes, I feel it." he said.

I felt sick to my stomach, so much so that I honestly thought I might throw up, right there in the examining room. And I did, so what? Breast cancer is such a MESS, anything else pales by comparison, particularly a little vomit sloshing about the room. I didn't.

He continued palpating in silence, then said, after what seemed like an eternity, "It's probably nothing more than scar tissue, but we do need to follow up on it."

All I heard was the "...nothing more than scar tissue." "Oh thank You God!" I exclaimed to myself in silence, although I felt the whole world somehow could hear me.

Dr. Shapiro then asked Suanne to lie down so he could continue the examination. After finishing with the right breast he moved to left and gazed off into space as his fingers "played" over the contour of Suanne's "good" breast. He continued to poke, paw and prod, saying nothing. I was going out of my freaking mind. The silence was deafening. His fingers finally stopped at about 12:00 o'clock, about an inch and a half above the nipple, circled, pressed down and finally he looked toward me and asked Suanne, "Have you felt anything here?"

"No," she responded in a tone of utter dismal resignation, "do you feel something?"

"Yes," he replied, "I think there's a very small lump. Give me your hand." He took Suanne's hand and directed her fingers to the spot where he had found the lump. "Do you feel it?"

"Yes," Suanne said, "I feel it."

"We'll need to schedule a mammogram." Dr. Shapiro said in a monotone.

All the relief, the exuberance, the thankfulness, the solace that comes with the flush of victory, evaporated in an instant. All the answers we had heard to our most fervent prayers, all of the toasts to health, to life and to living, were but empty mocking echoes in face of the specter of a recurrent, a new or previously undetected lump.

I was frozen in my chair, almost oblivious to everything that was going on around me. The terrible refrain began again: Run, Fly, Hide... Search Find Kill,/ In desperation... Run Fly Hide... Search, Find, Kill,/ in desperation.

It was like being in a dream, where hours can be compressed into fractions of seconds and the bizarre, the mystical and the unfathomable nonchalantly mingle with the iron-cold-deer-in-the-headlights reality. It all comes flooding back in to your mind, in torrents, in enormous waves, in earthshaking magnitudes; all of the unspeakable horror, the paralyzing terror, the self-pity, the hopelessness, the helplessness.

"Scott, let's go", I heard Suanne's voice declaim. Then, "everything will be okay, it's probably nothing."

I cursed myself - again - for all of my past failings and misdeeds, pushed up from the chair and took her hand and walked out to the car. Nary a word was spoken by either of us, not then, not all the way back to the house. Somehow it struck me that words between the two of us would prove feckless anyhow. What was needed now, more than ever, were words of prayer, words between a human mortal and his Supreme Being.

When we arrived at home, I made some excuse to absent myself and went out back into our sideyard. There I sat down on an oak round and, as I have heard women phrase it, "had myself a good cry." I didn't care if Suanne or anybody else heard me or not, I just didn't want to infect her with my morbid fears. As I buried my face in my hands, sitting next to the wood pile, the tears poured down my face. I wanted God to see and hear my pain...and how searingly real it was.

I said out loud, "No, God, don't let this happen. Not again. Not to her. She doesn't deserve this. Please God, don't let this happen. Do anything to me, but spare Suanne. I began to think that maybe this was how Job felt. Maybe this WAS God's "answer." If so, I'd just have to get ready...again.

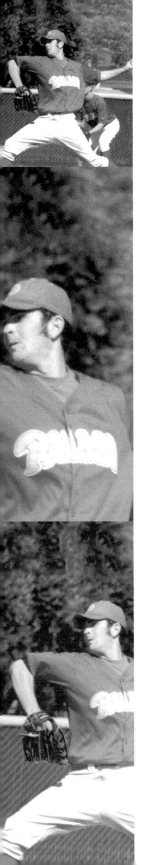

CHAPTER 32
The Impossible Fight

March 18, 1997

Suanne's annual visit to her Ob/Gyn (including a mammogram), was only a few days after the appointment with Dr. Shapiro. If the first time waiting for the appointment we were scared, this time it was shear terror.

The human mind, has a certain independence to it, a mind of its own, if you will. Which in this context is to say that I seemed to have very little control over my thinking about what the appointment might hold in store and what paths we might be headed down. Simply put, there is no way to sugar coat or put a positive spin on the way the mind reacts to the prospect of an impending disaster, actual or potential, and over which you have absolutely no control.

When the battle is one you think you've already fought and won the sense of helplessness is infinitely expanded. In "wars," literal or figurative, at least you can fight. Even if the fight is against all odds, you can throw yourself into the fray with total abandon and raise abstractions like personal honor, fortitude and courage to a very real but ever-elusive quest for the Holy Grail.

Even victims of terrifying diseases like breast cancer can commit themselves to the battle with such complete uncom-promised dedication and resolution that the catharsis that accompanies, or results from the struggle compensates in part for the knowledge of their lost cause. But for me, experiencing utter and complete powerlessness in the face of an equal desire to contribute, to help, to intervene, is at once maddening and profoundly humiliating. All I could do was wait and sit at my computer and joust at windmills by recording my thoughts, in a futile effort to be a part of the process that I knew was one of the most important ordeals of my life. But even while withdrawing into the shelter of my personal pathos, I vowed to myself to redouble my efforts in the service of the queen of my heart and hearth.

The last thing that Suanne needed, indeed that I needed, was for either one of us to lose faith and drop out of the race.

When Suanne returned from the mammogram appointment, she issued the report: it was part good news, part bad news. The latter was that both the lump on the right breast near the old excision site and the new one on the left breast were deemed as somewhat suspect. As a result, Dr. Andrews asked Suanne to go back for more mammogram views of the right breast. The additional views are intended to expose the suspicious lump from different angles. We were aware that what can look suspicious from one angle can disappear from another. The good news was that there could be an entirely benign explanation for the lumps in both breasts, including the angles of the mammogram..

After getting the extra views and having them reviewed by the diagnostic radiologist, came the really good news. The consensus was that the "lumps" did not present themselves in the mammograms as indicative of malignant tumors. Needlessly to say, we received this as joyous news of the highest order. But however comforting, we took pause, reminding ourselves that we had heard a similar refrain a year earlier. It was impossible, given the history, not to say, "Whoa there, let's not get too excited. Haven't we been given this same story before?"

A few days thereafter Suanne went to see Dr. Mahoney, who after reviewing the results of the mammograms and doing her own physical examination, weighed in with a "second opinion" that corroborated that of Dr. Andrews and Dr. Randol. Still, we didn't have the comfort level that we needed.

By the same token, Dr. Mahoney, is the kind of physician who engenders (I'm tempted to say, "radiates" here, but in the context it seems ill-fitting, except perhaps among crepehangers), in her patients the confidence that we would all like to have in our physicians. You'll recall that after the first meeting, Suanne told me that she "instantly liked" the doctor. Having been through the experience of the year, that "instant like" had become more akin to a respectful love, or maybe a loving respect. I too, was beginning to take, undemurringly and at face value, whatever it was that Dr. Mahoney said.

Dr. Mahoney's opinion, after physically examining Suanne and reviewing the mammogram films, including the ones from last year, was that the anomalies in both breasts were not cancerous tumors. I repeat, NOT CANCEROUS!

Waxing the same confidence she had displayed from the start, Dr. Mahoney opined that what we were seeing and feeling in the right breast was scar tissue left over from the first operation. The new suspicious area in the left breast, she concluded, was just part of the architecture of Suanne's breast and entirely consistent with her prior tests and treatment. That said, she also cautioned us that, notwithstanding her unqualified opinion, if either of the suspicious areas were going to be a source of ongoing concern to Suanne, we might want to consider doing biopsies.

In discussing her findings, Dr. Mahoney treated Suanne almost like a medical resident on grand rounds to whom she was explaining the basis of her medical judgment. She put Suanne's mammogram films up on the view box and described the distinctions she saw between the current set of mammograms and those taken back in April of last year. She invited questions and offered to provide her with medical literature.

On the one hand, we were enormously relieved to hear an unqualified verdict in our favor from a doctor we had complete faith in. On the other, given what we had come to learn about breast cancer in general, we remained skeptical and deeply concerned with leaving the unidentified "lumps" in Suanne's breasts without knowing beyond a reasonable doubt, what they were.

We had learned from hard personal experience that which ought to be self-evident to anyone with half a brain. Ultimately the patient must take a certain amount of responsibility for the decisions that are made in managing their own health care. The key word here is "decisions." Leaving ultimate medical decisions (such as whether or not to obtain a definitive answer to the "suspicious lump" issue) unquestioningly in the hands of others - no matter how caring or competent the hands may be - is tantamount to a cop-out. We knew it, both of us, from first-hand experience. It required no discussion on our part. Even if on the surface they seemed redundant and unnecessary, further biopsies would have to be done. The fact that we made this decision in the face of countervailing medical advice is not to suggest, however, that patients should not be entitled to expect their physicians to captain the ship of their healthcare. Furthermore, patient responsibility for decision making should not be confused with physician responsibility for medical management. Let there be no mistake about it, physicians do make mistakes.

As a board certified professional malpractice attorney I had been around the track more than a few times in dealing with physicians and knew with absolute certainty, that all of them perform the same constitutional ritual that the rest of us do when we get up in the morning. I knew with complete confidence that they have the same or similar problems with their adolescent kids the rest of us have; that they divorce and re-marry, abuse drugs, experience financial and health problems, and even kick their dogs on occasion. In other words, I knew that physicians are fallible, that they experience common human frailties, and that they make mistakes (like the rest of us), no matter how loath some of them (like the rest of us), are to admit it.

Even as a plaintiffs' attorney suing physicians on behalf of injured patients, however, I have found the majority of defendant physicians to be intelligent, thoughtful and genuinely caring people. But I have also found that many of them, actually most, are not inclined to fess up to mistakes even under the most clear-cut and flagrant of circumstances, such as in Doug Yancy's case.

The reasons for this reluctance to acknowledge mistakes are not so simple as an inflated ego or the much ridiculed doctor "god-complex." Oftentimes it is simply a business decision. Like all liability insurance companies, those that insure physicians are profit driven enterprises in which non-medical executives are even more loath than the doctors to pay out settlements if they think there is any possible way to defense the case or to cough up substantially less than the injured victim is demanding. As has been uttered by the famous corporate raider, Warren Buffett, "Insurance companies are not in the business of indemnifying against liability, they're in the business of the float." In other words, keep the money in an account drawing interest for as long as possible. But this certainly isn't the complete answer.

Owing to the complexity of the issues involved in medical negligence cases, far more often than not, the doctors can claim that regardless of what they did or did not do to the patient, they were simply exercising medical judgment and did nothing that violated the accepted standard of care. If this doesn't wash, they can claim that the outcome was a foreseeable risk of the treatment. Or, they can claim that if they did do something wrong, it didn't cause the damage that the plaintiff claims it did.

Jurors empaneled to hear medical malpractice cases (not surprisingly, many of whom have been treated successfully by their own doctors for one malady or another), sit there and listen to the defendant's expert witnesses (all of whom are fellow physicians that share a disdain, no, make that hatred, for medical malpractice cases), explain why black is white and up is down, and why it is a mortal sin to question the judgment of the poor defendant physician who was just trying to heal the patient. And, of course, how the patient didn't adequately participate in his or her own medical care.

In pointing this out, I do not intend to imply by any means that every claim of medical malpractice has merit, or that all physicians are taught to cook the books (alter records), and never cooperate in any way with a plaintiffs' attorney that sues doctors. I am suggesting however, that unique problems exist for patients seeking justice from the legal system when the defendant is a physician.

In short, it's a different set of rules. When all is said and done, juries do in fact, consider doctors to be "more equal," regardless of their oath to the contrary. I have seen it time and time again.

In my own practice, I turn down easily 99% of the medical malpractice cases that are presented to my office. It is axiomatic among most experienced medical malpractice lawyers that an untoward outcome for the patient doesn't mean the doctor was negligent. In other words, a bad result doesn't mean bad medicine. Any procedure on any patient can go awry for an infinite number of reasons that are unrelated to negligence on the part of the physician. Its only when the injury to the patient is the result of the physician violating the accepted standards of care that medical malpractice occurs.

What this means is that in each and every case, the jury is required to understand and literally define the standard of care, based on the testimony of expert witnesses, and then make a factual determination whether the defendant violated the standard of care. A heady task for the layman, for people unfamiliar with any aspects of the practice of medicine.

Suanne, in contrast to the average patient, had the rare privilege and experience of having listened to literally hundreds of people calling in to our office with horror stories about medical malpractice. In addition to her background on the administrative side of professional malpractice litigation, by the time the "déjá vu" second round of suspicious "lumps" appeared, Suanne had the experience of having followed her own instincts to seek a surgical consultation in the face of, at best, some equivocal medical advise regarding the necessity to do so. This time, the debate of, yes, I'll have the test/no I won't have the test, didn't even come up. For her the questions answered themselves. It was a classic textbook, no-brainer.

Why? Because she was unwilling to live every day not knowing what might or might not be growing in her breasts. She opted, without so much as a nanosecond of hesitation, for having both newfound suspicious masses in her breasts biopsied.

All of this had an incredible air of déjà vu. Until the demon was expelled, or metaphorically speaking, exorcised, it would plague us both with dark and morbid images of the extraordinary power that breast cancer had held over our lives for the past year and a half.

CHAPTER 33
Say It Now

May 11, 1997.

It might be surmised from the fact that I am writing this book that I am highly expressive about my feelings and like to say (and sometimes write about) whatever is on my mind. I have certainly never been accused of being timid about expressing myself. Whether it be over the dinner table, in opening statements or closing arguments, or in quiet repose whispering sweet nothings in Suanne's ear, words and language have always flowed freely from my lips or my pen or now my keyboard.

Capturing things in writing (events, emotions, ruminations) has always made a lot of sense to me. Ever since I was a little kid I have been fascinated by the remarkable power of words and language and by the capacity of our species to make an abstraction out of anything that impinges on our senses. That averred, I must ask (rhetorically), when are we ever really confident that we have conveyed in words and language or even by our deeds, all that we might really feel and want to convey, especially when the time to convey those feelings may suddenly be over or dramatically shortened. There are times, I'm sure, when each of us wishes we had more fully or more clearly our feelings toward another, especially I suspect, in communications between husbands and wives and parents and their offspring.

I remember ever so vividly, when I was eleven years old sitting alone in the tack room behind our house on the farm listening to the sirens scream and the clatter of emergency vehicles arriving and leaving the ranch. Horrific, petrifying, God-awful scenes of my brother being dragged through the orchard by his horse kept replaying over and over in my mind.

I found him lying up against a tree unconscious with one bare foot showing and a look of unbearable pain on his

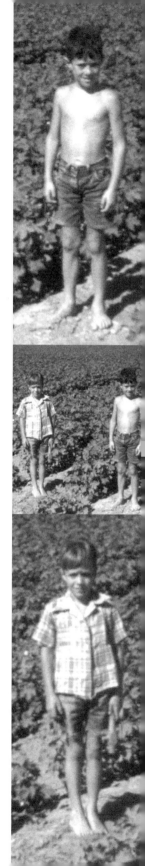

face. Even his sock was gone. For several moments the utter panic and terror I felt was totally paralyzing. I finally jumped back on my horse Amber and raced in a headlong panic-stricken sprint back to the house screaming at the top of my lungs and crying all the way. When I reached the house, through my terror and tears, I managed to convey to my mom and dad that Jerry had been dragged by his horse and was hurt very badly. My dad, horrified at what he was hearing, ran out to the date grove while my mom called for an ambulance. In the confusion and panic that followed, I retreated to the tack room where I waited in silence for word on my brother.

A short while later, Dad summoned me from outside the tack room. Hoping against hope, and fearing the worst, a bewildered little boy, stripped of every illusion and fantasy he had about being a big cowboy, got up from his bunk and walked outside. Dad put his big strong arm around my skinny little shoulders and said, "Scotty, your brother is gone. He couldn't be saved. You're all we have left now." Later that day I was sent to stay with my cousin Frank for a few days while my mom and dad grieved together.

After about a week I went home to a changed world. Not a word was ever spoken about those dark days following my brother's death until nearly three decades later. Today psychotherapists speak of the need for "closure." Did I ever find closure over the loss of my brother? The answer is both yes and no.

Yes, at some point I think I did, but not because of anything explicit that was said. Maybe on my fiftieth birthday after receiving from my mom and dad a personal photo collage that they entitled "A Picture Study in the Life of A Winner." But then there are times when the answer is no, I never did get over the loss of my brother and perhaps I never will. To this day I still will occasionally wallow in my own personal little Hell, over the events of that September so long ago. Growing up, I tried my best, time and time again, to sort it all out, all to no avail. Usually, just blotting it out seemed like the best solution. At some point I came to the conclusion, as previously alluded to, that the answer is that there is no answer. Life hands us what it hands us - some good, some bad, some indifferent - and we each have to deal with the challenges as best we can.

Funny how themes tend to reprise in one's life. Back then, in 1953, at the age of eleven, I mused to myself hour upon hour why it was my brother Jerry and not me who was taken away. I remember telling God that it should have been me he'd taken instead of my brother, that it wasn't fair and how the heck was a kid supposed to deal with losing his one and only brother whom he looked up to and all that. Now, nearly half a century later, I find myself asking the same question about Suanne and her disease. Why her? Why not me? I'd have gladly taken her place. In both instances I found the issue of why bad things happening to good people to be more than a little troubling. Yet, I don't ascribe any design to it, other than the complicated mix of genetic and environmental factors discussed above.

Then, there was the night not too many years ago when Suanne and I had just returned home from visiting some friends and the phone rang. Suanne's mom and dad were at our house visiting. Suanne answered the phone and in just a few moments I could see an anguished expression darkening her face. All she said was "Oh God, no!" It was my cousin Frank's wife, Sylvia.

Frank and I grew up together on the ranch; our fathers were identical twins. We explored the same deserts and mountains on horseback, drove the same tractors down the same long corn rows in the summertime; we attended the same schools, and had the same teachers. Decades before it was Frank who did his mightiest to help an aggrieved, distraught eleven-year-old little boy named Scotty cope with the loss of his brother by becoming his new big brother. He went away to Stanford for college and encouraged me to follow in his footsteps.

"It's Sylvia," Suanne finally said, looking at me with that sickening glazed-over pall of tragedy, "Frank died of a heart attack today." He was only 49 years old.

If only I could have had one more day or even one more hour with my brother Jerry and my cousin Frank. All the things I would like to have said to Jerry have remained with me throughout my life. He was a star in every aspect of his life and my hero. I would like for him to have known that for certain. I would like to have said similar things to Frank. I would have told Frank how much I appreciated the way he tried to take Jerry's place in my life and how he inspired me to achieve in a way that maybe I wouldn't have otherwise. Perhaps words don't exist to explain or say such things, but we must try. We miss out on so much, I think, by not exposing ourselves and our deepest feelings to those we love and care about. We're afraid that maybe the words won't come out right, so no words come out at all. We cheat ourselves by our silence. Even when we feel completely tapped in a bottomless pit of our own insecurities and fears, it is my belief that expression and revelation is our only hope of finding light, hope and terra firma.

On Mother's Day, 1997 I wrote the following to Suanne:

My Dearest Love,

I was thinking this morning how appropriate your Mother's Day presents are. A teak bench for us to sit on together outside our bedroom for the rest of our lives, and a gardening easel for you to do your art at.

Of course, your art goes far beyond gardening, your needlework, your decorating, or your cooking. Your art has always been the creation of beauty and harmony in our lives and in the life of our family. And if I may wear the hat of an art critic for a moment, I would like to say that you are truly a master artist.

Beauty and harmony exude from your pores like warmth and light from the sun, like romance from the harvest moon.

What I'd like to do on this Mother's Day, in this little missive, is express to you how I feel about sitting beside you on "your" teak bench and watching you stand, working at your easel.

Almost everyone can admire great art, great love stories, great lives, great heroism, and some can even aspire to participate in some of all of these moments of greatness.

But precious few, oh so few among us, can live such lives by simple inclination, with never a thought given to reward or recognition.

So few, oh so few of us, spend our time in thoughtful reflection of even the ones we love, as do you.

I marvel at your deep unquestioning commitment to what we all are taught to understand as "goodness". You walk through life spreading acts of love, consideration, devotion and goodness as if putting in a load of laundry.

I marvel at you, My Love, at your mastery of the Art of Living.

On this Mother's Day I want you to know that of all the events of my life, when all is said and done, it is our union, the picture of our lives together that I most treasure and forever will.

It is our moments together, in quiet reflection of our successes and failures that I truly feel pride in the canvas upon which the picture of our family has been painted.

It is in the passion of my love for you and our family that I have come to know life's most profound and enduring meaning.

So stand, My Sweet Love, at your gardening easel, painting the colors, hues, and shapes of our lives together; molding and nurturing the family that issued from you. Sit upon the bench in the cool shadows of our late summer's afternoons, and know that I know who you truly are. I love you Suanne, deeply, passionately, and endlessly. JSL

The biopsies of the new lumps in Suanne's breasts was scheduled for Monday May 19th at Stanford.

CHAPTER 34
More Surgery

May 19, 1997

Being a member of the troops in the war against breast cancer means you're never alone; you always have a lot of company and that, I'm sure, will continue until the war is finally won. Which eventually I am confident it will be.

There are events and activities taking place almost every day ranging from walks and runs to sailboat regattas and sales to raise money for education and research. The main battle front nowadays is in medical research that is delving into the depths of the molecular biology and genetic roots of the disease. But even with all this intensified activity, the funds devoted to fighting cancer are but a fraction of what is needed to defeat cancer, so we are always looking for new recruits and vehicles.

On this day, Senators Dianne Feinstein of California and Alfonse D'Amato of New York introduced a bill that would raise millions of dollars for breast cancer research by selling a special 33 cent breast cancer stamp through the United States Postal Service. This makes the second time the bill has been introduced. The first time it was defeated based on the Postal Service's opposition to using stamps to support particular causes. I tell myself it will fare better this time.

I didn't sleep much Sunday night, although I really didn't expect to. Mostly I laid awake in my bed trying to fend off the tricks my mind was playing on me all night, such as answering questions that I refused to ask myself, creating scenarios that guilt and fear prevented me from considering, and recounting the tens of thousands of scenes from the life that I had shared with Suanne. I knew the drill and this time, instead of fighting it, I just went along for the ride.

As a young man and for much of our marriage, I always thought of myself as the star of all those thousands of scenes with Suanne. It was only later, when a delinquent maturity finally permitted, that I learned I was the one in the supporting role and it was Suanne who was the real star. Now, looking back over the years, I think most of my friends recognized it long before I did. Some probably even tried to gently break the news to me a time or two only to find that I couldn't comprehend what they were saying. Pete, my partner, even wrote letters wherein he drew pictures for me. It wasn't that I was deaf or blind - it was more like I could only see and hear what I wanted to see and hear. I wish that I could have been able view and assess things more clearly, sooner. But how many times has that been said? Why are the pitfalls of self-absorption and selfishness such difficult lessons to learn? Are the blinders of youth and hubris so intractable that it takes a catastrophe like cancer to remove them? For some people this is not the case - for most of us it apparently is.

We had gone to the spring sports awards banquet at Josh's high school on Sunday afternoon. I watched Suanne more than I did the master of ceremonies who was giving out the awards. Even when Josh was given the most valuable player award by the coaches of his baseball team, I couldn't help but watch her reactions, and my own. At times I allowed my imagination to fade her in and out of the scene. Behind the calm, even serene mask she wore, behind even her deep felt pride in Josh's many accomplishments, I knew that she was entertaining some of the same dark foreboding thoughts that would plague me throughout the night. I knew she was fading herself in and out of the scene just like I was. Having gone through it all before, only made it worse. No matter how high and how bright glow the fires of hope and optimism, no matter how positive and secure Dr. Mahoney sounded in her prognosis, the cruel hand of fate could always trump the promising hand we had come to believe we had been dealt.

I reached over and shut off the alarm before it announced the five o'clock hour. Suanne, of course, was already awake. I turned on Fox News. Jurors in the Timothy McVeigh Oaklahoma City bombing trial were shown pictures of some of the victims. There was Leora Lee Sells smiling in a church picture, Randolph Guzman standing tall in his Marine Corps uniform and a laughing picture of Baylee Almon at one year and one day old. The jurors were also shown the better known picture of the bloodied lifeless body of little Baylee being carried from the rubble of the Alfred Murrah Federal Building by a firefighter on April 19, 1995.

Everything is relative. All you have to do is look around for things to be thankful for and they appear in droves. I suppose the opposite is also true.

We were scheduled to check into the ambulatory surgery center at 8:00 a.m. The drive from Santa Cruz to Stanford took the same time as it did before. The risk of traffic congestion was always the same on a weekday so we left early to give ourselves the same margin of error as before. We drove in silence most of the way listening to the news. Fortunately, no traffic tie-ups; we arrived at the Medical Center at about the same time as before. I offered to drop Suanne off, then go park, but she preferred walking with me. We found a parking place, gathered her things and walked hand in hand into the hospital. We recognized the person at the check-in desk as the same woman that was there last year. The familiarity of the scene did not feel good to either one of us.

A woman checking in ahead of us had an expired insurance card and they were trying to get her to call home to get somebody to bring the current one. The patient wanted the receptionist to make the call but the receptionist kept directing the patient to the phones over near the elevators with the explanation that she had other check-in patients to attend to. But the patient was persistent, saying she didn't have any change. The receptionist retorted that she didn't have any change either. I reached into my pocket and gave the woman a quarter for the call.

After getting Suanne checked in, including being given the wrist band ID to (better) insure that the right procedure is done on the right patient, we went into the waiting room and sat down to await Suanne's name to be called.

I scanned an article in the San Jose Mercury News about 1st Lieutenant Kelly Flinn who accepted a general discharge from the Air Force in lieu of facing a court martial on charges of adultery, disobeying orders and lying. I'm sure Lt. Flinn probably shared many of my thoughts about the difficulties we all face in dealing with our own personal blinders.

I brought my laptop to do some work, as I had in the past, but after opening up a file, I felt absolutely no energy to continue. Instead, I picked up the first magazine my hand fell upon. I anticipated that by the time I looked at the cover the receptionist would call Suanne to go into the prep room. It was GQ, one with David Duchovny on the cover. Finding no interest there I put it down and fumbled through *People, U.S. News* and *World Report,* and *Sunset,* before alighting on a magazine called *US.* Still no call.

The *US* magazine was a whoopdeedoo special "Summer Movie Preview" edition. On the cover was a montage of Harrison Ford, Julianne More, Julia Roberts, Sandra Bullock, Jodie Foster, Alicia Silverstone, Mel Gibson, Tim Robbins, Will Smith and Sly Stallone. I wondered if any of the women depicted on the cover had been diagnosed with breast cancer. I wondered how many of them might someday be sitting in the same chair Suanne was now sitting in, awaiting the same procedure. Statistically, the odds are good that at least one of them will be before the war is won.

I was contemplating the dour aspect of a Van Gogh in a Metropolitan Museum of Modern Art poster when a nurse finally came out and called Suanne's name. She got up to follow the nurse through the door beside the receptionist. I followed behind again, as I had last year, until the nurse again told me to wait until I was called. I explained that I wasn't a patient but Suanne's husband and she explained that she knew that but that I'd have to wait until she was changed and on the prep table before they'd call me in. I couldn't believe that I had done the same thing twice. Memory lapse? Incipient Alzheimer's? Hello Scott!

I returned to another six-ounce Sweetheart cup of coffee (yuck!) by Associated Services Company and choked it down under the watchful eye of Van Gogh in St. Remy and Auverges. About the time I finished the barely passable brew, I was called into the prep room. I tossed the Sweetheart cup into the first available trash can and left my computer sitting unattended on the magazine table. Wake up, Scott.

By this time, of course, the prep-room, had become familiar territory. There are nine bays suitable for gurneys, barely affording enough room for one person to walk around the sides with the curtains closed. Suanne was the only patient in the entire prep-room at the time. The nurse attending to Suanne explained that we were at the end of the first "seating" and at the start of second, so it would be filling up shortly. While we were waiting for the anesthesiologist to arrive I picked up the chart and started reading it. "Bilateral breast biopsy, post lumpectomy one year ago with radiation therapy." It sounded like the sub-title to a horror movie, maybe starring Jodie Foster.

The anesthesiologist arrived, unceremoniously stuck his hand out for the chart, and asked Suanne the usual battery of questions: "Why are you here? What procedure is going to be performed? Who is your doctor? What was the last thing you had to drink? When?" Satisfied with the answers, he started the anesthesia dripping into one of the needles sticking in the back of Suanne's right hand.

Dr. Mahoney arrived scarcely acknowledging my presence, maybe even averting her eyes a bit. I ask about the length of time of the surgery.[45] "An hour and a half to two hours." she answered. Same as before. That was it.

The room began filling up with other patients as Suanne was wheeled on her gurney into the OR. I went back to the waiting room where I set up my undisturbed laptop (thankfully it was still there!) for an extended stay.

After pretending for a few minutes that I was concentrating, I gave up on doing any work and wandered around the halls for a while instead. I had no appetite for the "O" or an LA Hot. I had a bad premonition that everything we had been told would be proved untrue this time.

After about an hour Dr. Mahoney emerged declaring that the surgery was over and that Suanne was greatly relieved. We had a brief discussion about how the surgery went in the course of which Dr. Mahoney mentioned that she felt that Suanne had a "problem" with the medical establishment but that this operation should help allay her concerns. The doctor seemed buoyant regarding the results but said that we would have to await the outcome of the pathology studies.

---

45 - I think this was the OR game face again – I have no recollection of any negative thought about Scott – just all business and trying to get through the day and please all constituents in the OR. Maybe I was a little abashed because I was so sure that this was an unnecessary trip. This is another example of why family members need to establish a good relationship with the surgeon early on. **EM**

I felt compelled to parry the doctor's comment about Suanne's putative "problem" with the medical community.**46**

"Suanne really doesn't have a problem with the medical community at all. Her problem, if you want to call it that, is that she was given medical advice back in 1996 that was extremely equivocal as to the need for any follow up on the hard pea-sized lump she had felt in her breast. And despite this equivocal advice, which many women would have simply accepted, she opted to follow up. To my way of thinking, if it were not for Suanne, we could very well be having the biopsy now for the first time and Suanne would probably have a very short life expectancy."

I was feeling very emotional at this point, perhaps even a bit panicky. It doubtless showed in the tone (if not volume) of my voice. I could feel the aggression percolating up, but recognized that this was neither the time nor place for an extended discourse on the care and feeding of my anxieties.

Although she did not openly counter anything I said, Dr. Mahoney pointed out, "for the record," she had nothing to do with the events that could have sent Suanne home last year without the benefit of a follow-up appointment.

I acknowledged that if it were not for her decisive intervention, the outcome probably would have been profoundly different (which I strongly felt to be true). We discussed the results of the mammogram and I asked Dr. Mahoney what would happen if there is a malignancy? She said that we would cross that bridge when we got to it.

"Thank you doctor," I said, "We appreciate everything you have done."

She smiled, shook my hand and said, "Suanne will be ready to leave in about thirty minutes; a nurse will come get you." The doctor then turned and headed in the direction of the operating room to attend to another patient, another surgery. As she walked toward the big swinging double doors leading back to the OR, I thought about the burden physicians like her must bear.

I take my responsibility very seriously when I decide to take a case against a physician. They are under tremendous pressure and stress, often times with life or death hanging in the balance. If anybody thinks that there is a lot of pressure on a pitcher in the seventh game of the World Series with the score two to one in the bottom of the ninth with two outs and the bases loaded, they should think about what it's like to cut people open in an effort to save their lives.

I vaguely wondered if the doctor knew about the type of law I practice and

---

46 - What I meant to say was that Suanne felt betrayed due to her previous experience, and that trust came hard to her, even with me. I was saying that it is too bad that we had to go this far to prove that these areas were benign – if she had more trust maybe she could have believed my reassurances at least long enough to do serial exams and watch the areas blend. But I wanted her to have piece of mind and this was the only way to do it. I live my whole life to avoid mistakes, and the expense of my other valuable aspects of my life – and I like it when others recognize this and realize that there is no way I would advise an action or inaction in a slipshod way to save my ego. I extracted a promise from Sue that if I was right this time that she would trust me in the future - again, not for ego, but as one mechanism to try to control that fear Scott speaks of so eloquently. **EM**

whether she considered me part of the "problem." I walked back to the waiting room, packed up my things and went to get the car.

Friday May 23, 1997

The call came in the early afternoon at the office. Because Suanne was gone for the day, the call was transferred to me. On the line was a nurse from Dr. Mahoney's office. She announced exuberantly, "The biopsies were clear! Completely clear!" As you would expect, she seemed to take considerable pleasure in relating this information. I had calmed down a lot since the surgery and thanked her effusively for the call. If I could have I would have leapt through the phone line and planted a giant smooch on the nurse's lips. Hallelujah! Victory is ours!

I flashed a giddy thumbs-up to my legal assistant, Carolyn, signifying that everything was okay with Suanne. She beamed back a response with her own thumbs-up and a broad smile.

The long journey that began some seventeen months before in Suanne's shower seemed finally to be drawing to a happy ending, that is at least insofar as a journey in the company of breast cancer ever really ends.

CHAPTER 35
Epilogue

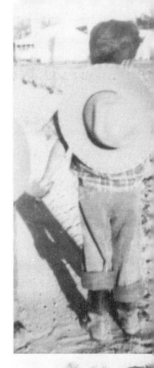

January 1998

It is two full years since Suanne first found the malignant lump in her breast. Not long enough to celebrate the "cure" that Dr. Mahoney had prognosticated, or even to rid ourselves of the daily drill of uncertainty that the breast cancer diagnosis had imposed on our lives, but more than enough time to fully appreciate our great good fortune in having a) discovered the cancer early and b) taken remedial action immediately.

Suanne still allows her hand to examine the tumor site in her breast several times throughout the day, but it is more a subconscious habit now rather than a compulsion driven by anxiety over a recurrence of her breast cancer.

The hot flashes from the tamoxifen therapy remain in full bloom. Almost every night she will break out in a sweat two or three times, throw off the covers and wait for her body to cool. She does have quiescent periods when the hot flashes go away, but they are short-lived, lasting only a day or two. Along with the hot flashes there are periods of emotional slumps - I would not raise these "slumps" to the level of depression - likewise attributable to the tamoxifen therapy. On more than an occasion or two Suanne and I have talked about the necessity of the long-term tamoxifen therapy, but her conclusion is always the same, stoic to the core, she views the tamoxifen as a personal challenge to herself to do everything within her power to beat her breast cancer, regardless of the stress, the discomfort or the inconvenience.

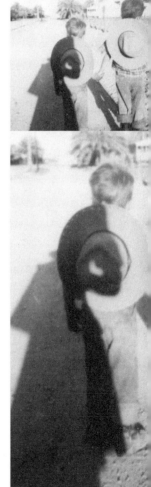

The visits with Doctors Mahoney, Shapiro and Mann are down to only once every three months, but Suanne actually looks forward to seeing them because of her tremendous regard and admiration for these remarkable and caring people. Consequently, instead of the appointments being a reminder of her disease, she treats them as an opportunity to remain in contact with the people that probably saved her life; not a difficult metamorphosis if you think about it.

For Suanne, and me, experiencing breast cancer has changed our lives forever. I know that for the next few years every time Suanne has a doctor's appointment, a blood test, a mammogram, or even a prescription filled, her thoughts will turn to breast cancer.

Likewise, I know that very time she has a headache, a bruise, muscle pain, a colon spasm or any other unexplained physical symptom, the cancer grooves in her neurons would light up like the night sky on the Fourth of July. We are both resigned to be living on this fault line, as are all cancer patients and their loved ones. Only the passage of time will further quiet these fears.

But, as I have previously noted, Suanne is one very tough and very resilient woman. She managed, in the darkest hours of her breast cancer experience, to retain her sense of humor and to focus her attention on our family, our home, our business and all the other things that give texture and meaning to our lives. She has never been one to focus on the negatives, never let on that she was down in the mouth. A woe-is-me kind of person Suanne is not; indeed, she is the very antithesis.

The usual course for patients that fit in Suanne's breast cancer profile is for the "fixation" (worry, stress what-have-you), on the disease to taper off over a period of a year or two. With each passing medical appointment with her medical oncologist, each test that shows negative for evidence of a recurrence, each unexplained ache or pain that goes away, the fear of finding a new lump or tumor somewhere in her body will recede, but it will never go away entirely. The breast cancer experience, I'm sure, is so ingrained, so imprinted that it will always be a part of her very being - of who she is - just like being a mother, a wife, a daughter.

For me, there is a bittersweet aspect to my experience as a breast cancer husband. The "bitter," on a personal level, fills many of the pages of this memoir. The feeling of sympathetic pain and total helplessness (and also in my case guilt) that all cancer victims and their families go through defy description. Unless you've been there yourself, you cannot fully comprehend, you cannot fully appreciate how it all tears like a high-revving Sawzall, at your mind, your gut, your soul, your very being.

In dealing with almost any kind of cancer words like terror, panic, desperation, and despair are applicable, but not necessarily apropos. But experiencing cancer is not something that is devoid of potentially positive ends. The "sweet" in the bittersweet, consists of the opportunity this experience gave me to learn more about myself, to think about my role as a husband and as a father, as well as the subject of breast cancer in particular and cancer in general and the millions of people afflicted by it, most of whom meet with a much less salubrious outcome than Suanne's.

The extraordinary power and complexity of the biological process that is the hallmark of cancer presents medical science with challenges that just a few years ago were thought to be insurmountable. Suanne and I were among the most fortunate of those who find themselves facing the scourge of cancer. Basically, we "lucked out." As Dr. Mahoney notes in her Introduction, breast cancer is the most egalitarian of all female diseases. Most cancers strike everyone and anyone indiscriminately. There are enough different forms of cancer to run one's pen dry just attempting to list them all. There's bladder cancer, bone cancer and brain cancer; there's colorectal cancer, prostate cancer and testicular cancer; there's liver cancer, lung cancer, and stomach cancer; there's cervical cancer, ovarian cancer, and uterine cancer; there's mouth cancer, skin cancer and tongue cancer. And let's not forget about the blood family: leukemia, multiple myeloma and lymphoma, among others. Small wonder that the disease is often referred to simply as "the Big C." Big indeed!

If your chances of getting one is relatively low (lung cancer in non-smokers versus smokers), the damnable statistical likelihood is that there's another variety that will "like" you better. The Big C strikes people of all ages, all races, and in all time zones. It cares not a whit about democracy or autocracy or plutocracy; about capitalism or socialism or communism. Laying awake at night and thinking about the different avenues cancer can and does take is an experience not unlike hitting oneself in the head with a hammer. It feels so good when you stop.

The obituary columns of daily newspapers in every city and town in the country, and indeed around the world, are eloquent testimony to the power and pervasiveness of cancer. It kills, maims and cripples locally, nationally and globally. In the isolated context of my own life I have seen not only my wife stricken with breast cancer, but no less than two dozen people I have personally known have died from the disease. In the past five years I myself have had two skin cancers removed and a suspicious lesion in my colon that thankfully turned tested benign.

At a professional level, my medical malpractice office receives, on average, as many as ten calls a week dealing with cancer cases, or as many as 500 calls a year. And my office is tucked out of the way in the relative hinterlands of Santa Cruz County, removed from the nearest city of any consequence by a mountain range. San Francisco is two hours away.

In any given issue, jury verdicts will list one or two trials arising out of the care and treatment of cancer patients. As I write this concluding chapter, I am preparing to go to trial on a prostate cancer case wherein the general practitioner failed to follow up on a PSA (prostate specific antigen) test that was positive for prostate cancer and as a result, my client, who was fifty-four years of age and eminently curable when he was originally tested, is now diagnosed as terminal. His life expectancy? Ten years max.

Meanwhile, I find myself perforce rescheduling the depositions set for next Tuesday to attend the funeral of the son of a colleague that died at the age of twenty-eight from inoperable brain cancer. He had been in remission for several years and was engaged to be married when the disease suddenly reappeared; six months later he succumbed. Yes, there are many heart-wrenching outcomes that remind us that cancer remains largely beyond our control.

On the good-news front, Mendy, mentioned in the early pages of this book, has also remained cancer free, as do Karen and Sandy from Chapter 13. But we have no room for arrogance or overconfidence.

I'm going to let Diary rest now for a while. The time is not yet ripe, not yet appropriate for sending it to the publisher. We have a ways yet to go.

January 1999

Turns out that breast cancer was not the top story of 1998. President Clinton and his sexual liaison in the Oval Office with a twenty-three year old intern named Monica Lewinsky managed to sweep it under the rug. I had intended to finish this book before now, but for reasons probably rooted in trepidation and respect (for both Suanne and the craftiness of the disease), I haven't.

We're only three years out and Suanne stills allows her hand to explore her breasts searching out the signs of a new lump every day. I've continued to do research for the book and regularly investigate cancer cases for prospective clients. There always seems to be something more to say, a new twist to add, or new reports of progress or complications in the war on breast cancer. At least that's the excuse I've given myself for why the book isn't done and gone.

The reality is that three years of being free of breast cancer just isn't enough time. I've thought a lot about how we would feel if I had to explain to everyone that has been so supportive and optimistic that there was a recurrence of Suanne's breast cancer. It hasn't happened yet, and we certainly don't expect it, but I say this with my fingers and toes crossed. We are three years "out" and Suanne is enjoying a lifestyle not terribly dissimilar to the one she had "B.C.," other than the intractable side-effects of the tamoxifen.

She works out at Charlie's World (her fitness club), three days a week. She runs our office, takes care of the house (with Richie's help), and now has a granddaughter named Helena Rae who lights up her life in a way that our three grandsons, loved as they are, just couldn't.

My dad died on February 17th of 1998 from heart failure, probably due to complication from aortic aneurysm surgery. The last words he heard spoken at his bedside were from me, his lone surviving Son No. 2. "I love you Daddy," I said.

I could tell from the look in his eyes that he knew how much I meant it. I had the great good fortune of having my dad as my greatest hero in life and I think he knew it. He also contributed mightily to that illusive image of the real person down deep I've always wanted to be. With him too I wish I would have had more time to say a few more things that may have remained unsaid.

Josh, our Son No. 3 graduates from high school this year and before long, it will be just Suanne and me and our dog Shasha (an Airdale Wheaton cross) at home. Ah yes, the endless circle of life.

Mendy, from Chapter 1 and Chapter 12, also remains disease free of breast cancer and her beautiful little girls are now three and six years old. I concluded the case where the doctor failed to follow-up on the high PSA (prostate specific antigen) test. Karen and Sandy also remain breast cancer success stories. Carol also has remained in remission. My PSA client has remained in remission, married his sweetheart and is hell-bent-for-leather pursuing a successful career with a major stock brokerage house.

Owing to a variety of commitments, Suanne and I were unable to sail in the San Juans in 1998, but we managed to spend more than a few weekends tending to Suanne's rose garden and the never-finished chores any house demands of its tenants. Just a short time ago, having contemplated a future so different from the one that we are living, things like cleaning the garage, working in the yard, and doing long toss with Josh, seems very much like being on a vacation. There are so many things to be thankful for. All one needs do is look. Make no mistake, they are all about.

January 2000

Diary has remained dormant, sitting ever so benignly on my hard drive and in probably a half dozen disks strewn about my study. I work on it when I have the urge, which hasn't been much this year. Every time I return to it, I feel compelled to change something. At times I ask myself, am I making a contribution in writing this "story" or is it perhaps strictly a self-serving (cathartic) exercise. In either case, it has managed to tire me out. I've decided that I need to wait for a while longer before we proclaim final victory. Five years is generally considered the milestone. It's not that far off.

As I write this, I am investigating the case of a thirty-year-old LVN that discovered a lump in her breast in late January of 1999, had a mammogram in March and was not biopsied until September. By then the tumor had grown from less than one centimeter to ten centimeters and spread to both breasts, necessitating a double mastectomy. Her prognosis is extremely poor. Regrettably, I probably will have to turn the case down because of the lack of evidence that the outcome would have been materially changed in any way by an earlier diagnosis. In other words, it appears that the delay just didn't make that much difference in her prognosis. While this isn't usually the case, remember this woman was extremely young to have breast cancer.

I am investigating another case involving a forty-two-year-old woman who reported that she felt a lump on self examination and immediately went to her HMO clinic for an examination. The physical examination was inconclusive/questionable and a follow-up mammogram was ordered and taken about a month later. The mammogram showed a suspicious area in the left breast, which was reported back to the primary care physician for follow-up. Unexplainably, neither the radiologist nor the primary care physician at the HMO followed up.

Six months later the tumor had grown from approximately one centimeter to six to seven centimeters from about the size of a pea to the size of a small tangerine. Along with the exponential growth of the tumor they found lymphnodes matted together by metastasized cancer cells. On the TNM (Tumor size, Node involvement, Metastasis) scale this is a Stage IV cancer with a life expectancy of less than five years. The woman had undergone a double mastectomy, radiation and chemotherapy - the works. Yet the experts I have consulted with on this case have told me that due to the virulence of this woman's particular form of breast cancer, statistically, it is unlikely that the outcome would have been different had the tumor been removed when first discovered. A lousy situation, yes, but the hard cruel unvarnished truth nonetheless.

As we approach anniversary number four, Suanne remains free of any signs of cancer. She no longer sees Dr. Mahoney or Dr. Mann and her appointments with Dr. Shapiro have now extended to six-month intervals. All signs are favorable that she has, in fact, been literally (and clinically) "cured."

That said, it must be understood and recognized that as is true for any cancer patient, there remains lurking in the background of every new pain or malady the fear and threat of the cancer returning. Until there is a screening test that can effectively identify a cancer cell anywhere in our bodies, this is the lot of cancer victims. But we have come to accept this as a permanent part of the cancer experience, at least until medical detection technology provides us with the sought after ability to determine from a drop of blood whether a microscopic tumor exists anywhere in the body.

Mendy remains in remission. Only a year to go for both her and Suanne before each is declared statistically, "out of the woods!" I'll start looking for a publisher after the five year anniversary. I know that Sandy too, remains cancer free, but I haven't checked on Carol and Karen, which I need to do.

January 2001

We're close enough to the five year anniversary that I feel comfortable with Diary reawakening from my computer hard drive and going to press. I've found a publisher and we've agreed that a professional edit is in order. Thanks to the arrival of that welcome breeze known as the Writer's Second Wind, and with a literary and moral boost from Doctors Mahoney and Mann (bless them both), I have now revised and expanded sections of the book that need more work. Tom Black, my editor has done nothing short of a spectacular job of editing the latest draft of Diary. Dr. Susan Love has graciously allowed me to incorporate the appendices from her wonderfully learned, informative tome, *Dr. Susan Love's Breast Book* into Diary for which I owe her (and her charming assistant, Connie Long), a debt of heartfelt gratitude.

I continue to hear about many women with palpable lumps that have questionable mammograms but are told not to worry about what they are feeling. Some reports claim this phenomenon happens on an epidemic scale. CNN, the cable news channel, aired a special on breast cancer and misdiagnoses that hit home with a bang: It involved one of their own correspondents, Jill Dougherty, chief of CNN's Moscow bureau.

After having been cleared to return to Moscow, she was more than a little upset when she learned from a second opinion that she indeed had breast cancer. I understand that Jill's tumor was similar to Suanne's and she expects a similar outcome, but clearly there remains a great deal to do before we can even think about this war being won.

Whether as friend or author, I could not, in good conscience conclude this book without letting the reader know the outcome of Mendy's case. Mendy, you will recall is the daughter-in-law of a former neighbor. It was Mendy's being diagnosed with breast cancer that was the red flag prompting Suanne to do the self-examination in January of 1996 that got the Saga of Suanne and Breast Cancer rolling.

Without having had the conversation with Nancy, would Suanne have done a thorough breast examination the next morning in the shower? Not a chance. Without the alarm generated by her self-examination that January morning would she have simply awaited her annual examination in April? Absolutely; there's no good reason to think otherwise. Would the mammogram readings been interpreted as negative by the radiologist when she had her mammogram in April? They were anyway, even with the report of a lump on self-examination, so there's no reason to doubt that she would have been cleared for another year. Would it have been April or May of 1997, more than a year hence, when her breast cancer would have been discovered? Again, there's no reason to think otherwise. Would Suanne be in the same position as the young Stage IV LVN with the double mastectomy whose case I am now investigating? Almost certainly.

To say that but for the wake-up call regarding Mendy, Suanne might not be alive today is no exaggeration. So to Mendy and the red flag her diagnosis raised, Suanne and our family and I owe an eternal debt of gratitude. But, as is often the case with young women diagnosed with breast cancer, Mendy's prognosis was always guarded.

As reported in this final chapter, Mendy's breast cancer seemed to be under control for a period of over three and a half years. Then in early 2000 she began to experience headaches. At first, they didn't seem particularly out-of-the-ordinary; nothing an Excedrin wouldn't cure. But as they increased in frequency and intensity, she and her husband Rob did grow alarmed. An MRI revealed a suspicious lesion in her brain. Further tests showed that her breast cancer had metastasized not only to the brain, but the bones and lungs as well. The ultimate horror story for breast cancer patients was unfolding.

The brain tumors were deemed inoperable, although chemotherapy had seemed to cause the lung and bone tumors to go into remission. A gallant and wonderful person, a devoted and loving wife and mother, Mendy died in November 2000 at the age of thirty-eight. Her little girls are only six and eight years old.

Dr. Stone's wife Sandy remains in good health, as does Richard's wife Karen. Carol's story is less sanguine. Like Mendy, Carol's breast cancer has recurred with a vengeance. The disease has metastasized in her bones throughout her body and is now classified as a Stage IV cancer patient. She has been given about 21 months to live. But like so many of the foot soldiers in the war on breast cancer, Carol doesn't know the meaning of the words quit or give up. She continues to battle every day. She gets up and goes to work with a smile on her face. She exercises, watches her diet and scrupulously follows her therapeutic regimen. She now has a roommate that is both dear friend and caretaker and has gone to hospice classes. Her commitment is total and complete - she will fight to survive until the moment she draws her last breath. From all accounts, like Mendy, Carol is a Medal of Honor winner. If only there would have been a way to catch the disease earlier.

Getting a phone call from a neighbor in distress is not the type of alarm that anyone wants to receive or rely upon to become aware of the very real and immediate threat of cancer. No woman, no matter how healthy she feels or is told she is, should wait until they receive the type of phone call Suanne did to become sufficiently motivated to do a thorough self-examination and generally be on heightened alert against breast cancer. No one should ever underestimate the extraordinary power of mutant cancer cells to confound health care providers and elude the best efforts of researchers to find a cure.

In the United States alone, over 550,000 people die from cancer each year. It is estimated that, absent an extraordinary medical breakthrough, roughly four Americans in ten now living will eventually be stricken with the Big C. While all this makes for a startlingly grim picture, there is an upside that has come to me from my roller-coaster ride as a breast cancer husband.

In the course of dealing with my wife's breast cancer I have learned that the tide of battle in the worldwide war against cancer may now be turning. In doctors' offices, research institutes, hospitals, pharmaceutical companies, and among cancer patients, there are reports of dramatic successes.

Suanne's is but one such example among tens of thousands wherein early detection coupled with a personal dedication and resolve to bring every weapon to bear, resulted in a positive outcome. From minor skirmishes to massive engagements, new discoveries and advancements are being made in our under-standing of the biology of cancer, detection and diagnostic technology, surgical procedures for excision and conservation, chemotherapy and genetic and molecular engineering. To paraphrase the published report of one medical researcher: These discoveries are solid and robust - they will survive the scrutiny of future generations of research scientists and clinicians, and they will form the foundation for extraordinary new approaches to diagnosis, treatment and ultimately a cure for cancer. No one can predict exactly when the research and clinical trials now underway will find expression at the practice level, but help is on the way.[47] Heady stuff; but there is yet more reasons for hope for winning this war.

I want to end this tale of one breast cancer husband's experience by giving the last word to Dr. Steven Mann, radiation oncologist, neighbor, friend and the person who inspired me to begin this literary journey:

In 1896 Wilhelm Roentgen discovered the X-ray and within 18 months attempts were made to use it to treat skin cancer. In 2000, simultaneous reports from Francis Collins of the International Human Genome Project and Celera Biotechnology described the identification of the entire human genome. A map, or chemical description of each of the DNA strands in the 46 human chromosomes had been worked out. With this knowledge the function of each of the genes in each of the chromosomes will eventually be identified. Genes whose function is to make the enzymes that drive biochemical reactions that lead to aging, that lead to errors in metabolism and that lead to a cell's inability to control its capacity to replicate - all will eventually be mastered. There are probably dozens of genes involved in the determination of whether a cell will start dividing, continue to divide, stop dividing, or die. Once the mechanisms that control the process are identified, ways to interfere with those mechanisms will be developed. We have reached a point at the beginning of the 21st Century that it is possible to claim not if there will be a cure for cancer, but only when it will arrive.

The crowning success for the radiation oncologist in the 21st Century will be to see himself out of work, and his treatment machine for sale.

---

47 - Robert A. Weinberg, "How Cancer Arise," *Scientific American,* September 1996.

APPENDIX A
- Dr. Ellen Mahoney's Breast Self-Examination -

One of the purposes of breast self-examination is to acquaint yourself with your "baseline breast texture," in order that should a lump ever you will know, "beyond a reasonable doubt,"that it is different from anything that ordinarily and "normally" forms in your particular breasts (every breast is unique, including each of the two per human body).

First and foremost, practice preventive medicine. (Truth is, most of us women and men alike do more preventive maintenance on their automobiles than on their own bodies.)

Without fail, do a thorough self-examination monthly. Ideally it should be at a time of the month when the breasts are least swollen and tender, that is, if they change cyclically (due to menses). Otherwise, just pick a day.

Look at yourself in the mirror unclothed with your hands at your side, then with hands on hips, and finally with hands in the air. Look carefully for changes in the skin, nipples, superficial veins, and/or dimpling of the skin.

While showering or bathing, when the skin is soapy and wet, with fingers together and using the flats of the fingers, cover the surface of the breast in any comfortable manner, applying light to moderate pressure. Breast tissue can extend from the collarbone down to the abdominal wall, out to the armpit and across the breastbone (sternum). Be sure to cover the entire area. Ideally, this should be repeated when you are reclining, perhaps at another time of the day or in bed. Your mind can be "idling"while performing the self-examination; you do not need to memorize every lump or determine whether the lump is larger this month. Chances are that you are probably very "lumpy" on both sides. This is okay, so long as no one area stands apart as being noticeably, markedly different. After you cover the territory, ask yourself if you are basically made of the same stuff (feel the same as "usual"),on both sides. If the answer is yes, then you are done. If you feel something different or unusual from all of the rest of your breast tissue, something that causes you to halt the finger movement, be it the size of a grain of rice or a walnut, by all means go seek medical attention, and without undue delay. Time can be, and often is, of the essence, as this book has clearly illustrated. If, however, you are menstruating at the time, it is prudent and reasonable to wait through one more cycle, and then report it if it persists. Get into the habit of practicing this self-examination on a fixed schedule. It could save your life.

APPENDIX B
- Resources* -

PLASTIC SURGERY

American Society of Plastic and Reconstructive Surgeons, 444 East Algonquin Road, Arlington Heights, IL 60005. (312) 228-9900 or (800) 635-0635 (referral message tape). Will provide written information and mail a list of certified reconstructive surgeons by geographical area after caller provides details on above (800) message tape.

Command Trust Network, Inc. The Breast Implant Information Network. For information, call (800) 887-6828; for attorney settlement information, call (513) 651-9770. A network established to provide assistance and information to women with or considering implants.

Breast Implants: An Information Update (US Food and Drug Administration). Information on silicone and saline implants for reconstruction and augmentation. Call (800) 532-4440 or www.fda.gov/oca/breastimplants/bitac.html.

Silicone Breast Implants: Why has Science been Ignored? (1996) Prepared for American Council on Science and Health by Michael Fumento, order from ACSH, 1995 Broadway, 2nd floor, New York, NY 10023-5860. (212) 362-7044.

Marcia Angell, *Science on Trial: The Clash of Medical Evidence and the Law in the Breast Implant Case.* (New York: Norton, 1996). Examines litigation and scientific studies following 1992 FDA ban on silicone implants.

Karen Berger and John Bostwick, *What Women Want to Know about Breast Implants* (St. Louis: Quality Medical Pub, 1998). (800) 348-7808. Highlights from their larger book: A Woman's Decision: Breast Care, Treatment & Reconstruction (St. Martin's Press, 1998). Very good on reconstruction.

Nancy Bruning, *Breast implants: Everything You Need to Know* (Alameda, CA: Hunter House, 1995). Paperback. Valuable resource for any woman considering breast implants or for those who already have implants.

Amy J. Goldrich, *Command Trust Network's Introduction to the Legal System*

* Appendix B is taken from *Dr. Susan Love's Breast Book* with the kind permission of Dr. Susan Love.

(1992). Available for $18 from Command Trust Network, 256 South Linden Drive, Beverly Hills, CA 90212. (310) 556-1738. Reference booklet for women with implants who are pursuing lawsuits against implant manufacturers.

John B. Tebbets. ***The Best Breast: The Ultimate, Discriminating Woman's Guide to Breast Augmentation*** (CosmetXpertise, 1999). Hardcover.

COMMON PROBLEMS OF THE BREAST

American College of Surgeons, 95 Past Erie Street Chicago, IL 60611 (312) 664-4050. Will provide information on certified surgeons specializing in breast surgery by geographical area.

Questions and Answers about Breast Calcifications (P199, 1995). Fact sheet, NCL (800) 4-CANCER.

Understanding Breast Changes: A Health Guide for All Women (P051, 1998). Booklet from NCL (800) 4-CANCER. Explains how to evaluate breast lumps and other normal breast changes that often occur and are confused with breast cancer. It is for all asymptomatic women.

When you Can't Feel It—Needle Localization and Breast Biopsy (Beth Israel Medical Center, NY, 1991). Video describes the procedure. 28 minutes. Single copies free from marketing department (800) 825-8257.

Kerry A. McGuinn, The Informed Woman's Guide to Breast Health (Palo Alto: Bull Publishing, 1992). Paperback. A thorough review of breast lumps and benign conditions.

Kirby I. Bland, Edward M. Copeland (Eds.), ***The Breast: Comprehensive Management of Benign and Malignant Diseases*** (WB Saunders, 1998) Textbook.

Cushman Haagensen, (Ed.), ***Diseases of the Breast, third edition*** (Philadelphia: Saunders 1986). This textbook is the ultimate reference for benign breast tumors. However, his approach to breast cancer is dated.

Judy C. Kneece, RN , OCN, ***Solving the Mystery of Breast Pain*** (EduCare Publishing, 1996). $7.95 plus $4.50 shipping. This handbook provides straight-forward answers to many questions about breast pain. EduCare Publishing, P.O. Box 280305, Columbia, SC 29228. (800) 849-9271.

Judy C.Kneece, ***Solving the Mystery of Breast Discharge*** (EduCare Publishing, 1996) $7.95 plus $4.50 shipping. This handbook provides straightforward answers to many questions about breast discharge. EduCare Publishing, P.O. Box 280305, Columbia, SC 29228. (800) 849-9271.

GENETICS, RISKS, PREVENTION, AND DETECTION OF BREAST CANCER

Genetics, Risk, and Prevention: The Family Cancer Risk Counseling and Genetic Testing Directory (found on CancerNet, NCI's website, http://cancernet.nci.nih.gov /www.prot/genetic/genesrch.shtm) . Offers a listing of cancer risk counseling resources and genetic testing providers across the country. The Directory is searchable by name, state, country, and type of cancer or cancer gene.

FORCE (www.facingourrisk.org), Groups organized around women who are at high risk for breast and ovarian cancer especially those with BRCA1 or 2.

National Society of Genetic Counselors (www.nsgc.org). To find a genetic counselor to help you understand your risks and explore your options.

The Alliance of Genetic Support Groups (www.geneticalliance.org).

The National Cancer Institute's Breast Cancer Risk Assessment Tool. The "Risk Disk" (September 1998) is free from the NCI and serves as an interactive patient education tool to help assess an individual's risk of developing breast cancer. NCI (8OO) 4-CANCER.

National Women's Health Network Hearts, Bones, Hot Flashes and Hormones (2000). $1, National Women's Health Network, 514 10th St NW Suite 400, Washington, DC 20004. (202) 347-1140. An excellent review of the current state of knowledge about postmenopausal hormone therapy.

Committee on the Relationship Between Oral Contraceptives and Breast Cancer, Institute of Medicine, Oral Contraceptives and Breast Cancer (Washington, DC: National Academy Press, 1991).

Cancer and Genetics: Answering Your Patients Questions. Booklet produced jointly by the American Cancer Society and PRR, Inc. It answers patients' questions about inherited cancer syndromes, identifies individuals and families that may be at higher than average risk due to alterations in cancer susceptibility genes, and familiarizes the reader with the social and clinical implications of decisions to seek genetic testing.

American Cancer Society. (800) ACS-2345. Cancer Facts Questions and Answers: The Breast Cancer Prevention Trial (1999). This fact sheet answers common questions about The Breast Cancer Prevention Trial including its design, results and significance for women. Available at no charge from the National Cancer Institute. (800) 4-CANCER.

DES Exposure: Questions and Answers for Mothers, Daughters and Sons (1990). DES Action, Oakland, CA 94612. (800) DES-9288. Authoritative booklet. 20 pages, $2.50. They also have free literature on DES.

Diet Nutrition and Cancer Prevention: A Guide to Food Choices (87-2878) National Cancer Institute. This booklet describes what is known about diet nutrition and cancer prevention.

Understanding Breast Changes: A Health Guide for All Women (97-3536, 1997). Booklet explains various type of breast changes that women experience, and outlines methods that doctors use to distinguish between benign changes and cancer. NCI's CIS, (800) 4-CANCER.

Understanding Gene Testing (97-3905,1997). This easy-to-understand guide provides readers with basic information and addresses issues raised when considering testing under managed care. 30 pages. Order from NCI's CIS, (800) 4-CANCER.

Understanding Genetics of Breast Cancer for Jewish Women (American Jewish Congress and Hadassah, 1997). As follow-up to the First Leadership Conference on Jewish Women's Health Issues, this brochure was compiled to answer questions about hereditary risk of breast cancer and deciding if genetic testing is right for you. Available by calling the Hadassah Health Education Department, (212) 303-80094.

Genetic Testing for Cancer Risk: It's your Choice (National Action Plan on Breast Cancer). Hosted by Cokie Roberts, this video gives an overview of the risks and benefits of being tested for genetic susceptibility to breast and ovarian cancer. Companion brochure available. 14 minutes. A free copy of the tape can be obtained for NCI, (800) 4-CANCER.

Testing for Hereditary Risk of Breast and Ovarian Cancer—Is it Right for You? (MY8447, Myriad Genetics 1999) a video from Myriad, a for-profit company marketing gene-testing, designed to answer questions and suggest topics to be discussed with a physician or counselor. Order by calling (800) 469-7423 or visit www.myriad.com.

Nancy C. Baker, ***Relative Risk: Living with a Family History of Breast Cancer*** (New York). Discusses risk factors as well as women's reactions to being at "increased risk."

Kevin Davies and Michael White, ***Breakthrough: The Race to Find the Breast Cancer Gene*** (New York: John Wiley, 1996). A history of the discovery of the BRCA1 gene, including information on current treatments and future research directions.

Patricia T. Kelly, ***Assessing Your True Risk of Breast Cancer*** (New York: Henry Holt, 2000). Her latest book tells you how to calculate your own personal risk.

M. Margaret Kemeny and Paula Dranov, ***Breast Cancer and Ovarian Cancer: Beating the Odds*** (Reading, MA: Addison-Wesley, 1992). Reviews risk factors.

Earl Mindell, ***Earl Mindell's Vitamin Bible*** (New York: Warner, 1994).

Prevention Magazine (Ed.), ***The Complete Book of Cancer Prevention: Foods, Lifestyle and Medical Care to Keep You Healthy***

Carol Rinzler, ***Estrogen and Breast Cancer: A Warning to Women*** (Order from BCA Bookstore, 1280 Columbus Avenue, Suite 204, San Francisco, CA 94133).

Basil Stoll (Ed.), ***Reducing Breast Cancer Risk in Women*** (Norwell, MA: Kluwer Academic Publishers, 1995). Review what is currently known about prevention, limited as it is.

Laurie Tarkan, *My Mother's Breast, Daughters Face their Mothers Cancer* (Taylor Publishing, 1999). Paperback.

DETECTION

Agency for Health Care Policy and Research, Quality Determinants of Mammography Guidelines for consumers and health care professionals on what is necessary for the best possible test. For a copy of the consumer or professional guidelines, call (800) 358-9295.

National Consortium of Breast Cancers, c/o Barbara Rabinowitz, RN, MSW, ACSW, Comprehensive Breast Center, Robert Wood Johnson Medical School, One Robert Wood Johnson Place, CN19, New Brunswick, NJ 08903-0019. Will send you a list of breast centers throughout the entire country registered with them. Many are diagnostic only and others are involved in diagnosis only and others are involved in both diagnosis and treatment.

The Older You Get, The More You Need a Mammogram (5020, 1993). (800)522-2345.

Questions and Answers About Choosing a Mammography Facility (94-3228, 1994). This four-page brochure should accompany Are You Age 50 or Over? A Mammogram Could Save Your Life, from NCI. (800) 4-CANCER.

CANCER IN GENERAL

American Cancer Society, (800) ACS-2345 or www.cancer.org. National toll-free hotline provides information on all forms of cancer, referrals for the ACS sponsored "Reach to Recovery" program.

AMC Cancer Research Center's Cancer Information Line, 1600 Pierce St, Denver CO 80214. (800) 525-3777. Professional cancer counselors provide answers to questions about cancer, support, and advice and will mail instructive free publications upon request. Equipped for deaf and hearing impaired callers.

Cancer Information Service of the National Cancer Institute (www.nci.nih.gov). This information service can be reached toll-free at (800) 4-CANCER. They give information and direction through their national and regional network on all aspects of cancer. Spanish-speaking staff members are available on request.

Cancer Information Service of the Canadian Cancer Society. Information service in English and French. For calls from Canada only (888) 939-3333, or www.cancer.ca.

Cancercare, Inc. (800) 813- HOPE or www.cancercare.org. Support services, education, information, referrals and financial assistance.

Vital Options TeleSupport Cancer Network, the GroupRoom Radio Talk Show, P.O. Box 19233, Encino, CA 91416-9233. (818) 788-5225. A weekly syndicated call-in cancer talk show linking callers with other patients, long-termed survivors, family members, physicians, researchers, and therapists experienced in working with cancer issues.

BREAST CANCER IN GENERAL

Community Breast Health Project (www.med.Stanford.EDU:80/CBHP). One of the first community breast cancer resource centers. Information from Ellen Mahoney, MD (founder and breast surgeon).

Department of Defense Decision Guide (www.bcdg.org). An interactive guide through the decisions a newly diagnosed women needs to make.

Faces of Hope (www.facesofhope.net). Nationally recognized not-for-profit educational breast cancer program that focuses on the importance of early detection and prevention. The program features a portable radio exhibit of breast cancer survivors.

ibreast (www.ibreast.com) Website of Dr. Marisa Weiss, radiation oncologist gist, and author of Living Beyond Breast Cancer.

Mothers Supporting Daughters with Breast Cancer (www. mothersdaughters.org) MSDBC is a national nonprofit organization co-founded by a mother and her daughter. The support services provided by this organization are by signed to help mothers who have daughters battling breast cancer.

National Action Plan on Breast Cancer (www.napbc.org): The National Action Plan is a public private partnership which sprung out of the demands of advocates.

SusanLoveMD.com (www.susanlovemd.com) Provides breast cancer chats for baby boomer women.

MAMM Magazine covers issues helpful to women who have been diagnosed with breast and reproductive cancer, their partners and their families. Published ten times a year. Subscription, $17.95 per year. Contact MAMM Magazine, 349 West 12th Street, New York, NY 10014-1796, (888) 901-MAMM or subscription@mamm.com.

Judges arid Lawyers Breast Cancer Alert, 50 King Street , Suite 6D, New York, NY 10014. Confidential hotline for judges, lawyers and law students who have been diagnosed with breast cancer.

National Alliance of Breast Cancer Organizations (NABCO), 9 East 37th Street, 10th Floor, New York, NY 10016. (888) 80NABCO; (212) 719-0154 or www.nabco.org. Membership organization is a central source of information about breast cancer and provides up-to-date information packets. Their annual resource list is available for $5; guide to Regional Support Groups is available for $2 from their office, or free at www.nabco.org.

National Breast Cancer Coalition, 1707 L Street NW, Suite 1060, Washington, DC 20036, (202) 296-7477 or www.natlbcc.org. Coalition of over 500 groups involves women with the disease and those who care about them in changing public policy as it relates to progress against breast cancer. The NBCC welcomes individuals and organizations as members.

Susan G. Komen Breast Cancer Foundation, Occidental Tower, 5005 LBJ Freeway, Suite 370, Dallas, TX 75244. (800) I'M AWARE, (972) 855-1600, or www.breastcancerinfo.com. Largest private funder of breast cancer research in the U.S. as well as organizers of Races for the Cure.

Women's Information Network Against Breast Cancer (WIN ABC) 19325 East Navilla Place, Covina, CA 91723, (626) 3322255, or www.winabc.org. National non-profit organization offering resources, peer support, and referral sources through telephone counseling, mail support and community outreach.

Y-ME National Breast Cancer Organization, 212 West Van Buren Street,

Chicago, IL 60607. Provides support and counseling through their national toll free hotline. (800) 221-2141 (24 hours; Spanish language line, (800) 986-9505); www.yme.org. Trained peer counselors are matched by background and experience to callers whenever possible. Y-ME offers information on establishing local support programs, and has 23 chapters nationwide. Y-ME also has a hotline for men whose partners have had breast cancer

YWCA Encore Plus Program ENCOREplus, (800) 95-EPLUS or www.ywca.org. Provides early detection outreach, education, post diagnostic support, and exercise services to all women.

Inflammatory Breast Cancer (www.ibcsupport.org). Good information regarding the relatively rare inflammatory breast cancer.

Lymphedema Network (www.lymphnet.org). Support for all kinds of lymphedema although that caused by breast cancer surgery is the most prominent.

Male Breast Cancer (interact.withus.com/interact/mbc/). Information on male breast cancer.

Young Survivor Coalition (www.youngsurvival.org). Young breast cancer survivors.

Pregnant with Cancer Support Group, P.O. Box 1243, Buffalo, NY 14220, (800) 743-6724 ext.308 or www.pregnantwithcancer.org. For women who are facing a diagnosis of cancer while pregnant, this group will match a new patient with someone who once faced cancer while pregnant.

Breast Cancer Facts and Figures 1999/2000 (American Cancer Society). A booklet containing statistics including incidence, survival and trends. Order from American Cancer Society (800) ACS-2345 or www.cancer.org.

A Helping Hand-The Resource Guide for People with Cancer (Cancer Care, Inc., 1997). Cancer Care, (800) 813-HOPE, or www.cancercare.org.

If You've Thought about Breast Cancer Rose Kushner Breast Cancer Advisory Center, (Summer 1998 edition). Updated general pamphlet on breast cancer detection and treatment, including definitions and resources. Order multiple copies from The Rose Kushner Breast Cancer Advisory Center, PO Box 224, Kensington, MD 20895, (301) 949-2531. Single copies free of charge from Y-ME.

Understanding Breast Cancer Treatment (July 1998). This booklet contains lists of questions that will help a patient talk to her doctor about breast cancer. Topics covered include early detection, diagnosis, treatment, adjuvant therapy, and reconstruction. 72 pages. NCI's CIS, (800) 4-CANCER or rex.nci.nih.gov.

What You Need to Know about Breast Cancer (98-1556, August 1998). NCI's most comprehensive pamphlet on breast cancer, this updated booklet covers symptoms, diagnosis, treatment, emotional issues, and questions to ask your doctor. Includes an index of terms. 44 pages. NCI's CIS, (800) 4-CANCER or rex.nci. nih.gov. (Note: A 1999 version is expected to be available mid-year).

Your Breast Cancer Treatment Handbook by Judy C. Kneece, RN, OCN (EduCare Publishing, 1998). This easy to use book contains useful information about managing treatment decisions and addresses sensitive emotional issues in an insightful manner. 210 pages. EduCare Publishing, P.O. Box 280505, Columbia, SC 29228, (800) 849-9271 or www.cancerhelp.com/ed.

Initial Discovery and Diagnosis (1999) Video. In this first of a planned series of 12 videos for breast cancer patients, seven breast cancer survivors share how they learned of their breast cancer diagnosis and how they learned to cope with their disease. Also includes a resource guide. 15 minutes, $15.00.

Contact Woman to Woman (877) 85-WOMAN or www.womantowoman-videos.org.

Roberta Allman and Michael J Sarg, ***The Cancer Dictionary*** (NY: Fact File, 1992). Includes acronyms for chemotherapy protocols and simple anatomical illustrations. Order from Facts on File (800) 322-8755.

Larry and Valerie Althouse, ***You Can Save Your Breast: One Woman's Experience with Radiation Therapy*** (New York: WW Norton, 1982).

Suzanne W. Braddock, et al., ***Straight Talk About Breast Cancer: From Diagnosis to Recovery: A Guide for the Entire Family*** (Addicus Books, 1996).

Paperback.

Linda Brown Harris, ***Breast Cancer Handbook: A Basic Guide for Gathering Information, Understanding the Diagnosis, and Choosing the Treatment*** (1992). A great booklet on breast cancer with many questions you should pose to your doctors. Melpomene Institute for Women's Health Research, 1010 University Avenue, St. Paul, MN 55104 (612) 642-1951.

Yashar Hirshaut, Peter Pressman. ***Breast Cancer: The Complete Guide*** (Baintam Books, 1997). Paperback. An easy-to-follow resource written by an oncologist and a surgeon.

Vladimir Lange, ***Be A Survivor: Your Guide to Breast Cancer Treatment*** (Lange Productions, 1998). Has great graphics.

Kathy LaTour, ***The Breast Cancer Companion*** (NY. William Morrow & Co, 1994). Guidebook offers useful tips, insights of 75 survivors and background information about advocacy and politics of breast cancer.

John Link. ***The Breast Cancer Survival Manual: A Step-by-Step Guide for the Woman with Newly Diagnosed Cancer*** (Owl Books, 2000). Paperback. Another step-by-step guide by a medical oncologist.

Rosie O'Donnell and Deborah Axelrod with Tracy C. Semler, ***Bosom Buddies: Lessons and Laughter on Breast Health and Cancer*** (Warner Books, 1999). Answers frequently asked questions about breast cancer in an easy-to-read manner.

Swirsky and Barbara Balaban, ***The Breast Cancer Handbook: Taking Control After You've Found a Lump 2nd edition*** (NY. Power Publications, 1998). Easy to read guide takes you step-by-step through diagnosis and treatment.

M.J. Silverstein, editor. ***Ductal Carcinoma in Site of the Breast*** (Baltimore, MD: Williams, and Wilkins, 1997).

J.R. Harris, S. Hellman, 1. C.Henderson, D.W.Kinne, ***Breast Diseases*** (Philadelphia, Lippincott 1991). Medical textbook with a very comprehensive treatment of breast cancer.

EMOTIONAL ASPECTS

Wellness Community-National, 35 East 7th Street, Cincinnati, OH 45242. (888) 793-WELL; www.wellness-community.org. Started in California with many centers across the Country, its facilities provide free psychosocial care to cancer patients and their families.

The Wellness Community, 1235 Fifth Street, Santa Monica CA 90401 (310) 393-1415. Extensive support and education programs which encourage emotional recovery and a feeling of wellness.

Cancer Care, Inc. and the National Cancer Care Foundation, 1180 Avenue of the the Americas, New York NY 10036. (800) 813-HOPE, www.cancercare.org. A social service agency which helps patients and their families cope with the impact of cancer. Direct services are invited to the greater New York area but callers will be referred to similar assistance available in their areas.

Cancer Hope Network, 2 North Road, Suite A, Chester, NH 07930, 877-HOPENET Offers one-on-one support to cancer patients and their families undergoing cancer treatment from trained volunteers who have survived cancer.

The Cancer Wellness Center/The Barbara Kassel Brotman House, offers free emotional support on its 24-hour hotline and through support groups, relaxation groups, educational workshops, and library. Revere Northbrook, IL 50062. (708) 509-9595.

Gilda's Club, 195 W.Houston Street, New York, NY 10014. (212) 647-9700. A free, nonprofit program where people with cancer and their families and friends join with others to build social and emotional support as a supplement to medical care in a nonresidential, home-like setting. Twenty-five locations nationwide.

The National Self-Help Clearinghouse, c/o Graduate School and University Center of City University of New York, 33 West 42 Street, Room 620N, New York, NY 10036. Will refer written inquiries to regional self-help services.

Reach to Recovery Program of the American Cancer Society. Trained volunteers visit newly-diagnosed patients. (800) ACS-2345.

Coping Magazine. A bi-monthly magazine for cancer patients and survivors. Subscription $18/year. Media America, Inc., 2019 North Carothers, Franklin, TN 37064. (615) 790-2400 (copingmaggaol.com).

Actions People with Cancer Can Take to Join with their Physicians in the Fight for Recovery This brochure is free of charge from Wellness Community, 2716 Ocean Park Blvd, Santa Monica CA 90405 (310) 334-2555.

Breast Cancer and Sexuality (Cancer Care, NY, 1998). Booklet on sexuality, intimacy and menopausal symptoms. Free from (800) 813HOPE or www.cancercare.org.

For Single Women with Breast Cancer (1994). Y-ME booklet offers practical guidance and emotional support for women without partners or those who live alone. Single copies available FREE (800) 221-2141.

Facing Forward, A Guide for Cancer Survivors (9302424, 1992). Addresses the special needs of cancer survivors and their families. 43 pages NCI (800)4-CANCER.

Taking Time: Support for People with Cancer and the People Who Care About Them (National Cancer Institute, P126, 1996). Booklet addresses the feelings and concerns of others in similar situations and how they have coped. 68 pages. Call NCI's CIS, (800) 4-CANCER.

Talking with your Doctor (American Cancer Society, 4638-CC, 1997 edition). Suggestions for effective doctor/patient communication. Six pages. Call the ACS, (800) ACS-2345.

Teamwork The Cancer Patients—A Guide to Talking with Your Doctor (National Coalition for Cancer Survivorship, $3.00 for members of the NCCS, $4.00 for non-members). Useful suggestions on how to best begin and maintain a working relationship with a physician. 32 pages. Contact NCCS, 1010 Wayne Avenue 5th Floor, Silver Spring, MD 20910, (888) 937-6227 or www.cansearch.org.

Anne Fogelsanger, *See Yourself Well: For People with Cancer* (Brooklyn NY.

Equinox). Audiocassette, $10.95. May be helpful to use while under treatment.

Barbara Bergholz and Eva Shaw, Diana's Gift. (La Jolla, CA: Gentle Winds Press, 1992).

Helene Davis, **Chemo-poet and Other Poems** (Cambridge, MA: Alice James Books, 1989).

Wendy Schlessel Harpham, **Diagnosis Cancer: Your Guide Through the First Few Months** (NY. 1992). Guide for newly-diagnosed cancer patients, written by an internist who is also a cancer survivor.

Danette G. Kauffman, **Surviving Cancer** (Washington, D.C.: Acropolis Books, 1989). A practical guide to experiencing cancer and its treatment, with an emphasis on lists of resources for managing the medical, emotional, and financial aspects of this disease.

Ronnie Kaye, **Spinning Straw into Gold: Your Emotional Recovery from Breast Cancer** (NY: Fireside,1991). Paperback. Excellent guide to the emotional aspects of this disease from a psychologist who is also a survivor.

L. LeShan, **Cancer as a Turning Point: A Handbook for People with Cancer, Their Families and Health Professionals** (NY. E.P. Dutton, 1989).

Leatrice Lifshitz, **Her Soul Beneath the Bone: Women's Poetry on Breast Cancer** (Urbana: University of Illinois, 1988).

Raymond A. Moody, M.D., **The Light Beyond: New Explorations by the Author of Life After Life** (Bantam, 1988).

Susan Nessim and Judith Ellis, **Cancervive: The Challenge of Life after Cancer** (Boston: Houghton Mifflin, 1992, $8.95). Addresses the practical and emotional issues faced by cancer survivors such as insurance, relationships, infertility and long-term side effects of treatment.

Hester Hill Schnipper, Joan Feinberg Berns. **Woman to Woman: A Handbook for Women Newly Diagnosed with Breast Cancer** Wholecare Paperback, 1999).

Midge Stocker, editor, **Confronting Cancer, Constructing Change: New**

Perspectives on Women and Cancer Essays confronting cancer myths.

Rebecca Zuckweiler. ***Living in the Postmastectomy Body: Learning to Live in and Love Your Body Again*** (Andrews Mcmeel Publishing, 1998). Paperback. The author, a nurse and psychotherapist who had a double mastectomy, focuses on regaining confidence in your body.

Practical Advice: Complements to Breast Cancer Therapy-Treating the Body and Soul
Retreats and getaways designed for cancer survivors are increasingly available.

Casting for Recovery offers weekend retreats that teach survivors how to fly-fish and focus on emotional and physical well-being. Contact Casting for Recovery, (888) 553-3500 or cfrprogram@aol.com.

The Colorado Outward Bound School offers a course specifically for women surviving cancer, (MM) 837-5204. Healing Adventures sponsors outdoor adventures for people challenged by cancer and for their friends and families, (510) 2378291.

Wilderness Bay Wellness Foundation designs and delivers therapeutic wilderness programs for female cancer patients and survivors, (773) 334-0809.

Women in Nature is an annual outdoor adventure in northern Minnesota for cancer survivors, (612) 520-1704.

Life Choices Wellness Center seven day retreat includes meditation and empowerment activities, (800) 439-0083.

Two other programs are **Summits-Inner Mountain Wilderness Education Center,** (907) 766-2074, lifechoices@lewcenter.com, and **Expedition Inspiration** at (208) 726-6456 co

FAMILIES AND CHILDREN

Caringkids (http://oncolink.upenn.edu/forms/listsev.html). Internet support group for children who know someone who is ill. Monitored, open forum where children may exchange information, share their feelings, and make friends with other children dealing with similar issues.

Helping Children Cope Program of Cancer Care, Inc. (800) 813-HOPE or www.cancercare.org. Offers support groups and telephone counseling for children who have a parent with cancer.

Kids Count Too is a six session program of the American Cancer Society for preschool through teenage children who are coping with a parent's cancer. To find the program nearest you, contact the ACS, (800) ACS-2345 or www.cancer.org.

Kids Konnected, 27071 Cabot Road, Suite 102, Laguna Hills, CA 92653. (800) 899-2866. Provides friendship, education, understanding, and support to kids who have a parent with cancer.

The National Family Caregivers Association, 51 National Family Counseling Assn, 10400 Connecticut Avenue #500, Kensington, MD 20895-3944, (800) 896-3650 or www.nfcacares.org. Offers information, education, support, public awareness, and advocacy to address the common needs of family caregivers.

It Helps to Have Friends (American Cancer Society, 4654.00). A pamphlet for children with a parent who has cancer. Call the ACS, (800) ACS-2345.

Helping Children Cope When a Parent Has Cancer 12 pages American Cancer Society. A booklet to help you help your children.

Handbook for Mothers Supporting Daughters with Breast Cancer (1999). 26 pages. Contact Mothers Supporting Daughters with Breast Cancer, 21710 Bayshore Road, Chestertown, MD 21620-4401, (410) 778-1982, msdbc@dmv.com or www.mothersdaughters.org.

A Shared Purpose: A Guide for Daughters Whose Mothers Have Advanced Breast Cancer (Cancer Care, 1998). Answers questions about advanced breast cancer, and addresses feelings and emotions that mothers and daughters may face. 18 pages. Contact Cancer Care, (800) 813-HOPE or www.cancercare.org.

Journaling Through the Storm" and "Silver Linings: The Other Side of Cancer (Oncology Nursing Press, 1998). Companion volumes: an illustrated journal that invites the patient and her family to chronicle events, thoughts and feelings, and a collection of inspirational essays and poems. Contact ONS Customer Service, (412) 921-7373, customer.service@ons.org or www.ons.org.

Taking Time: Support for the People with Cancer and the People Who Care About Them (92-2059) National Cancer Institute. Booklet for persons with cancer and their families. 69 pages. NCI (800) 4-CANCER

When Someone in Your Family Has Cancer (National Cancer Institute, P619, 1995). Written for the young person whose parent has cancer. This booklet describes what cancer is, its treatment, and its emotional impact on family relationships. Includes a glossary of cancer-related terms. 28 pages. Call the NCI's CIS, (800)4-CANCER

BOOKS FOR PARENTS

My Mom Has Breast Cancer-A Guide for Families (1996) A KIDSCOPE, Inc. A video for parents and children about coping with a mother's breast cancer diagnosis. Structured as interviews with six breast cancer survivors and their young children. Contact KIDSCOPE, 3400 Peachtree Road, Suite 703, Atlanta, GA 30326, (404) 233-0001 or www.kidscope.org.

Talking About Cancer: A Parent's Guide to Helping Children Cope (Fox Chase Cancer Center). A video that helps parents with cancer explain their diagnosis to their children, 18 minutes. Call the Fox Chase Cancer Center, (888) FOX-CHASE.

Kathleen McCue, MA, CCLS with Ron Bonn, ***How to Help Children Through a Parent's Serious Illness*** (NY. St. Martin's Press, 1994). Explains a child's special needs when a parent is seriously ill. Provides guidelines advice and real-life examples to help parents and other caregivers help children during this stressful time.

Elizabeth Winthrop and illustrated by Betsy Lewin, ***Promises*** (NY: Clarion Books, 2000). Book addresses the range of emotions that children can experience when a parent has cancer.

BOOKS FOR CHILDREN

Claire Blake, Eliza Blanchard, and Kathy Parkinson, ***The Paper Chain*** (Health

Press, 1998). For children ages three to eight. This book relays the emotions of two young boys whose mom has breast cancer. 32 pages. Bookstores or call Health Press, (800) 643-BOCK.

Pat Brack and Ben Brack, **Moms Don't Get Sick** (Aberdeen, SD: Melius Publishing, 1990). One woman's story as told through her eyes and those of her ten year old son. Excellent for women with children.

Christine Clifford, **Our Family Has Cancer Too!** (Duluth MN: Pfeifer-Hamilton Pubs, 1997). For children ages five to 14, this book talks about one child's struggle to understand and cope with his mother's cancer. Illustrated with cartoons. 64 pages. Bookstores or contact The Cancer Club, 6533 Limerick Drive, Edina, MN 55439, (800) 586-9062 or www.cancerclub.com.

Judylaine Fine, **Afraid to Ask, A Book for Families to Share about Cancer** (NY Lothrop, Lee and Shepard Books, 1986).

Wendy S. Harpham, **When a Parent has Cancer: A Guide to Caring for Your Children with Becky and The Worry Cup.** (Harper Collins Publishers, 1997). The author, a lymphoma survivor, presents sensitive and practical advice to help children understand and cope with a parent's diagnosis of cancer. An illustrated children's book is included that tells the poignant story of Becky, a seven-year-old girl and her experiences with her mother's cancer.

H. Elizabeth King, **Kemoshark** (1995). A colorfully illustrated booklet to help children understand chemotherapy when their parent is undergoing treatment. 14 pages. Contact KIDSCOPE, 3399 Peachtree Road, Suite 2020, Atlanta, CA 30326, (404) 233-0001 or www.kidscope.org.

Sherry Kohlenberg, **Sammy's Mommy Has Cancer** (NY: Magination Press, 1993). The author, who was diagnosed with breast cancer when she was 34 and her son was 18 months old, offers parents a thoughtful and sensitive way to explain breast cancer to a child. (800) 374-2721 or www.maginationpress.com.

Laura Numeroff and Wendy S. Harpham, **Kid's Talk—Kids Speak Out About Breast Cancer** (Samsung Telecommunications America and Sprint PCS, 1999). For children aged ten and younger, short stories told by children about living with a mother with breast cancer. Call the Susan G. Komen Foundation (800)I'MAWARE.

Carolyn Steams Parkinson, *My Mommy Has Cancer* (TN: Cope/Coping Books).

Deborah Weinstein-Stem, *Mira's Month* ($5.00). When the author's breast cancer recurred, she wrote this book for her four year old daughter. 38 pages. Contact the Blood and Marrow Transplant Information Network, 2900 Skokie Valley Road, Suite B, Highland Park, IL 60035, (888) 597-7674.

HUSBANDS AND PARTNERS

The Well Spouse Foundation, 30 East 40th Street, P.H., New York, NY 10016, (800) 838-0879 or www.wellspouse.org. A national, non-profit membership organization that gives support to husbands, wives, and partners of the chronically ill and/or disabled. Support groups and a bi-monthly newsletter are available.

Y-ME National Breast Cancer Organization has trained male volunteers who provide support and counseling to other male partners of women with breast cancer through their national toll-free hotline, (800) 221-2141 (9:00 am to 5:00 pro CST, Monday through Friday).

Sexuality and Cancer: For the Woman Who has Cancer, and Her Partner (1999 edition) 64 pages. American Cancer Society. A booklet that gives information about cancer and sexuality in areas that might concern the patient and her partner. ACS (800) ACS-2345.

When the Woman You Love I Has Breast Cancer (Y-ME, 1994). A booklet that helps partners give emotional support to their loved ones. Single copies available free, bulk orders available on request, Call Y-ME, (800) 221-2141 or www.y-me.org.

The Breast Cancer Companion Tapes: Diagnosis and Decision-Making/The Male Perspective (1994, two tapes, $35.00 each). Offers couples two separate videotapes, one for the patient and one for her partner and includes insight into how other couples have dealt with the medical and emotional issues surrounding a breast cancer diagnosis. 30 minutes each. Contact the Breast Cancer Companion Tapes, P.O. Box 141182, Dallas, TX 75214.

Larry T. Eiler. ***When the Woman You Love Has Breast Cancer*** (Queen Dee Publishing Ann Arbor, ME 1994). Issues faced by a man whose wife or friend has the disease, suggesting steps he can take to be supportive. Queen Bee Publishing, 900 Victors Way, Suite 180, Am Arbor, MI 48108, (734) 761-3399.

Judy C. Kneece. ***Helping Your Mate Face Breast Cancer Tips for becoming an effective support partner for the one you love during the breast cancer experience*** (Edu Care, Inc., 1999). Paperback. Offers helpful suggestions on coping strategies and how to support the physical and emotional recovery of a partner

Andy Murcia and Bob Stewart, ***Man to Man: When the Woman You Low has Breast Cancer*** (NY.St. Martin's Press, 1990).

Leslie R. Schover, ***Sexuality and Fertility after Cancer***, (John Wiley and Sons, Inc., New York, NY, 1997). Paperback. Explains how treatment may emotionally and physically interfere with male and female sexual function and fertility.

Bruce Sokol, et al. ***Breast Cancer: A Husband's Story.*** (Crane Hill Publishing, 1997). Paperback.

LESBIANS

The Lesbian Community Cancer Project 4753 North Broadway, Suite 602, Chicago, IL 60640-4907, (773) 561-4662 or www.iccp.org. Gives support, information, education, advocacy, and direct services to lesbians and women living with cancer and their families.

The Mautner Project for Lesbians with Cancer, 1707 L Street NW, Suite 500, Washington, DC 20036, (202) 332-5536, mautner@mautnerproject.org or www. mautnerproject.org. A volunteer organization dedicated to helping lesbians with cancer, as well as their partners and caregivers. The pamphlet, Lesbians and Cancer, provides early detection information; available at no cost in English or Spanish.

The National Lesbian and Gay Health Association, (202) 939-7880, nlgha@aol .com or www.nlgha.org. Provides general health information and resources, including cancer.

Seattle Lesbian Cancer Project, 1122 E. Pike Street, #1333, Seattle WA 98122 (206) 286-0166 Grassroots organization provides advocacy, education and referrals, with an emphasis on the medically underserved.

Wendy's Hope: Reaching Out to lesbians with Cancer and Other Life Threatening Diseases City of Hope,1055 Wilshire Blvd, 12th Floor, Los Angeles CA (310) 798-9085 or corewellness.com Offers education, assistance and support groups.

Sandra Butler and Barbara Rosenblum, Cancer in Two Voices (Spinsters Book Company, MN, 1996, expanded edition). A particularly moving and honest account of the authors' identity as Jewish women and as lesbians as they live with advanced breast cancer.

Cancer in Two Voices   This video complements the book described above. (16mm /video, rental $140/$90, plus $22.00 shipping; VHS $275.00, plus $15 00 shipping). 43 minutes. Contact Women Make Movies, Sales and Rental Department 462 Broadway, Suite 500-C, New York, NY 10013 or (212) 925-0606.

Roz Perry, *Rose Penski* (Tallahassee, FL: Naiad Press). A novel about a lesbian and her lover going through diagnosis and initial treatment of breast cancer.

PERSONAL STORIES

SHOW ME: A Photo Collection of Breast Cancer Survivors' Lumpectomies, Mastectomies, Reconstructions and Thoughts on Body Image. Fantastic resource created by a Breast Cancer Support Group which shows what your body will look like after different surgeries. Order from Penn State Geisinger Health System Women's Center, Box 850, Code H306, Hershey PA 17033, (717) 531-5867 or view at SusanLoveMD.com.

Victories: Three Women Triumph over Breast Disease (MBM Communications, San Francisco, CA 1989). Videotape of three personal stories (mastectomy/ reconstruction, benign disease, lumpectomy/chemo/RT, recurrence). Includes group discussions, husband/wife counseling and mammography. To order call (415) 642-0460. 23 minutes, $195.00/$45.00 rental.

Not Alone-Women Coping with Breast Cancer (Adelphi Oncology Support

Program, Garden City, NJ, Fall 1988). Filmed during actual sessions, a group of breast cancer patients accompanied by a social worker discuss their concerns and offer mutual support. 22 minute video, $150.00. Order from Adelphi (516) 877-4444.

Voices of Healing: You're Not Alone-Conversations with Breast Cancer Survivors and Those Who Love Them (Voice Arts Publishing, Madison, WI, 1998). This two hour audiotape package narrates the experiences and insights of breast cancer survivors, their partners, and children. Covers physical, emotional, social and spiritual aspects of the disease $7.95 To order, call (800) 267-1705,

Cathy Saved Her Life (1989). Videotape of televised story of Cathy Masamitsu, an ABC "Home Show" staff member who had breast cancer. 90 minutes, $7.50. Order from Woody Fraser Productions, PO Box 7548, Burbank, CA 91510-7548.

Elizabeth Berg, ***Talk Before Sleep*** (New York: Dell, 1997). Paperback. A fictional account of how a group of women face the diagnosis of breast cancer in one of their friends.

Judy Brady, ***One in Three: Women With Cancer Confront all Epidemic*** (Pittsburgh: Clei's press, 1991) Collection of essays by women involved in grassroots cancer activism.

Nancy Brinker with Catherine McEvily Harris, ***The Race is Ran One Step at a Time, My Personal Struggle and Everywoman's Guide to Taking Charge of Breast Cancer*** (NY. Simon & Schuster, 1990) Also available on audio cassette, account Of the battle against breast cancer by the author and her sister, Susan Kamen.

Sue Buchanan. ***I'm Alive and the Doctor's Dead: Surviving Cancer with Your Sense of Humor and Your Sexuality Intact.*** (Zondervan Publishing House, 1998). Paperback,

Rita Busch (editor), et al. ***Can You Come Here Where I Am? The Poetry and Prose of Seven Breast Cancer Survivors*** (E M Pr Paperback, 1998)

Donna Cederberg, Daria Davidson, Joy Edwards, Carol Hebestreit, Betsy Lambert, Amy Langer , Cathy Masamitsu, Sally Snodgrass, Carol Stack and Carol

Washington, ***Breast Cancer? Let Me Check my Schedule***. (Vancouver, WA: Innovative Medical Education Consortium, 1994). Ten professional women share their wisdom and experience about living with breast cancer. Order from IMEC, 500 W. 8th Street, Suite 100A, Vancouver. WA 98660.

Katlyn Conway. ***Ordinary Life: A Memoir of Illness***. (W.H. Freeman and Company, New York, NY, 1997). Written by a Psychotherapist, this book details the author's struggle through her breast cancer diagnosis and treatment,

Linda Dackman, ***Up Front: Sex and the Post-Mastectomy Woman*** (NY: Viking 1990). A personal account, with frank details about the intimate challenges faced by a single woman in her 30's.

Laura Evans, ***The Climb of My Life***. (Harper San Francisco, 1996). The author traces her experience from the time she was diagnosed with breast cancer in 1990 to 1995, when she led sixteen other breast cancer survivors in a climb to the summit of the highest mountain in the Western Hemisphere.

Gayle Feldman, ***You Don't Have to Be Your Mother*** (NY. W.W. Norton, 1994). Courageous account of a 40 year old pregnant woman's struggle to deal with breast cancer and to come to terms with the death of her mother, who died of breast cancer.

Nora Feller and Marcia Stevens Sherrill, ***Portraits of Hope***. (NY. Southmark Publishers, 1998). Fifty-two inspirational survivors are profiled by Ms. Sherrill and their color portraits are photographed by Ms. Feller. The two-volume set includes a journal for thoughts and notes.

Robert C. Fore, Ed and Rorie E. Fore, RN. ***Survivor's Guide to Breast Cancer***. (Macon, GA: Smyth & Helwys Pub, 1998) A couple's story of faith, love and hope, it describes their experience with Rorie's diagnosis of breast cancer.

Andrea Gabbard. ***No Mountain Too High- A Triumph Over Breast Cancer: The Story of the Women of Expedition Inspiration***. (Seal Press, 1998). Paperback.

Amy Gross and Dee Ito, ***Women Talk about Breast Surgery, from diagnosis to recovery*** (NY. Clarkson Potter, 1990). Women's stories describing the range of situations and treatments. Better for its support aspects than the accuracy of the medical information.

Judy Hart, Love, ***Judy - Letters of Hope and Healing for Women with Breast Cancer***. (Berkeley, CA: Conari Press, 1993).

Lois Tschetter Hjelmstad, ***Fine Black Lines: Reflections on Facing Cancer, Fear, and Loneliness***. (Mulberrry Hill Press, 1993). Paperback.

Carolyn Ingram, et al. ***The Not-So-Scary Breast Cancer Book: Two Sisters' Guide from Discovery to Recovery*** (Impact Publication, 1999). Paperback.

Deborah Kahane, ***No Less a Woman, Ten Women Shatter the Myths about Breast Cancer*** (Prentice Hall Press, 1990). A cross-section of women with breast cancer tell their own stories.

Jane Lazarre, ***Wet Earth and Dreams: A Narrative of Grief and Recovery***. (Duke University Press, 1998). Moving cancer journal.

Audre Lorde, ***The Cancer Journals*** (San Francisco: Aunt Lute Books, 1980). Reflections on her breast cancer by an extraordinary black, lesbian poet. Available from Aunt Lute Books (415) 558-8116.

Christina Middlebrook. ***Seeing the Crab: A Memoir of Dying Before I Do***. (NY. Doubleday, 1998). Paperback.

Jacque Miller, ***The Lopsided Cat - The Humor, Blessings and Trials of Breast Cancer***. (Colorado: Parker Printing, 1987).

Musa Mayer, ***Examining Myself: One Woman's Story of Breast Cancer Treatment and Recovery*** (Winchester, MA: Faber and Faber, 1993). Exploration of the emotional aspects of disease and recovery. Faber and Faber is donating a portion of the book's proceeds to the National Breast Cancer Coalition.

Madeleine Meldin, ***The Tender Bud: A Physician's Journal Through Breast Cancer*** (Hillsdale, NJ: Analytic Press, 1993). Written from the point of view of a psychiatrist attempting to keep her professional life intact during breast cancer treatment.

Deena Metzger, *Tree* (Oakland, CA: Wingbow Press, 1983). Written by the woman pictured in the well-known poster of an exultant woman with a mastectomy and a tattoo of a tree on her scar. The poster can be obtained from Tree, PO Box 186, Topanga, CA 90290.

Cynthia Ploski. ***Conversations with My Healers-My Journey to Wellness from Breast Cancer*** (Council Oak Books, Tulsa, OK 74210, 1995). Paperback. Upbeat personal narratives offer help and hope to those facing breast cancer.

Margit Esser Porter (Editor). ***Hope is Contagious: The Breast Cancer Treatment Survival Handbook*** (Fireside, 1997). Paperback. Collection of quotes from women who responded to a questionnaire on how to cope with breast cancer treatment.

Hilda Raz (Editor). ***Living on the Margins: Women Writers on Breast Cancer*** (Persea Books, 1999).

Katherine Russell Rich, ***The Red Devil: To Hell with Cancer-And Back*** (NY: Crown Books, 1999). This woman has been through every imaginable breast cancer treatment and tells the tale with great wit.

Allie Fair Sawyer and Noma Suzette Jones, ***Journey: A Breast Cancer Survival Guide*** (Alexander, NO WorldComm Press, 1992). Authors share their personal experiences.

Lillie Shockney, ***Breast Cancer Survivor's Club: A Nurse's Experience***. (Windsor House, 1999). Paperback.

Melissa Springer, ***A Tribe of Warrior Women: Breast Cancer Survivors***, (Crane Hill, 1996). Contains photographs and personal vignettes of 32 breast cancer survivors.

Claudia Sternbach. ***Now Breathe: A Very Personal Journey Through Breast Cancer***. (Whiteaker Press, 1999). Paperback.

Barbara Stone, ***Cancer, An Initiation-Surviving the Fire***. A Guide for Living with Cancer for Patient, Provider, Spouse, Family or Friend (Open Court Publishing, 1994). Paperback.

Carolyn Walter and Julienne Oklay, ***Breast Cancer in the Life Course: Women's Experiences*** (Springer, 1991).

Ken Wilber, ***Grace and Grit: Spirituality and Healing in the Life and Death of Treya Killam Wilber*** (Boston: Shambala, 1993).

Susan Winn, ***Chemo and Lunch—One Woman's Triumph Over Hereditary Breast Cancer*** (Fithian Press, 1990).

Juliet Wittman, ***Breast Cancer Journal. A Century of Petals*** (Golden, CO: Fulcrum Publishing, 1993). Paperback. Wellwritten, honest, personal story by a journalist.

Ina Yalof. ***Straight from the Heart: Letters of Hope and Inspiration from Survivors of Breast Cancer*** (NY: Kensington Books, 1996). Women from all walks of life discuss their experiences with breast cancer.

NOTE: Several other notable personal stories are out of print but can be found in libraries, including: ***Getting Better***, ***Conversations with Myself and Other Friends***, by Anne Hargrave; ***Life Wish*** by Jill Ireland; ***My Breast: One Woman's Cancer Story*** by Joyce Wadler; ***Of Tears and Triumphs: The Family Victory That Has Inspired Thousands of Cancer Patients***, by Georgia and Bud Photopulos; and ***Exploding into Life*** by Dorothea Lynch.

TREATMENT OPTIONS

Cancerfax. This service allows access to NCI's Physician's Data Query (PDQ) system (see entry below) via fax machine, 24 hours/day, 7 days/week, at no charge. Two versions of the treatment are available: one for health care professionals and the other for lay people. Information is also available in Spanish. For information and list of necessary codes, call (301) 402-5874 or call (800) 4-CANCER or on the web, cancernet.nci.nih.gov (no 'www' is needed).

PDQ (Physician Data Query). The cancer information database of NCI, providing prognostic, stage and treatment information and more than 1,500 clinical trials that are open to patient access by computer equipped with a modem, and by fax (see above). For more information, call NCI at (800) 4-CANCER.

CANHELP. Will research patient's treatment options (including alternative therapies) based on your medical records. A personalized 10-15 page packet will be mailed within seven working days for $400.00. Contact CANHELP 3111 Paradise Bay Road, Port Ludlow, WA 98365-9771 (206) 437-2291.

National Comprehensive Cancer Network (www.nccn.org). Provides accepted treatment guidelines for breast cancer care. 50 Huntington Pike, Suite 200; Rockledge, PA 19046. (215) 728-4788; patient information service (888) 909NCCN.

NIH Consensus Conference Statement: Treatment of Early Stage Breast Cancer (June, 1990, Vol.8, No.6). Still the current standard, the treatment recommendations of the expert panel convened by the National Institutes of Health. On the web: www.odp.od.nih.gov/consensus.

International Cancer Alliance (ICA), 4853 Cordell Avenue, Suite 11, Bethesda MD 20814. (800) I-CARE-61. Provides a free cancer therapy review that includes information on a specific type of cancer (description, detection and staging, treatment, diagnostic tests and clinical trials), cancer breakthroughs. Report is sent quarterly.

SURGERY

Mastectomy: A Treatment for Breast Cancer (87-658 8/87) 24 pages. National Cancer Institute. Information about different types of breast surgery.

Standards for Breast-Conservation Treatment (3405, 1992). ACS booklet, call (800) ACS-2345.

The Surgical Management of Primary Breast Cancer (3493, 1991). ACS booklet, call (800) ACS-2345.

Rosalind Dolores Benedet, *Healing: A Woman's Recovery Guide to Recovery After Mastectomy* (San Francisco: R.Benedet Publishing, 1993). Guide to postoperative care after a mastectomy. To order, send $10 plus $1 shipping to R. Benedet Publishing, 220 Montgomery Street Penthouse #2, San Francisco, CA 94104.

RADIATION

Radiation Therapy: A Treatment For Early Stage Breast Cancer (87-659 9/ 1987). 20 pages. National Cancer Institute, (800) 4-CANCER. This booklet discusses the treatment and side effects of primary radiation therapy.

Radiation Therapy and You: A Guide to Self-Help During Treatment (97-2227, 1997). 52 pages National Cancer Institute, (800) 4-CANCER. Written for the patient receiving radiation,

The Role of Radiation Therapy in the Management of Primary Breast Cancer (3492,1991). ACS booklet, (800) ACS2345.

SYSTEMIC THERAPY

American Society of Clinical Oncology (ASCO), 435 North Michigan Avenue, Suite 1717 Chicago, IL 60611. (312) 644-0828. Will mail a list of member oncologists by geographical area to medical professionals.

Chemotherapy and You: A Guide to Self-Help During Treatment (97-1136, 1997). A question-and-answer booklet, including glossary and guide to side effects. 56 pages. NCI (800) 4-CANCER.

Chemotherapy: Your Weapon Against Cancer (1998 edition). Explanation of the benefits and side effects of chemo. One copy free from The Chemotherapy Foundation, 183 Madison Ave, Suite 403, NY, NY 10016. (212) 213-9292.

Chemotherapy: What it is, How it Helps (1990, 4512). Brief introduction to chemotherapy. (800) ACS-2345.

Community Clinical Oncology Program ("CCOP") (April 1993, updated periodically). List of the 48 medical centers in 36 states and Puerto Rico selected by, NCI to participate in newest clinical protocols and to accrue patients to clinical trials. (800) 4-CANCER.

Coping with the Side Effects of Chemotherapy (1992). 19 page booklet. Order from Wyeth-Ayerst (800) 395-91938.

Helping Yourself During Chemotherapy: 4 steps for Patients (94-3701, 1994). This easy-to-read brochure suggest four steps to follow during chemotherapy,

NCI (800) 4-CANCER.

Questions and Answers About Tamoxifen (1994). Fact sheet on tamoxifen (Nolvadex) and its side effects. 4 pages. NCI (800) 4-CANCER.

The Role of Chemotherapy in the Management of Primary Breast Cancer (3356, 1991). Booklet from ACS (800) ACS2345.

Robert Bazell. ***HER-2: The Making of Herceptin, A Revolutionary Treatment for Breast Cancer***. (NY. Random House, 1998). Written by NBC's chief science correspondent, the story of Genentech's Herceptin, the first gene-based therapy for breast cancer.

Nancy Bruning, ***Coping with Chemotherapy*** (Ballantine Books, 1993). Overview of medical and emotional effects of chemotherapy.

Michael W.DeGregorio, Valeria J. Wiebe, ***Tamoxifen and Breast Cancer.*** (Yale University Press, 1999). Paperback.

Marylin J. Dodd, ***Managing the Side Effects of Chemotherapy and Radiation Therapy: A Guide for Patients and their Families.*** (UCSF Nursing Press, 3rd edition, 1996). Suggestions for managing each side effect. Order from UCSF Nursing Press, 521 Parnassus Ave, Room 535, San Francisco, CA 94143 (415) 476-4992.

V.Craig Jordan, et al. ***Tamoxifen for the Treatment and Prevention of Breast Cancer***. (Publisher Research and Representation, 1999).

John F. Kessler MD, et al. ***Tamoxifen: New Hope in the Fight Against Breast Cancer*** (Wholecare Mass Market Paperback, 1999).

Judith McKay, and Nancee Hirano, ***The Chemotherapy and Radiation Survival Guide*** (Oakland: New Harbinger Pub, 1998). Written by two oncology nurses about physical and psychological issues. Call (800) 748-6273 or www. newharbinger.com

Joyce Slayton-Mitchell, ***Winning the Chemo Battle*** (NY. WW Norton, 1991). Personal account of chemotherapy treatment from a woman who has "been there."

National Bone Marrow Transplant Link. 20411 West 12 Mile Road #108,
Southfield MI 48076 (9-00) LINK-BMT or http://comnet.org/nbmtlink.
Information clearinghouse on bone marrow transplants which also links patients
or family with former patients or family.

Blood and Marrow Transplant Newsletter, Blood and Marrow Transplant
information Network, 2900 Skokie Valley Road, Suite B, Highland Park, IL 60035,
(888) 597-7674, (947) 433-4599 (fax) or www.bmtnews.org. Quarterly newsletter
for patients who have had or who are considering bone marrow, peripheral stem
cell or cord blood transplantation; also attorney referral service to help resolve
insurance problems.

COMPLIMENTARY AND ALTERNATIVE THERAPIES

The Alternative Medicine Homepage (wwwpitt.edu/-cbw/altm.html). Links to
information sources about complementary and alternative therapies.

The National Center for Complementary and Alternative Medicine
(http://nccam.nih.gov). Good place to find research alternatives.
   The Osher Center for Integrative Medicine (www.ucsf.edu/ocim.research/
breastcancer.html). University of California San Francisco Center studies alternatives in women with breast cancer.

The Rosenthal Center for Complementary and Alternative Medicine
(www.cpmcnet.columbia.edu/dept/rosenthal/women.html). Columbia
University's center does research on alternatives and women's health.

American Botanical Council/HerbalGram (www.herbalgram.org). Herbal
information on the internet.

Herbal Research Foundation (http://sunsite.mc.edu/herbs.hrinfo.html).

IBIS, Interactive BodyMind Information System (unomteleport.coml-ibis).
Everything you want to know about the alternative options for any one disease.

The Cancer Club, 6533 Limerick Drive, Edina, MN 55439. (800) 586-9062,
www.cancerclub.com. Markets humorous and helpful products including a

quarterly newsletter, books and videos.

Center for Mind-Body Medicine, 5225 Connecticut Ave NW, Suite 414, Washington DC 20015 or www.cmbm.org. A leader in promoting complementary cancer care (treatments that combine standard treatments with alternative approaches).

The Institute for the Advancement of Health, 16 East 53rd Street, New York, NY 10022. (212) 832-8282. A national organization devoted to promoted awareness of mind body health interactions. Supplies information on behavioral techniques to promote comfort and health.

National Center for Complementary and Alternative Medicine, NIH. Investigates alternative medical treatments, offers information packages. NCCAM Clearinghouse, Box 8218, Silver Spring, MD 20907, (888) 644-6226, http:// nccam.nih.gov.

The Planetree Health Resource Center. A non-profit, consumer-oriented resource for health information, including material and relaxation and visualization techniques. Write or call for a catalogue and price list: 2040 Webster Street, San Francisco, CA 95115. (415) 923-3680.

Unproven Methods of Cancer Management (3028 /88) American Cancer Society. The local Division Offices have statements providing details on each of 27 treatment methods listed in this brochure.

The National Council Against Health Fraud. Call the Council's Resource Center (800) 821-6671 or write to Dr. John Renner, Consumer Health Information Research Institute, 3521 Broadway, Kansas City, MO 64111.

German Commission E Monograph. Translated and made available by the American Botanical Council. (PO Box 201660, Austin, TX 78720). This is the German government's analysis of indication and safety of commonly used herbs.

Harold H.Benjamin, *The Wellness Community Guide to Fighting for Recovery* (revised and expanded edition of From Victim to Victor) (NY.- Putnam, 1995). Herbert Benson, The Relaxation Response (NY. Avon Books, 1985).

John Boik, *Natural Compounds in Cancer Therapy.* (Princeton, MN - Oregon Medical Press, 2000). Thoroughly reviews the potential of selected natural compounds in cancer treatment, including mechanisms of action, activity, pharmacology, and toxicology.

Joan Borysenko, *Minding the Body, Mending the Mind* (Menlo Park: Addison Wesley, 1987).

Christine Clifford, illustrated by Jack Lindstrom, *Not Now ... I'm Having a No Hair Day: Humor and Healing for People with Cancer* (Pfeifer-Hamilton, Duluth, MN, 1996, $9.95). Author shows how the power of laughter and positive thinking can promote recovery and growth. Contact The Cancer Club, 6533 Limerick Drive, Edina, MN 55439, (800) 586-9062 or www.cancerclub.com.

Norman Cousins, *The Healing Heart* (NY: Avon Books 1983).

Norman Cousins, *Anatomy of an Illness* (NY: Bantam Books, 1986).

Linda Dackman, *Affirmations Meditations, and Encouragements for Women Living with Breast Cancer* (San Francisco: Harper, 1992). Uses quotes and anecdotes to provide insight into the process.

Larry Dossey, M.D., *Healing Words: The Power of Prayer and the Practice Of Medicine* (San Francisco: Harper-Collins, 1993).

Ron Falcone, Lynn Sonberg. *Natural Medicine for Breast Cancer* (Dell, 1997). Paperback. Includes herbal and other alternative remedies for fatigue, loss of appetite, nausea, and liver toxicity due to breast cancer treatment.

Neil Fiore, *The Road Back to Health* (NY.Bantam Books 1984). Good explanation on how to make your own visualization tapes, by a psychologist and former cancer patient. Book is out of print but may be found in some libraries.

Anne Fogelsanger, *See Yourself Well: For People with Cancer* (Brooklyn: Equinox, 1994). Audiocassette provides series of mental exercises to encourage relaxation.

The Humor Project. A resource for humorous materials; free catalogue available. Quarterly magazine, Laughing Matters, available for $16/year. Conferences are held on using humor to cope with illness. 110 Spring Street, Saratoga Springs, NY 12866-3397. (518) 587-8770.

Jon Kabat-Zinn, *Full Catastrophe Living: Using the Wisdom of Your Body and Mind to Face Stress, Pain and Illness* (Delta Press, 1990).

Michael Lerner, *Choices in Healing: Integrating the Best of Conventional and Complementary Approaches to Cancer* (Cambridge, MA: MIT Press, 1994). A wonderful book on ways to integrate alternative approaches to traditional medicine.

Ellen Michaud and Editors of Prevention Magazine, *Fighting Disease: The Complete Guide to Natural Immune Power.*

Ralph Moss, *Cancer Therapy: The Independent Consumer's Guide to Non-Toxic Treatment and Prevention* (NY: Equinox Press, 1992). Discusses nearly 100 nontoxic modes of cancer prevention and treatment.

Bill Moyers, *Healing and the Mind* (NY: Doubleday, 1993).

P.C. Rood, *Making Miracles: An Exploration into the Dynamics of Self-Healing* (NY: Warner Books, 1990).

Ellen Schaplowsky, Nan Lu. *Traditional Chinese Medicine: A Woman's Guide to Healing from Breast Cancer* (Avon Books, 1999).

Bernie Siegel, M.D., *Love, Medicine, and Miracles* (NY: Perennial Library, 1987 $8.95). Promotes visualization, meditation, discussion, and positive thinking.

David Spiegel, *Living Beyond Limits: New Hope and Help for Facing Life-Threatening Illness* (NY. Times Books, 1993).

Susan Weed, *Breast Cancer? Breast Health! The Wise Woman Way* (Ash Tree Publication, 1997). Paperback.

Honora Lee Wolfe, Bob Flaws. *Better Breast Health Naturally with Chinese Medicine*. (Blue Poppy Press, 1998).

LIVING WITH BREAST CANCER

The National Coalition for Cancer Survivorship (NCCS), 1010 Wayne Avenue, Suite 505, Silver Spring, MD 20910, (877) 622-7937 or www.cansearch.org. Raises awareness of cancer survivorship through its publications, quarterly newsletter, education to eliminate the stigma of cancer, and advocacy for insurance, employment, and legal rights.

National Cancer Survivors Day Foundation, PO Box 682285, Franklin TN 37068-2285 (615) 794-3006 or www.ncsdf.org. National Cancer Survivor's Day is America's nationwide, annual celebration of life for cancer survivors, their families, friends, and oncology teams. It is celebrated on the first Sunday in June each year.

Facing Forward: A Guide for Cancer Survivors (NCI, P119, 1994). Booklet focuses on maintaining physical health, emotions, managing insurance, and employment. Call NCI's CIS 9800) 4-CANCER.

Karen M Hassey, ***Pregnancy and Parenthood After Treatment for Breast Cancer Oncology Nursing Forum, Vol. 15*** (4)439-444 1988 You will probably have to get this from a hospital or medical library. A very good review of all that has been published on the subject.

The Cancer Survivor's Tool A self-learning audio program also available in Spanish and Chinese. Free to survivors and professionals, call (877) TOOLS-4-U. Susan Kuner, et al.

Speak the Language of Healing: Living with Breast Cancer Without Going to War (Conari Press, 1999). Paperback.

Carolyn Runowicz and Donna Haupt, ***To Be Alive: A Woman's Guide to a Full Life After Cancer*** (New York: Henry Holt, 1996) Written by an oncologist and breast cancer survivor.

Mansa C. Weiss, Ellen Weiss. ***Living Beyond Breast Cancer A Survivor's Guide for When Treatment Ends and the Rest of your Life Begins*** (New York Times Books, 1998) Paperback.

APPEARANCE AND COMFORT

Look Good...Feel Better is a public service program from the Cosmetic Toilet and Fragrance Association Foundation in partnership with ACS and the National Cosmetology Association. It is designed to help women recovering from cancer deal with changes in their appearance resulting from cancer treatment. The program's print and videotape materials are designed for both patients and health professionals. Call (800) 395-LOOK or your local ACS office.

Look Good...Feel Better—Caring for Yourself Inside and Out (CTFA Foundation, 1988). The LGFB Program's video for cancer patients undergoing chemotherapy and radiation therapy. Women discuss their experiences and beauty professionals review ways to look and feel better during treatment; including makeup, nail care and wigs. 16 minutes. Order from CTTA (800) 395-LOOK.

PRACTICAL ADVICE-HOW TO FIND POST MASTECTOMY PRODUCTS

Prostheses: The lingerie areas in some department stores employ professionals who will fit you with a prosthesis and a bra to wear with it. Smaller lingerie boutiques in major cities often perform this function as well. Check your local yellow pages under "Lingerie" or "Brassieres," or in larger cities under "Breast Prosthesis." Prostheses may also be ordered from selected surgical supply stores, often listed under "Surgical Appliances and Supplies." Temporary prostheses can be ordered by mail. Women who cannot afford a prosthesis may wish to contact the **Y-ME Prosthesis Bank** (see listing below).

Bathing suits and lingerie—Contact the sources mentioned above. In addition, a number of specialty boutiques sell clothing with post-mastectomy needs in mind, although there is not yet a national chain. Consult your yellow pages under lingerie.

If you have difficulty locating a local retailer, contact the Reach to Recovery volunteer at your **American Cancer Society** office, call a local breast cancer support group, or contact the social work department of your hospital.

Becoming, Inc. is a catalog of clothes and prostheses where 20% of profits go to breast cancer programs. (800) 980-9085.

Breast Cancer Resource Center of the Princeton YWCA offers free wigs and prostheses to women in need. Paul Robeson Place, Princeton, NJ 08540. (609) 2522003.

Buyer's Guide to Wigs and Hairpieces Two page summary from Ruth L. Weintraub, Inc., 420 Madison Avenue, Suite 406, NY 10017 (212) 838-1333.

Camp Health Care offers breast forms and lingerie. (800) 788-2267.

Charming with Dignity. Supplies fashion-designed turbans and the "Sollee Comfort Form" prosthesis for use immediately following breast surgery. Call for catalog. 112 West 34 Street, Suite 1617, NY 10120. (800) 477-8188. External Reconstruction Technology, Inc.

The **"Third Alternative"** is a nonsurgical procedure that sculpts a breast from a cast of your body and then colors it to match your skin tone. 4535 Benner Street, Philadelphia, PA 19135. (215) 333-8424.

Hat & Soul. Sells hats by mail order. (719) 991-HATS or e-mail tahmed@ix. netcoin.com.

Intimate Image. Offers full line of prostheses, lymphedema sleeves, lingerie. (888) 948-7965.

ISA Designs. Line of headware. For catalog call (888) ISA-HATS.

Ladies' First Choice. Post-breast surgery boutique, Medicare accepted, newsletter published. Mail orders accepted. 6465 Sunnyside Road SE, Salem, OR 97306. (503) 363-3940 or (800) 300-3940.

Ladies First, Inc. Wholesale manufacturer of Softee Comfort form and mastectomy lingerie. Accepts Medicare. For provider near you (800) 497-8285 or www.wvi.com/ladies1.

Lady Grace Stores. Chain of post-breast surgery stores with locations in Massachusetts, New Hampshire, Florida, and Maine. Mail orders and Medicare accepted, they publish a newsletter. (800) 922-0504.

Lands' End. Five different styles of specially designed mastectomy swimwear. Order a catalog from (800) 356-4444.

New Beginnings. Post-mastectomy, fashion service that takes phone orders. 1556 Third Avenue, Room 603, NY 10128 (212) 369-6630.

Schwartz' Intimate Apparel. Post-surgery boutique. Phone orders, Medicaid and Medicare accepted. 108 Skokie Blvd., Wilmette, IL 60091 (708) 251-1118.

"TLC" is a catalog created by the American Cancer Society. Medicare reimbursement available. For catalog, call (800) 850-9445.

Y-ME Prosthesis and Wig Bank. Y-ME maintains a prosthesis and wig bank for women with financial need. If the appropriate size is available, Y-ME will mail anywhere in the country for a nominal handling fee. (800) 221-2141.

"Beauty of Control" (1995) with Jill Eikenberry, videotape created by Laurie Feldman about cosmetic and emotional side effects of treatment. Medical Video Productions, 450 North New Ballas Rd, Suite 266 St. Louis MO 63141 (800) 822-3100.

Best Look Forward (Graduate Hospital, 1991). Videotape in which a makeup artist and hairdresser give advice and demonstrations, including on eyebrows and lashes. 30 minutes, $45.00. Order from The Graduate Hospital Cancer Program, 1840 South Street, Philadelphia, PA 19146 or call Eileen Murphy at (215) 893-7298

Maintaining a Positive Image with Breast Cancer Surgery Videotape covering prosthetic, lingerie, and swimsuit choices following breast cancer surgery. $19.95 plus $2 postage. Johanna's on Call to Mend Esteem, 199 New Scotland Avenue, Albany, NY 122208. (518) 482-4178.

Maintaining a Positive Image with Hair Loss and Cancer Therapy Videotape providing useful tips for maintaining self-esteem during treatment. $19.95 plus $2 postage. Johanna's on Call to Mend Esteem, 199 New Scotland Avenue, Albany, NY 122208. (518) 482-4178.

RECONSTRUCTION

Breast Reconstruction Following Mastectomy American Society of Plastic and

Reconstructive Surgeons 444 East Algonquin Road, Arlington Heights, IL 60005. (312) 228-9900. For referrals call the Society's message tape at (800) 635-0635.

RENU Breast Reconstruction Counseling. Einstein Medical Center, Philadelphia (215) 456-7387. A support program staffed by trained volunteers who have had post-mastectomy reconstruction. Hot-line counseling and written materials are available.

A Sense of Balance: Breast Reconstruction $29.95 videotape. To order call (617) 732-3379. An interactive videotape developed by the staff at the Breast Evaluation Center of the Dana Farber Cancer Institute to inform about the pros and cons of various types of reconstruction.

Breast Reconstruction After Mastectomy (1991, 4630). Describes types of surgery with photographs and drawings and answers to commonly asked questions. 20 pages. ACS (800) ACS-2345.

Marilyn Snyder, *An Informed Decision: Understanding Breast Reconstruction* (NY Evans/Little, Brown, 1989). Paperback $12.95. An informative mixture of one woman's account and clearly presented illustrated information about breast reconstruction after mastectomy.

LYMPHEDEMA

The National Lymphedema Network and Network Hotline, 2211 Post Street, Suite 404, San Francisco, CA 94115. (800) 541-3259; nln@lymphnet.org;www.lymphnet.org. Nonprofit organization that provides patients and professionals with information about prevention and treatment, physical therapy, general information and support in your area. They will send an information packet.

Breast Cancer Physical Therapy Center, 1905 Spruce Street, Philadelphia, PA 19103. Provides a booklet on exercises to help manage lymphedema. Cost is $8.95 which includes shipping.

Jeannie Burt, et al. *Lymphedema: A Breast Cancer Patient's Guide to Prevention and Healing.* (Hunter House, 2000). Paperback. Covers preventing lymphedema, and reducing lymphedema through professional therapy and self-massage.

Joan Swirsky and Diane Sackett Nannary. ***Coping with Lymphedema.*** (Garden City Part, NY: Avery, 1998). Practical guide to understanding, treating and living with lymphedema. (800) 548-5757x123.

DIET

American Institute for Cancer Research, 1759 R. Street NW, Washington DC 20009. Provides information on cancer and nutrition, publishes a newsletter and cookbooks, offers a hotline for nutrition-related cancer inquiries. (800) 843-8114, www.aicr.org

Eating Hints for Cancer Patients (98-2079, 1998). Suggestions and recipes. NCI 4-CANCER

Saundra N. Aker and Polly Lennsen, ***A Guide to Good Nutrition During and After Chemotherapy and Radiation*** (3rd edition, 1988). Practical approach to nutrition. Order from The Fred Hutchinson Cancer Research Center Clinical Nutrition Program, 1124 Columbia Street, Room E211, Seattle, WA 98104. (206) 667-4834.

Daniel W. Nixon, ***The Cancer Recovery Eating Plan: The Right Foods to Help Fuel Your Recovery*** (NY: Random House, 1996). Paperback. Includes a three-month eating plan and recipes.

Donna Weihofen, Christina Marino, ***The Cancer Survival Cookbook*** (Minneapolis, MN: Chronimed Pub, 1997). Paperback. Nourishing recipes and advice on overcoming eating problems. Bookstores or (800) 848-2793.

EXERCISE

The YWCA ENCOREplus Program. Designed to provide supportive discussion and rehabilitative exercise for women who have been treated for breast cancer. Call your local YWCA for more information, or contact the YWCA Office of Women's Health Initiatives, 624 9th Street, NW, Washington, DC 20001. (202) 628-3636.

Beginning Ballet for the Post-Mastectomy Woman (First Position Productions, 1990). Videotape of a class of women who have had mastectomies. 50 minutes, $39.95. First Position Productions, Star Route Box 472, Sausalito, CA 94965. (415) 381-9034.

Better than Before Fitness video with exercises designed to restore muscle tone and range of motion. 50 minutes, $49.95 plus $5.95 shipping. Order from (800) 488-8354 or www.breastfit.com.

Focus on Healing Through Movement & Dance (Sherry LeBed Davis/Albert Einstein Medical Center, PA). Movement program and 14-day plan for breast cancer survivors of all ages and fitness levels. Video $29.95 plus tax and shipping (800) 366-6038 or www.enhancementinc.com

Get Up and Go: After Breast Surgery (ACS/University of Michigan, Oak Park, MI, 21989). Order from health tapes Inc., (888) 225-5486. Total body exercises demonstrated by five women who have had a mastectomy, lumpectomy or reconstructive surgery. Increasingly challenging levels. 60 minutes, $39.95

One Move at a Time: Exercise for Women Recovering from Breast Cancer (Minneapolis: Green Light Productions, 1996). Video with simple, gentle exercise. $19.95 plus $4.45 shipping. Order from The Cancer Club, 6533 Limerick Drive, Edina, MN 55439, (800) 586-9062, or www.cancerclub.com.

Stretch Exercise Program (1988). An eight-week exercise/support program for women who have had surgery for breast cancer. Manual, video materials and sessions offered free through volunteer services. Call the Alabama Division of the ACS (205) 879-2242.

MENOPAUSE

Menomaven (www.menomaven.com): Source of a wonderful set of cards for sorting through menopause.

Powersurge (www.dearest.com) One of the first, and the best source of information for menopausal women.

National Women's Health Network, 1325 G Street NW, Washington DC 20005. Written packets and booklets on many aspects of women's health, including menopause, benign, and malignant breast diseases.

Women's Health Initiative. 1-800-54-WOMEN. This is the first controlled, national study to look at postmenopausal women and their health including hormone replacement therapy, diet, calcium, and exercise. If we do not participate, we will never know the answers. Call to find the center closest to you.

Women's Health in Midlife (www.cw.bc.ca/womens/midlife/). The women's health in midlife project (W.H.I.M) is a provincial initiative designed to help women make informed choices about managing key midlife health issues through health education and community action.

Sandra Coney, ***The Menopause Industry: How the Medical Establishment Exploits Women*** (Alameda, CA: Hunter House, 1994). May be ordered by calling 1-800-266-5592. This book describes the most accurate view of menopause I have seen. It will wake you up.

Paula Brown Doress, Diana Laskin Siegel, and The Midlife and Older Women Book Project, ***Ourselves, Growing Older*** (New York: Simon and Schuster, 1987). Good overview of midlife and beyond, written in cooperation with the Boston Women's Health Book Collective.

Paula Brown Dranov, ***Estrogen: Is it Right for You? A Thorough Factual Guide to Help You Decide.*** New York: Simon and Schuster, 1993). A short, balanced book on the pros and cons or hormone therapy.

Sadja Greenwood, M.D., ***Menopause Naturally: Preparing for the Second Half of Life*** (San Francisco: Volcano Press, 1989). Good discussion of menopause without hormone replacement therapy, and the dangers of hormonal replacement.

Dee Ito, ***Without Estrogen: Natural Remedies for Menopause and Beyond*** (New York: Random House, 1995). Paperback.

Carol Landau, Michele G. Cyr and Anne W. Moulton, ***The Complete Book of Menopause*** (New York: Berkeley, 1992). Written by two gynecologists and a psychologist, this book is a good overall guide to menopause in all of its aspects. It sticks to traditional medicine and lifestyle issues and doesn't discuss alternative therapies.

Susan M. Love, ***Dr. Susan Love's Hormone Book: Making Informed Choices***

About Menopause. (New York: Times Books, 1998). Paperback.

Janine O'Leary Cobb, ***Understanding Menopause: Answers and Advice for Women in the Prime of Life.*** (New York: Penguin, 1993). A very good and friendly book by the editor of the newsletter: 'A Friend Indeed'

Susan Perry and Katherine A. O'Hanlan, ***Natural Menopause: The Complete Guide to a Woman's Most Misunderstood Passage.*** (Reading, MA: Addison-Wesley, 1992). A good guide to all of the aspects of menopause with a friendly balanced approach (doesn't include alternatives).

Richard J. Santen, Margaret Borwhat, Sarah Gleason, ***Menopause*** (Bethesda: The Hormone Foundation, 1998). Summary of a 1997 meeting that discussed postmenopausal hormone deficiency after breast cancer. For a free copy, call The Hormone Foundation (800) HORMONE or www.hormone.org.

Ann M. Voda, Menopause, ***Me and You: The Sound of Women Pausing.*** (Binghamton, New York: Haworth Press, 1997). A wonderful book of women's experiences. It is especially strong in describing women's experiences of bleeding.

Ann M. Voda, Margaret Dennerstein, and S.R. O'Donnell, ***Changing Perspective on Menopause*** (Austin: University of Texas Press, 1982). Menopause from an anthropological, literary, psychological, and physiological perspective.

Honora Lee Wolfe. ***Menopause: A Second Spring*** (Boulder, CO: Blue Poppy, 1985). A good overview of traditional Chinese medicine and how it views menopause.

RECURRENCE AND METASTASIS

Free Wishes (www.agingwithdignity.org). An online living will that is legal in 33 states and DC. Website includes advice on establishing a surrogate, advance directives, free of charge.

Choice in Dying, 200 Varick Street, New York, New York 10014 (800) 989-WILL. A nonprofit educational organization which distributes the living will, a document that records a patient's wishes during treatment and in regard to terminal care.

Hospice Resources: National Hospice Organization, 1901 North Moore Street, Suite 901, Arlington, VA 22209 (800) 658-8898 or www.nho.org. Will provide a directory of hospice programs by state.

Hospice Foundation of America, 2001 S Street NW Suite 300, Washington DC 20009. (202) 638-5419 or www.hospicefoundation.org

Hospice Link, 190 Westbrook Road, Essex CT 06426-0713. (800) 331 1620 or (203) 767-1620 in Alaska and Connecticut,

Royal Victoria Hospital Palliative Care Service 687 Pine Avenue West Montreal QC 514) 843-1542. An independent national organization of groups Providing Palliative care and hospice in Canada.

After Breast Cancer: A Guide to Follow Up Care (87-2400) National Cancer Institute. 11 pages. Considers the importance of follow up, signs of recurrence, and the physical and emotional effects having had breast cancer.

Advanced Cancer: Living Each Day (85-856) National Cancer institute 30 pages. A booklet written to make living with advanced cancer easier.

Caring for the Patient with Cancer at Home—A Guide for Patients and Families (4656-PS 1988 edition) 40 pages. A guidebook providing detailed helpful information on how to care for the patient at home.

I Still Buy Green Bananas—Living with Hope, Living with Breast Cancer (Y-ME, 1997). Practical advice and personal stories. Single copies from Y-ME (800) 221-2141.

Managing Cancer Pain (1994). Still current, consumer booklet details US Government's Agency for Health Care Policy guidelines for treating cancer pain. Order from AHCPR Publications Clearinghouse (800) 358-9295.

Questions and Answers about Pain Control: A Guide for People with Cancer and Their Families (4518-PS 1995). Discusses pain control using both medical and non-medical methods. 76 pages. ACS (800) ACS-2345 or NCI (800)4-CANCER.

When Cancer Recurs: Meeting the Challenge Again (96-2709,1996). Booklet details the different types of recurrence, types of treatment. 30 pages. NCI (800)4-CANCER.

On with Life 1999 edition is NABCO's updated video about living with advanced breast cancer. Order free of charge from NABCO (888) 80-NABCO or nabcoinfo@aol.com.

Marcia Lattanzi-Licht with John Mahoney and Galen Miller. *The Hospice Choice: In Pursuit of a Peaceful Death* (Fireside, 1998). Coping with dying and providing comfort care rather than curative treatment.

Mum Mayer, Linda Lamb (Editor). *Advanced Breast Cancer: A Guide to Living with Metastatic Disease, 2nd edition* (patient-centered guides). (O'Reilly & Associates, 1998) Paperback. Updated, retitled edition of 1997 Holding Tight, Letting Go; excellent.

FINANCIAL AID, INSURANCE AND EMPLOYMENT

The viatical industry, which can provide a breast cancer patient with a portion of her life insurance benefits before death, has grown to more than 50 companies nationwide. For more information, contact your insurance for any.

Airlifeline (800) 446 1231(eww.airlifeline.org). A free, nationwide service that flies qualified patients to treatment centers nationwide.

The American Federation of Clinical Oncologic Societies has identified 15 basic criteria for choosing a health insurance plan to ensure coverage of high quality cancer care. Available at www.asco org.

American Preferred Prescription (800) 227-1195; Bio Logics (800) 850-4306; Community Prescription Service (800) 842-0502; Managed Rx Plans (800) 7998765 and Medi-Express RX (800) 873-9773 are services that ship medications by mail. Each has different policies regarding insurance and payment.

The Breast Health Access for Women with Disabilities Project, Alta Bates Medical Center, Dept. of Rehabilitation, 2001 Dwight Way, Berkeley CA 94704 (510) 204-4866. Provides direct services and public and professional education for this population.

HealthAllies.com will help you negotiate your medical bills.

ICI Pharmaceutical Nolvadex (Tamoxifen) Patient Assistance Program, Manager Professional Services-vices, ICI Pharmaceutical, Division of ICI Americas Inc, Wilmington Delaware 19897. (800)-456-5678. Provides tamoxifen to patients with financial need. Write for an application.

American Association of Retired People (AARP) Pharmacy Service. Catalog Dept., Box 19229, Alexandria, VA 22320. Members can use their non profit service to save on prescriptions delivered by mail. Good for tamoxifen (Novaldex). Write for free catalog.

Corporate Angel Network Inc (CAN), Westchester County Airport, Building 1, White Plains, New York 10604 (914)328-1313 (www.corpangelnetwork.org). A nationwide program designed to give patients with cancer the use of available seats on corporate aircraft to get to and from recognized treatment centers. There is no cost or any financial need requirement.

Mission Air Transportation Network (Canada), 77 Bloor Street West, Suite 1711, Toronto, ON M5S 3A1 (416) 9249333. Same as above.

National Cancer Institute, Bethesda, Maryland 20892-4200. (800)638-6694. Patients who are treated here as part of a clinical study receive their treatment free and may be housed free of charge at the hospital facilities of the NCI.

PRACTICAL ADVICE:
Pharmaceutical Company Breast Cancer Patient Assistance Programs

One of the most common concerns of women with breast cancer is obtaining adequate reimbursement for treatment, especially when drug therapy is ongoing. Some necessary drugs and treatments are not covered by Medicare and insurance plans—a source of frustration at a difficult and overwhelming time. The following is a listing of selected company reimbursement assistance programs for oncology-related products.

These programs are best accessed by a physician or nurse on the breast cancer patient's behalf. Eligibility requirements and application procedures vary with each program. Programs also vary by type of assistance, including reimbursement counseling, assistance with filing claims, appeal of denied claims and enrollment in State and Federal health insurance programs. Some companies offer free products for women who are uninsured and can demonstrate financial need. Since programs change, check the website of the **Pharmaceutical Research and Manufacturers of America** (PhRMA) at www.phrma.org for updates.

Adria Laboratories
ADRIA Pt. Assist Plan
Columbus OH
(614) 764-8100
Adriamycin, Vincristine, Vinblastine

ALZA Pharmaceutical
ALZA Oncology Connection Program
(800) 609-1083
Doxil (liposomal doxorubicin)

Amgen, Inc.
Amgen SAFETYNET(r) Program
(800) 272-9376
Epogen (epoetin alfa),
Neupogen (filgrastim)

AstraZeneca Pharmaceutical
Patient Assistance Program
(800) 424-3727
Nolvadex (tamoxifen citrate),
Arimidex (anastrozole),
Zoladex (goserelin)

Aventis Pharmaceutical
Aventis Oncology Program (PACT)
Providing Access to Chemotherapy
(800) 996-6626
Taxotere (docetaxel)

Bristol-Myers Squibb
Oncology/ Immunology
Patient Assistance Program

(800) 332-2056
BCNU (carmustine),
Cisplatin (plastinol),
Cytoxan (cyclophosphamide),
Megace (megestrol),
Taxol (paclitaxel)

Genentech, Inc.
Uninsured Pt Assist Prgrm
(800) 879-4747
Herceceptin (trastuzumab)

Glaxo Welcome, Inc.
Pt Assistance Program
(800) 722-9294
Wellcovorin (leucovorin),
Navelbine (vinorelbine tartrate)

Immunex Reimbursement Hotline
(800) 321-4669
Leucovorin Calcium (leucovorin),
Leukine (sargramostim),
methotrexate, Novantrone (mitoxantrone)

Eli Lilly Oncology
Lilly Cares
(800) 545-6962
Velban (vinblastine),
Oncovin (vincristine)

Merck and Co., Inc.
The Merck Patient Assistance Program
(800) 994-2111
Decadron (dexamethasone)

Novartis Pharmaceutical
Novartis Pt Asst Program
(800) 257-3273

Aredia (pamidronate disodium),
Femara (letrozole)

Ortho Biotech, Inc.
Procritline(tm)
(800) 553-3851
Procrit (epoetin alfa)

Pharmacia Oncology
RxMAP Prescription Medication
Assistance Program
(800) 242-7014
Adriamycin (doxorubicin),
Provera/Depo-Provera
(medroxyprogesterone), Zinecard (dexrazoxane)

Roche Laboratories, Inc.
Roche Medical Needs Program
(800) 443-6676
Xeloda (capecitabine),
5-FU (fluorouracil)

Roxane Laboratories, Inc.
Patient Assistance Program
(800) 274-8651
Roxanol (morphine),
Roxicodone (oxycodone)

Schering LaboratoriesKey Pharmaceutical
Commitment to Care
(800) 656-9485
Fareston (toremifine)

SmithKline Beecham Oncology
Access to Care Program
(800) 946-0420
Kytril (granisetron hydrochloride)

INSURANCE AND EMPLOYMENT

Information and Counseling about Cancer and the Workplace. Phyllis Stein, Radcliffe Career Services, Radcliffe College 10 Garden Street, Cambridge Mass 02138 (617) 495-8631; and Barbara Lazarus, Associate Provost for Academic Programs, Carnegie Mellon University Pittsburg, PA 15213 (412) 268 6994.

Patient Advocate Foundation (PAF) 780 Pilot House Drive, Suite 100C, Newport News, VA 23606. (800) 532-5274. Provides patient education relative to managed care terminology and policy issues flirt may affect coverage, legal intervention services, and counseling to resolve job and insurance problems.

The Job Accommodation Network provides information on employee's rights under the Americans with Disabilities Act. Call (800) ADA-WORK.

The National Insurance Consumer Helpline answers consumer questions, offers problem-solving support and printed materials on life and property casualty insurance. (800) 9424242.

Cancer Treatments Your Insurance Should Cover (April 1995). Brochure you can order from Association of Community Cancer Centers, 11600 Nebel St, Suite 201, Rockville MD 20852 (301) 984-9496

What You Should Know About Health Insurance (731,7/87)What You Should Know About Disability Insurance (733 10/87) Health Insurance Association of America, 1025 Connecticut Avenue, NW, Washington, DC 200043998. (202) 2237780.

Cancer: Your Job, Insurance and the Law (4585-ps /87) 6 pages. American Cancer Society. Summarizes cancer patients' legal rights regarding insurance and employment.

The Americans with Disabilities Act: Protection for Cancer Patients Against Employment Discrimination (4585, 1993). Brochure defines the ADA law by describing employment rights of the cancer patient. ACS (800) ACS-2345.

Cancer. Your job, Insurance and the Law (4585-PS, 1987). Summarizes cancer patient's legal rights; gives complaint procedure instructions. 6 pages. ACS (800) ACS-2345.

The Consumer's Guide to Disability Insurance (1995). A comprehensive guide to understanding disability insurance. Health Insurance Assn of America (HIAA) (202) 824-1600.

The Consumer's Guide to Long-Term Care Insurance (1995). HIAA, (202) 824-1600.

The Consumer's Guide to Medicare Supplement Insurance (1995). Instructions on using private insurance to supplement Medicare for maximum coverage. HIAA (202) 824-1600.

The Managed Care Answer Guide (1997). Reference handbook for cancer patients insured by managed care plans. Consumer publication of the Patient Advocate Foundation (757) 873-6668.

State Laws Relating to Breast Cancer (CDC, March 1998). The Centers for Disease Control and Prevention's summary of statutes across the country related to breast cancer. Available from the CDC at (770) 488-4751 or wwwcdc.gov.

Surviving the Legal Challenges: A Resource Guide for Women with Breast Cancer (California Women's Law Center, 1998). 85 page reference on women's legal rights. Free. (213) 637-9900 or wwwcw1c.org.

What Cancer Survivors Need to Know About Health Insurance (1995). Provides clear understanding of health insurance and how to receive maximum reimbursement on claims. 37 pages. Single copies available free from National Coalition for Cancer Survivorship at (888) 937-6227. The NCCS also publishes A Cancer Survivor's Almanac that contains useful information about insurance coverage.

Charles B. Inlander and Eugene I. Pavalon, *Your Medical Rights.*

CLINICAL TRIALS

NCJ Cancer trials (cancertrials.nci.nih.gov). This is a listing of all cancer clinical trials.

Center Watch: Clinical Trials Listing Service (www.centerwatch.corn): Lists all kinds of trials, not just breast cancer.

National Surgical Breast and Bowel Project (wwwnsabp.pitt.edu). The group responsible for most of the breast cancer clinical trials including the tamoxifen prevention trial, STAR trial and lumpectomy and radiation trial. 3550 Terrace Street Room 914, Pittsburgh, PA 15261 (412) 648-9720. Will let you know of physicians participating in their trials in your area.

Other regional websites include Eastern Clinical Oncology Group at ecog.dfci.Harvard.edu, Southwest Oncology Group at www.oo.saci.org and the CALGB at www.calgb.uchicago.edu

Community Clinical Oncology Program (CCOP). (April 1993, updated periodically).

National Cancer Institute (800 4CANCER). Network of 48 medical centers in 36 states and Puetro Rico that have been selected by the National Cancer Institute to participate in the introduction of the newest clinical protocols and to add patients to clinical trials.

Pharmaceutical Frontiers: Research on Breast Cancer (1993). Brochure providing overview of the latest research options. Lists the approved medications used in treating breast cancer and the drugs in clinical trials. One copy free from Editor, Pharmaceutical Frontiers, Pharmaceutical Manufacturer's Association, 1100 Fifteenth Street NW, Washington, DC 20005.

Patient to Patient: Cancer Clinical Trials and You (NIH No.V112) 15-minute videotape provides simple information. NCI's CIS (800) 4-CANCER.

Taking Part in Clinical Trials: What Cancer Patients Need to Know (981998). Booklet for patients considering participating in cancer treatment trials, includes glossary, also available in Spanish. NCI's CIS (800) 4-CANCER.

POLITICS
BREAST CANCER ADVOCACY SITES ON THE INTERNET
National

National Breast Cancer Coalition (wwwnatlbcc.org): The national advocacy group (I am one of the founders) responsible for increasing breast cancer funding to $900 million) Good source of advocacy opportunities.

Sister's Network (www.sistersnetworkinc.org). Sisters Network is the first nationwide Aftican-American breast cancer survivors organization targeting African-American Women.

Local Advocacy Groups (This is a selection; check susanloverad.corn or the NBCC for others in your area.)
Breast Cancer Action (www.bcaction.org): This San Francisco group's aim is to influence policy changes necessary to end the breast cancer epidemic.

Florida Breast Cancer Coalition (wwwbellsouthbuzz.cona): Grassroots organization advocating for increased funding for breast cancer research. Member of the NBCC.

Georgia Breast Cancer Coalition (wwwgabcc.org): Provides Georgians with an organizational platform from which to educate the public and increase research funding to eradicate breast cancer Member of NBCC.

Huntington Breast Cancer Action Coalition (www.hbac.org): New York group dedicated to promoting and providing breast cancer awareness, education and advocacy, involvement and support. Member of NBCC.

Linda Creed Breast Cancer Foundation (wwiv.libertynet.org/Icbf/Icbf. htrnl): Philadelphia group committed to empowering women and their families to practice breast health, foster the healing process and establish a public agenda for prevention and cure. Member of NBCC.

Massachusetts Breast Cancer Coalition (www.mbcc.org): Aims to stop breast cancer epidemic through activism, advocacy and education, our goal is the cure, prevention and ultimate eradication of breast cancer.

SHARE: Self-Help for Women with Breast and Ovarian Cancer (www.sharecancersupport.org): New York advocacy group with hotlines in English and Spanish. Aims to provide people with breast or ovarian cancer with opportunities to be more in control of their lives during and after diagnosis.

International Breast Cancer Advocacy
Brustlorebs-Initiative, Hilfe zur Brusthgesundheit (wwwbMstkrebs.net): A

German language Breast Cancer Activism site.

Canadian Breast Cancer Foundation (www.cbcf.org): Supports the advancement of breast cancer research, diagnosis and treatment.

Europa Dorma (wwwoncoweb.com/edoma): European Breast Cancer Coalition

PRACTICAL ADVICE:
How to Get Involved with Breast Cancer Organizations

Political Advocacy. Although each person can become active through contacting local and national elected officials, the most effective way to bring about change can be by taking part in a national movement. The National Breast Cancer Coalition was formed in 1991 to involve women with the disease in changing public policy as it relates to progress against breast cancer. The NBCC's goals include expanding breast cancer research funding; improving access to screening, diagnosis and treatment for all women, and increasing the degree of influence of survivors in guiding research, trials and medical policy. The NBCC welcomes individuals and organizations as members. Many of the NBCC's members are local Coalitions in more than 40 states. A list of current state coordinators can be obtained by calling the **NBCC: National Breast Cancer Coalition,** 1707 L Street NW, Suite 1060, Washington, DC 20036 (202) 296-7477, (202) 265-6854 (fax) or www.natIbcc.org.

Roberta Altman, ***Waking Up, Fighting Back: The Politics of Breast Cancer*** (Little, Brown, 1996). A journalist's survey of the issues and controversies of the breast cancer advocacy movement.

Artne Kasper and Susan Ferguson, **Breast Cancer: Society Constructs an Epidemic** (New York: St. Martin's Press, 2000).

Ellen Leopold, **A Darker Ribbon: Breast Cancer, Women, and Their Doctors in the Twentieth Century** (Beacon Press, 1999)

Karen Stabiner, **To Dance with the Devil: The New War on Breast Cancer** (Dell, 1998). Paperback.

Virginia M. Soffa, **The Journey Beyond Breast Cancer: From the Personal to**

the Political.

Alabama

Albert F LoBuglio, M.D.
Director, UAB Comprehensive Cancer Center
University of Alabama at Birmingham
1824 Sixth Avenue South, Room 237
Birmingham, Alabama 35293-3300
Tel: 205/934-5077
Fax: 205/975-7428
(Comprehensive Cancer Center)

Arizona

Daniel D. Von Hoff, M.D.
Director, Arizona Cancer Center
University of Arizona
1501 North Campbell Avenue
Tucson, Arizona 85724
Tel: 520/626-7925
Fax: 520/626-2284
(Comprehensive Cancer Center)

California

John S. Kovach, M.D.
Director, Cancer Research Center
Beckman Research Institute, City of Hope
Needleman Bldg., Room 204
1500 East Duarte Road
Duarte, California 91010
Tel: 626/301-8164
Fax: 323/865-0102
(Comprehensive Cancer Center)

Walter Eckhart, PhD.
Director, Cancer Center
Salk Institute
10010 North Torrey Pines Road
La Jolla, California 92037

Tel: 958/453-4100 X1386
Fax: 858/457-4765
(Cancer Center)

Erkki Ruoslahti, M.D.
President & CEO
The Burnham Institute
10901 North Torrey Pines Road
La Jolla, California 92037
Tel: 858/455-6480 X3209
Fax: 858/646-3198
(Cancer Center)

David Tarin, M.D., Ph.D.
Director, UCSD Cancer Center
University of California at San Diego
9500 Gilman Drive
La Jolla, California 92093-0658
Tel: 858/822-1222
Fax: 858/822-0207
(Clinical Cancer Center)

Judith C. Gasson, Ph.D.
Director, Jonsson Comprehensive Cancer Center
University of California Los Angeles Factor Building, Room 8-684
10833 Le Conte Avenue
Los Angeles, California 90095-1781
Tel: 310/825-5268
Fax: 310/206-5553
(Comprehensive Cancer Center)

Peter A. Jones, Ph.D.
Director, USC/Norris Comprehensive Cancer Center
University of Southern California
1441 Eastlake Avenue,
Rm. 815, MS #83
Los Angeles, California 90033
Tel: 323/865-0816

Fax: 323/865-0102
(Comprehensive Cancer Center)

Frank L. Meyskens, Jr., M.D.
Director, Chao Family Comprehensive Cancer Center
University of California at Irvine
101 The City Drive
Building. 23, Rt. 81, Room 406
Orange, California 92868
Tel: 714/456-6310
Fax: 714/456-2240
(Comprehensive Cancer Center)
Frank McCormick, Ph.D.
Director, UCSF Cancer Center & Cancer Research Institute
University of California San Francisco
2340 Sutter Street, Box 0128
San Francisco, California 94115-0128
Tel: 415/502-1710
Fax: 415/502-1712
(Comprehensive Cancer Center)

Colorado

Paul A. Bunn, Jr., M.D.
Director, University of Colorado Cancer Center
University of Colorado Health Science Center
4200 East 9th Avenue, Box B188
Denver, Colorado 80262
Tel: 303/315-3007
Fax: 303/315-3304
(Comprehensive Cancer Center)

Connecticut

Vincent T. DeVita, Jr., M.D.
Director, Yale Cancer Center
Yale University School of Medicine
333 Cedar Street, Box 208028
New Haven, Connecticut 06520-8028
Tel: 203/795-4371

Fax: 203/785-4116
(Comprehensive Cancer Center)

District of Columbia

Marc E. Lippman, M.D.
Director, Lombardi Cancer Research Center
Georgetown University Medical Center 3800 Reservoir Road, N.W.
Washington, DC 20007
Tel: 202/687-2110
Fax: 202/687-6402
(Comprehensive Cancer Center)

Florida

John C. Ruckdeschel, M.D.
Center Director & CEO
H.Lee Moffitt Cancer Center &
Research Institute at the University
of South Florida
12902 Magnolia Drive
Tampa, Florida 33612-9497
Tel: 813/979-7265
Fax: 813/979-3919
(Clinical Cancer Center)

Hawaii

Carl-Wilhem Vogel, M.D., Ph . D
Director, Cancer Research Center of Hawaii
University of Hawaii at Manua
1236 Lauhala Street
Honolulu, Hawaii 96813
Tel: 808/586-3013
Fax: 808/586-3052
(Clinical Cancer Center)

Illinois

Nicholas J. Vogelzang, M.D.
Director, Cancer Research Center
University of Chicago Cancer Research Center

South Maryland Avenue, MC 1140
Chicago, Illinois 60637-1470
Tel: 773/702-6180
Fax: 773/702-9311
(Comprehensive Cancer Center)

Steven Rosen, M.D.
Director, Robert H. Lurie Cancer Center
Northwestern University
303 East Chicago Avenue
Olson Pavilion 8250
Chicago, Illinois 60611
Tel: 312/908-5250
Fax: 312/908-1372
(Comprehensive Cancer Center)

Indiana

Richard F. Borch, M.D., Ph.D.
Director, Purdue University Cancer Center
Hansen Life Sciences Research Building
South University Street
West Lafayette, Indiana 47907-1524
Tel: 765/494-9129
Fax: 765/494-9193
(Cancer Center)

Stephen D. Williams, M.D.
Director, Indiana University Cancer Center
Indiana Cancer Pavilion
535 Barnhill Drive, Room 455
Indianapolis, Indiana 46202-5289
Tel: 317/278-0070
Fax. 317/278-0074
(Clinical Cancer Center)

Maine

Kenneth Paigen, Ph.D.
Director, The Jackson Laboratory

600 Main Street
Bar Harbor, Maine 04609-0800
Tel: 207/288-6041
Fax: 207/288-6044
(Cancer Center)

Maryland
Martin D. Abeloff, M.D.
Director, Johns Hopkins Oncology Center
North Wolfe Street, Room 157
Baltimore, Maryland 21287-8943
Tel: 410/955-8822
Fax: 410/955-6787
(Comprehensive Cancer Center)

Massachusetts
David G. Nathan, M.D.
President, Cancer Center
Dana-Farber Cancer Institute
44 Binney Street, Rm. 1828
Boston, Massachusetts 02115
Tel: 617/632-2155
Fax: 617/632-2161
(Comprehensive Cancer Center)

Richard 0. Hynes, Ph.D.
Director & Professor of Biology
Center for Cancer Research
Massachusetts Institute of Technology
77 Massachusetts Avenue,
Room E17-110
Cambridge, Massachusetts 02139-4307
Tel: 617/253-6422
Fax: 617/253-8357
(Cancer Center)

Michigan
Max S. Wicha, M.D.

Director, Comprehensive Cancer Center
University of Michigan 6302 CGC/ 0942
1500 East Medical Center Drive
Ann Arbor, Michigan 48109-0942
Tel: 734/936-1831
Fax: 734/615-3947
(Comprehensive Cancer Center)
William P. Peters, M.D., Ph.D.
Director & Chief Executive Officer

Barbara Am Karmanos Cancer Institute
Wayne State University
Operating the Meyer L. Prentis Comprehensive
Cancer Center of Metropolitan Detroit
4100 John R. Street
Detroit, Michigan 48201-1379
Tel: 313/993-7777
Fax: 313/993-7165
(Comprehensive Cancer Center)

Minnesota

John H. Kersey, M.D.
Director, University of Minnesota Cancer Center
Box 806, 420 Delaware Street, S.E.
Minneapolis, Minnesota 55455
Tel: 612/624-8484
Fax: 612/626-3069
(Comprehensive Cancer Center)

Franklyn G. Prendergast, M.D., Ph.D.
Director, Mayo Clinic Cancer Center
Mayo Foundation
200 First Sheet, S.W.
Rochester, Minnesota 55905
Tel: 507/284-3753
Fax: 507/284-9349
(Comprehensive Cancer Center)

Nebraska
Kenneth H. Cowan, M.D., Ph.D
Director, University of Nebraska Medical Center/
Eppley Cancer Center
600 South 42nd Street
Omaha, Nebraska 68198-6805
Tel: 402/559-7081
Fax: 402/559-4651
(Cancer Center)

New Hampshire
E. Robert Greenberg, M.D.
Director, Norris Cotton Cancer Center
Dartmouth-Hitchcock Medical Center
One Medical Center Drive, Hinman Box 7920
Lebanon, New Hampshire 03756 0001
Tel: 603/650-6300
Fax: 603/650-6333
(Comprehensive Cancer Center)

New Jersey
William N. Hait, M.D., Ph.D.
Director, The Cancer Institute of New Jersey
Robert Wood Johnson Medical School
195 Little Albany Street, Room 2002B
New Brunswick, New Jersey 08901
Tel: 732/235-8064
Fax: 732/235-8094
(Clinical Cancer Center)

New York
I. David Goldman, M.D.
Director, Cancer Research Center
Albert Einstein College of Medicine
Chanin Building, Room 209
1300 Morris Park Avenue
Bronx, New York 10461
Tel: 718/430-2302

Fax: 718/430-8550
(Comprehensive Cancer Center)

David C. Hohn, M.D.
President & CEO, Roswell Park Cancer Institute
Elm & Carlton Streets
Buffalo, New York 14263-0001
Tel: 716/845-2389
Fax: 716/845-7609
(Comprehensive Cancer Center)

Bruce W. Stillman, Ph.D.
Director, Cold Spring Harbor Laboratory
P.O. Box 100
Cold Spring Harbor, New York 11724
Tel: 516/367-8383
Fax: 516/367-8879
(Cancer Center)

Franco M. Muggia, M.D.
Director, Kaplan Cancer Center
New York University Medical 'Center
550 First Avenue
New York, New York 10016
Tel: 212/263-6485
Fax: 212/263-8210
(Comprehensive Cancer Center)

Paul A. Marks, M.D.
President, Memorial Sloan-Kettering Cancer Center
1275 York Avenue
New York, New York 10021
Tel: 212/639-6561
Fax: 212/717-3299
(Comprehensive Cancer Center)

Daniel W. Nixon, M.D.
President, American Health Foundation

320 East 43rd Street
New York, New York 10017
Tel: 212/953-1900
Fax: 212/687-2339
(Cancer Center)

Karen H. Antman, M.D.
Director, Herbert Irving Comprehensive Cancer Center;
College of Physicians & Surgeons
Columbia University
177 Fort Washington Avenue
6th Floor, Room 435
New York, New York 10032
Tel: 212/305-8602
Fax: 212/305-3035
(Comprehensive Cancer Center)

North Carolina
H. Shelton Earp, M.D.
Lineberger Professor of Cancer Research & Director, UNC Lineberger
Comprehensive Cancer Center
University of North Carolina Chapel Hill School of Medicine, CB-7295
102 West Drive
Chapel Hill, North Carolina 27599-7295
Tel: 919/966-3036
Fax: 919/966-3015
(Comprehensive Cancer Center)

0. Michael Colvin, M.D.
Director, Duke Comprehensive Cancer Center
Duke University Medical Center Box 3843
Durham, North Carolina 27710
Tel: 919/684-5613
Fax: 919/684-5653
(Comprehensive Cancer Center)

Frank M. Torti, M.D.
Director, Comprehensive Cancer Center

Wake Forest University
Bowman Gray School of Medicine
Medical Center Boulevard
Winston-Salem, North Carolina 27157-1082
Tel: 336/716-7971
Fax: 336/716-0293
(Comprehensive Cancer Center)

Ohio

James K. V. Willson, M.D.
Director, Ireland Cancer Center
Case Western Reserve University and
University Hospitals of Cleveland
11100 Euclid Ave., Wearn 151
Cleveland, Ohio 44106-5065
Tel: 216/844-8562
Fax: 216/844-7832
(Comprehensive Cancer Center)

Clara D. Bloomfield, M.D.
Director, Comprehensive Cancer Center
Arthur G. James Cancer Hospital
Ohio State University A455 Staring Loving Hall
300 West 10th Avenue
Columbus, Ohio 43210-1240
Tel: 614/293-7518
Fax: 614/293-7520
(Comprehensive Cancer Center)

Oregon

Grover C. Bagby, Jr., M.D.
Director, Oregon Cancer Center
Oregon Health Sciences University
3181 S.W. Sam Jackson Park Rd., CR145
Portland, Oregon 97201-3098
Tel: 503/494-1617
Fax: 503/494-7086
(Clinical Cancer Center)

Pennsylvannia

John H. Glick, M.D.
Director, University of Pennsylvania Cancer Center
16th Floor Penn Tower
3400 Spruce Street
Philadelphia, Pennsylvania 19104-4283
Tel: 215/662-6065
Fax: 215/349-5325
(Comprehensive Cancer Center)

Giovanni Rovera, M.D.
Director, The Wistar Institute
3601 Spruce Street
Philadelphia, Pennsylvania 19104-4268
Tel: 215/898-3926
Fax: 215/573-2097
(Cancer Center)

Robert C. Young, M.D.
President, Fox Chase Cancer Center
7701 Burholme Avenue
Philadelphia, Pennsylvania 19111
Tel: 215/728-2781
Fax: 215/728-2571
(Comprehensive Cancer Center.)

Carlo M. Croce, M.D.
Director, Kimmel Cancer Center
Thomas Jefferson University
233 South 10th Street
BLSB, Room 1050
Philadelphia, Pennsylvania 19107-5799
Tel: 215/503-4645
Fax: 215/923-3528
(Clinical Cancer Center)

Ronald B. Herberman, M.D.

Director, University of Pittsburgh Cancer Institute
3471 Fifth Avenue, Suite 201
Pittsburgh, Pennsylvania 15213-3305
Tel: 412/692-4670
Fax: 412/692-4665
(Comprehensive Cancer Center)

Tennessee

Arthur W. Nienhuis, M.D.
Director, St. Jude Children's Research Hospital
332 North Lauderdale
P.O. Box 318
Memphis, Tennessee 38105-2794
Tel: 901/495-3301
Fax: 901/525-2720
(Clinical Cancer Center)

Harold L. Moses, M.D.
Director, Vanderbilt Cancer Center
Vanderbilt University Medical Research Building II
Nashville, Tennessee 37232-6838
Tel: 615/936-1782
Fax: 615/936-1790
(Clinical Cancer Center)

Texas

John Mendelsohn, M.D.
President, University of Texas
M.D. Anderson Cancer Center
1515 Holcombe Boulevard, Box 91
Houston, Texas 77030
Tel: 713/792-6000
Fax: 713/799-2210
(Comprehensive Cancer Center)

Charles A- Coltman, Jr., M.D.
Director, San Antonio Cancer Institute
8122 Datapoint Drive, Suite 600

San Antonio, Texas 78229-3264
Tel: 210/616-5580
Fax: 210/692-9823
(Comprehensive Cancer Center)

Utah
Stephen M. Prescott, M.D.
Director, Huntsman Cancer Institute
University of Utah
15 North 2030 East, Rio 7410
Salt Lake City, Utah 94112-5330
Tel: 801/581-4330
Fax: 901 /585-3833
(Clinical Cancer Center)
Vermont

David W. Yandell, Sc.D.
Director, Vermont Cancer Center
University of Vermont Medical Alumni Bldg
Burlington, Vermont 05405
Tel: 802/656-4414
Fax: 802/656-8788
(Comprehensive Cancer Center)

Virginia
Charles E. Myers, Jr., M.D.
Director, Cancer Center
University of Virginia,
I Health Sciences Center Hospital Box 334
Charlottesville, Virginia 22908
Tel: 804/924-2562
Fax: 804/982-0918
(Clinical Cancer Center)

Gordon D. Ginder, M.D.
Professor of Medicine & Director
Massey Cancer Center
Virginia Commonwealth University

P.O. Box 980037
Richmond, Virginia 23298-0037
Tel: 804/828-0450
Fax: 804/828-8453
(Clinical Cancer Center)

Washington

Leland H. Hartwell, Ph.D.
President & Director
Fred Hutchinson Cancer Research Center
1100 Fairview Avenue, North
P.O. Box 19024, D1060
Seattle, Washington 98104-1024
Tel: 206/667-4305
Fax: 206/667-5268
(Comprehensive Cancer Center)

Wisconsin

John E. Niederhuber, M.D.
Director, Comprehensive Cancer Center
University of Wisconsin
600 Highland Ave., Rm. K4/610
Madison, Wisconsin 53792-O001
Tel: 608/263-8610
Fax: 608/263-8613
(Comprehensive Cancer Center)

Norman R. Drinkwater, Ph.D.
Director, McArdle Laboratory for Cancer Research
University of Wisconsin 1400
University Avenue, Room 1009
Madison, Wisconsin 53706-1599
Tel: 608/262-2177 or 7992
Fax: 608/262-2824
(Cancer Center)

Types of Centers:

Cancer Centers: 10

Clinical Cancer Centers: 12
Comprehensive Cancer Centers: 37
Total: 59

APPENDIX C
- Glossary -

abcess: Infection which has formed a pocket of pus

adenocarcinoma: Cancer arising in gland forming tissue. Breast cancer is a type of adenocarcinoma

adenine: A nucleotide base which pairs with thymine in forming DNA

adjuvant chemotherapy: Anticancer drugs used in combination with surgery and/or radiation as an initial treatment before there is detectable spread, to prevent or delay recurrence

adrenal gland: Small gland found above each kidney which secretes cortisone, adrenaline, aldosterone and many other important hormones

amenorrhea: Absence or stoppage of menstrual period

amino acid: The building block of proteins

androgen: Hormone which produces male characteristics

angiogenesis *(angiogenic)*: Stimulates new blood vessels to be formed

anorexia: Loss of appetite

apoptosis: Cell suicide

areola: Area of pigment around the nipple

aspiration: Putting a hypodermic needle into a tissue and drawing back on the syringe to obtain fluid or cells

asymmetrical: Not matching

ataxia telangectasia: Disease of the nervous system; carriers of the gene are more sensitive to radiation and have a higher risk of cancer

atypical cell: Mild to moderately abnormal cell

atypical hyperplasia: Cells that are not only abnormal but increased in number

augmented: Added to such, as an augmented breast augmented breast

augmented breast: one which has had a silicone implant added to it

autologous: From the same person. An autologous blood transfusion is blood removed and then transfused back to the same person at a later date

axilla: Armpit

axillary lymph nodes: Lymph nodes found in the armpit area

axillary lymph node dissection: Surgical removal of lymph nodes found in the armpit region

base pairs: Two nucleic acids which bind together in DNA and RNA

benign: Not cancerous

bilateral: Involving both sides, such as both breasts

biological response modifier: Usually natural substances such as colony stimulating factor that stimulates the bone marrow to make blood cells, that alter the body's natural response

biopsy: Removal of tissue. This term does not indicate how much tissue will be removed

bone marrow: The soft inner part of large bones that produces blood cells

bone scan: Test to determine if there is any sign of cancer in the bones

brachial plexus: A bundle of nerves in the armpit which go on to supply the arm

breast reconstruction: Creation of artificial breast after mastectomy by a plastic surgeon

bromocriptine: Drug used to block the hormone prolactin

calcifications: Small calcium deposits in the breast tissue that can be carcinoembryonic antigen

(CEA): Nonspecific (not specific to cancer) blood test used to follow women with metastatic breast cancer to help determine if the treatment is working

carcinogen: Substance that can cause cancer

carcinoma: Cancer arising in the epithelial tissue (skin, glands, and lining of internal organs). Most cancers are carcinomas

cell cycle: The steps a cell goes through in order to reproduce itself

cellulitis: Infection of the soft tissues

centigray: Measurement of radiation absorbed dose, same as a rad

checkpoint: Point in the cell cycle where the cell's DNA is checked for mutations before it is allowed to move forward

chemotherapy: Treatment of disease with certain chemicals. The term usually refers to cytotoxic drugs given for cancer treatment

chromosome: Genes are strung together in a chromosome

cohort study: Study of a group of people who have something in common when they are first assembled and who are then observed for a period of time to see what happens to them

colostrum: Liquid produced by the breast before the milk comes in: pro-milk

comedo: Type of DCIS where the cells filling the duct are more aggressive looking

comedon: Whitehead pimple

contracture: Formation of a thick scar tissue; in the breast a contracture can form around an implant

core biopsy: Type of needle biopsy where a small core of tissue is removed from a lump without surgery

corpus luteumn: Ovarian follicle after ovulation

cortisol: Hormone produced by the adrenal gland

costochondritis: Inflammation of the connection between ribs and breast bone, a type of arthritis

cribriform: Type of DCIS where the cells filling the duct have punched out areas

cyclical: In a cycle like the menstrual period, which is every 28 days, or chemotherapy treatment, which is periodic

cyst: Fluid filled sac

cystosarcoma phylloides: Unusual type of breast tumor

cytology: Study of cells

cytologist: One who specializes in studying cells

cytosine: A nucleotide base which pairs with guanine in DNA

cytotoxic: Causing the death of cells. The term usually refers to drugs used in chemotherapy

danazol: Drug used to block hormones from the pituitary gland, used in endometriosis and rarely breast pain diethylstilbesterol

(DES): Synthetic estrogen once used to prevent miscarriages, now shown to cause vaginal cancer in the daughters of the women who took it. DES is sometimes used to treat metastatic breast cancer

DNA: Deoxyribonucleic acid, the genetic code

double helix: The structure of DNA which allows it to be easily replicated

doubling time: Time it takes the cell population to double in number ductal carcinoma in situ

(DCIS): Ductal cancer cells that have not grown outside of their site of origin, sometimes referred to as pre cancer

edema: Swelling caused by a collection of fluid in the soft tissues

electrocautery: Instrument used in surgery to cut, coagulate or destroy tissue by heating it with an electric current

embolus: Plug or clot of tumor cells within a blood vessel

engorgement: Swelling with fluid, as in a breast engorged with milk erb

B2: Another name for the HER-2 neu oncogene

esophagus (esophageal): Organ carrying food from the mouth and the stomach

estrogen: Female sex hormones produced by the ovaries, adrenal glands, placenta, and fat

estrogen receptor: Protein found on some cells to which estrogen molecules will attach. If a tumor is positive for estrogen receptors, it is sensitive to hormones

excema: Skin irritation characterized by redness and open weeping

excisional biopsy: Taking the whole lump out

extracellular matrix: The material which surrounds the cells

fat necrosis: Area of dead fat usually following some form of trauma or surgery, a cause of lumps

fibroadenoma: Benign fibrous tumor of the breast most common in young women

fibrocystic disease: Much misused term for any benign condition of the breast

fibroid: Benign fibrous tumor of the uterus (not in the breast)

flow cytometry: Test that measures DNA content in tumors

fluoroscopy: Use of an x-ray machine to examine parts of the body directly rather than taking a picture and developing it, as in conventional x rays. Fluoroscopy uses more radiation than a single x ray

follicle stimulating hormone (FSH): Hormone from the pituitary gland which stimulates the ovary

follicles: In the ovaries, eggs encased in their developmental sacs

frozen section: Freezing and slicing tissue to make a slide immediately for diagnosis

frozen shoulder: Stiffness of the shoulder, which is painful and makes it hard to lift the arm over your head

galactocele: Milk cyst sometimes found in a nursing mother's breast

gene: A linear sequence of DNA that is required to produce a protein

genetic: Relating to genes or inherited characteristics

genome: All of the chromosomes that together form the genetic map

germ line: Cells that are involved in reproduction, i.e., sperm and eggs

ghostectomy: Removal of breast tissue in the area where there was a previous lump

guanine: One of the base pairs that form DNA; pairs with cytosine

gynecomastia: Swollen breast tissue in a man or boy

hemorrhage: Bleeding

hemangioma: A birth mark consisting of overgrowth of blood vessels

hematoma: Collection of blood in the tissues. Hematomas may occur in the breast after surgery

Her-2 neu: An oncogene which, when overexpressed, leads to more cell growth

heterogeneous: Composed of many different elements. In relation to breast cancer, heterogeneous refers to the fact that there are many different types of breast cancer cells within one tumor

homeopathy: System of therapy using very small doses of drugs, which can produce in healthy people symptoms similar to those of the disease being treated. These are believed to stimulate the immune system

hormone: Chemical substance produced by glands in the body which enters the bloodstream and causes effects in other tissues

hot flashes: Sudden sensations of heat and swelling associated with the menopause

HRT: Hormone replacement therapy

human choriogonadotropin (HCG): Hormone produced by the corpus luteum

hyperplasia: Excessive growth of cells

hypothalmus: Area at the base of the brain that controls various functions including hormone production in the pituitary

hysterectomy: Removal of the uterus. Hysterectomy does not necessarily mean the removal of ovaries (oophorectomy)

immunocytochemistry: Study of the chemistry of cells using techniques that employ immune mechanisms

immune system: Complex system by which the body is able to protect itself from foreign invaders

incisional biopsy: Taking a piece of the lump out

infiltrating cancer: Cancer which can grow beyond its site of origin into neighboring tissue. Infiltrating does not imply Ludt the cancer has already spread outside the breast. Infiltrating has the same meaning as invasive

informed consent: Process in which the patient is fully informed of all risks and complications of a planned procedure and agrees to proceed

in situ: In the site of. In regards to cancer, in situ refers to tumors that haven't grown beyond their site of origin and invaded neighboring tissue

intraductal: Within the duct. Intraductal can describe a benign or malignant process

intraductal papilloma: Benign tumor which projects like a finger from the lining of the duct

invasive cancer: Cancers that are capable of growing beyond their site of origin and invading neighboring tissue. Invasive does not imply that the cancer is aggressive or has already spread

lactation: Production of milk from the breast

latissimus flap: Flap of skin and muscle taken from the back used for reconstruction after mastectomy or partial mastectomy

lidocaine: Drug most commonly used for local anesthesia

lobules: Parts of the breast capable of making milk

lobular carcinoma in situ: Abnormal cells within the lobule which don't form lumps. They can serve as a marker of future cancer risk

lobular: Having to do with the lobules of the breast

local treatment of cancer: Treatment of the tumor only

lumpectomy: Surgery to remove lump with small rim of normal tissue around it

luteinizing hormone: Hormone produced by the pituitary which helps control the menstrual cycle

lymphatic vessels: Vessels that carry lymph (tissue fluid) to and from lymph nodes

lymphedema: Milk arm. This swelling of the arm can follow surgery to the lymph nodes under the arm. It can be temporary, or permanent and occur immediately, or any time later

lymph nodes: Glands found throughout the body which help defend against foreign invaders such as bacteria. Lymph nodes can be a location of cancer spread

macrophages: Blood cells that are part of the immune system

malignant: Cancerous

mastalgia: Pain in the breast

mastitis: Infection of the breast. Mastitis is sometimes used loosely to refer to any benign process in the breast

mastodynia: Pain in the breast

mastopexy: Uplift of the breast through plastic surgery

menarche: First menstrual period

metastasis: Spread of cancer to another organ, usually through the blood stream

metastasizing: Spreading to a distant site

methylxanthine: Chemical group to which caffeine belongs

microcalcification: Tiny calcifications in the breast tissue usually seen only on a mammogram. When clustered can be a sign of ductal carcinoma in situ

micrometastasis: Microscopic and as yet undetectable but presumed spread of tumor cells to other organs

micropapillary: Type of DCIS where the cells filling the duct take the form of 'finger' projections into the center

mitosis: Cell division

mutation: An alteration of the genetic code

myocutaneous flap: Flap of skin and muscle and fat taken from one part of the body to fill in an empty space

myoepithelial cells: The cells which surround the ductal lining cells and may serve to contain the cells

necrosis: Dead tissue

nodular: Forming little nodules

nuclear magnetic resonance (NMR or MRI): Imaging technique using a magnet and electrical coil to transmit radio waves through the body

nucleotide: One of the base pairs forming DNA

observational study: A study in which a factor is observed in a group of people

oncogene: Tumor genes are present in the body. These can be activated by carcinogens and cause cell to grow uncontrollably

oncogenes: Altered DNA which can lead to cancerous growth

oncology: Study of cancer

oophorectomy: Removal of the ovaries

osteoporosis: Softening of the bones, and bone loss, that occurs with age in some people

oxytocin: Hormone produced by the pituitary gland, involved in lactation

p53: A tumor suppressor gene

palliation: Act of relieving a symptom without curing the cause

pathologist: Doctor who specializes in examining tissue and diagnosing disease

pectoral's major: Muscle which lies under the breast

phlebitis: Irritation of a vein

pituitary gland: A gland located in the brain which secretes many hormones to regulate other glands in the body; the master gland

Poland's syndrome: A congenital condition in which there is no breast development on one side of the chest

polygenic: Relating to more than one gene

polymastia: Literally many breasts. Existence of an extra breast or breasts

postmenopausal: After the menopause has occurred

Premarin: Estrogen from pregnant horses' urine that is sometimes given to women after the menopause

progesterone: Hormone produced by the ovary involved in the normal menstrual cycle

prognosis: Expected or probable outcome

prolactin: Hormone produced by the pituitary that stimulates progesterone production by the ovaries and lactation

prophylactic subcutaneous mastectomies: Removal of all breast tissue beneath the skin and nipple, to prevent future breast cancer risk

prosthesis: Artificial substitute for an absent part of the body, as in breast prosthesis.

protein: Formed from amino acids, this is the building block of life

protocol: Research designed to answer a hypothesis. Protocols often involve testing a specific new treatment under controlled conditions

proto-oncogene: Normal gene controlling cell growth or turnover

Provera: Progesterone which is sometimes given to women in combination with Premarin after menopause

pseudolump: Breast tissue that feels like a lump but when removed proves to be normal

ptosis: Drooping, as in breasts which hang down

punch biopsy: A biopsy of skin done which just punches a small hole out of the skin

quadrantectomy: Removal of a quarter of the breast

rad: Radiation absorbed dose, same as centigray. One chest x ray equals 1/ 10 of a rad

randomized: Chosen at random. In regard to a research study it means choosing the subjects to be given a particular treatment by means of a computer programmed to choose names at random

randomized controlled study: A study in which the participants are randomized to one treatment or another

recurrence: Return of cancer after its apparent complete disappearance

remission: Disappearance of detectable disease

repair endonucleases: Enzymes that can repair mutations

RNA: Ribornucleic acid; carries the message from the DNA into the cell to make proteins

Cancer arising in the connective tissue

scoliosis: Deformity of the back bone which causes a person to bend to one side or the other

scleroderma: An autoimmune disease which involves thickening of the skin, difficulty swallowing among other symptoms

sebaceous: Oily, cheesy material secreted by glands in the skin

selenium: Metallic element found in food

SERM: Selective estrogen receptor modulator; a compound which is estrogenic in some organs and anti-estrogenic in others

seroma: Collection of tissue fluid

side effect: Unintentional or undesirable secondary effect of treatment

silicone: Synthetic material used in breast implants because of its flexibility, resilience and durability

somatic: A cell that forms the organs of the body but is not involved in reproduction

S phase fraction: A measure of how many cells are dividing at a time; if it is high it is thought to indicate an aggressive tumor

subareolar abscess: Infection of the glands under the nipple

subcutaneous tissue: The tissue under the skin

systemic treatment: Treatment involving the whole body, usually using drugs

tamoxifen: Estrogen blocker used in treating breast cancer

telomere: The end of a chromosome, a bit of which is clipped off every time a cell divides

telomerase: An enzyme which reattaches the end of a chromosome when it divides

thoracic: Concerning the chest (thorax)

thoracic nerves: Nerves in the chest area

thoracoepigastric vein: Vein that starts under the arm and passes along the side of the breast and then down into the abdomen

thymine: A nucleotide base which pairs with adenine in DNA formation

titration: Systems of balancing. In chemotherapy, titration means using the largest amount of a drug possible while keeping the side effects from becoming intolerable

trauma: Wound or injury

triglyceride: Form in which fat is stored in the body, consisting of glycerol and three fatty acids

tru-cut biopsy: Type of core needle biopsy where a small core of tissue is removed from a lump without surgery

tumor: Abnormal mass of tissue. Strictly speaking a tumor can be benign or malignant

tumor dormancy: Tumors which are present in a stable state

tumor suppressor gene: A gene that prevents cells from growing if they have a mutation

veg-f: Vascular epidermal growth factor; a protein which stimulates new blood vessels to grow

virginal hypertrophy: Inappropriately large breasts in a young woman

xeroradiography: Type of mammogram taken on a xerox plate rather than x-ray film

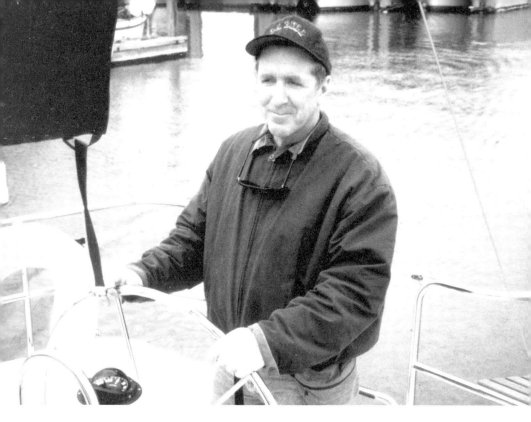

Author's Bio

J. Scott Lyman is husband, father of three sons and a professional negligence attorney in Santa Cruz County, California. Scott received his Bachelor of Arts in political science from Stanford University and his Doctor of Jurisprudence from Stanford Law School. Scott writes a syndicated column for the Aptos Times and is presently working on his second book, 1968: The Trip. Scott was a contributing editor to West Publishing Company's Civil Trial and Evidence and serves as a faculty member on the Trial Advocacy Workshop at Stanford Law School and the University of San Francisco Law School. Diary of A Breast Cancer Husband is Scott's first full length book.

raceoddysey@aol.com

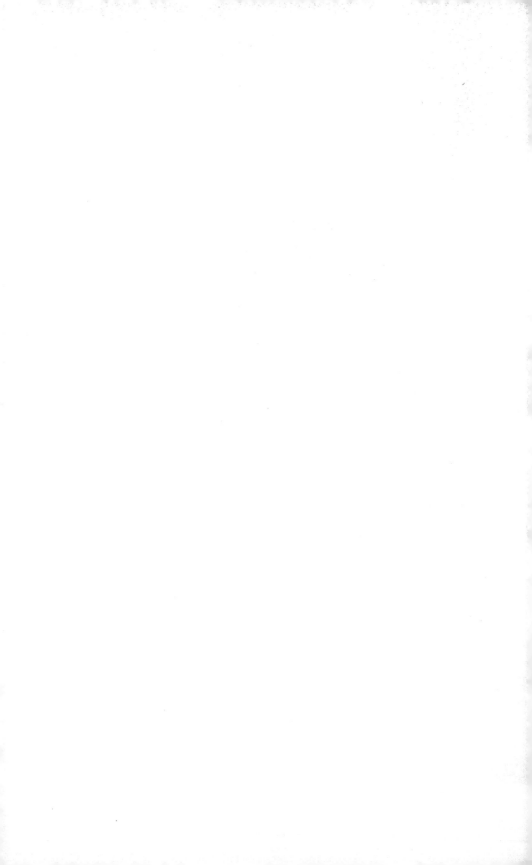